AF836471

MEDICINE AS THEATRE, THEATRE AS MEDICINE

Performance and Science: Interdisciplinary Dialogues explores the interactions between science and performance, providing readers with a unique guide to current practices and research in this fast-expanding field. Through shared themes and case studies, the series offers rigorous vocabularies and methods for empirical studies of performance, with each volume involving collaboration between performance scholars, practitioners and scientists. The series encompasses the modalities of performance to include drama, dance and music.

SERIES EDITORS

Amy Cook
Vice Provost for Academic Affairs and Professor of English
at Stony Brook University, USA

Nicola Shaughnessy
Professor of Performance at the University of Kent, UK

IN THE SAME SERIES

Affective Performance and Cognitive Science: Body, Brain and Being
Edited by Nicola Shaughnessy

An Introduction to Theatre, Performance and the Cognitive Sciences
John Lutterbie

Collaborative Embodied Performance: Ecologies of Skill
Edited by Kath Bicknell and John Sutton

Identity, Culture, and the Science Performance, Volume 1: From the Lab to the Streets
Edited by Vivian Appler and Meredith Conti

Identity, Culture, and the Science Performance, Volume 2: From the Curious to the Quantum
Edited by Meredith Conti and Vivian Appler

Performance and the Medical Body
Edited by Alex Mermikides and Gianna Bouchard

Performance, Medicine and the Human
Alex Mermikides

Performing Psychologies: Imagination, Creativity and Dramas of the Mind
Edited by Nicola Shaughnessy and Philip Barnard

Performing Specimens: Contemporary Performance and Biomedical Display
Gianna Bouchard

Performing the Remembered Present: The Cognition of Memory in Dance, Theatre and Music
Edited by Pil Hansen with Bettina Bläsing

Practice, Research, and Cognition in Devised Performance
Maiya Murphy

Theatre and Cognitive Neuroscience
Edited by Clelia Falletti, Gabriele Sofia and Victor Jacono

Theatre, Performance and Cognition: Languages, Bodies and Ecologies
Edited by Rhonda Blair and Amy Cook

MEDICINE AS THEATRE, THEATRE AS MEDICINE

Edited by
Marlene Goldman, Lawrence Switzky and Alice Flaherty

methuen | drama
LONDON • NEW YORK • OXFORD • NEW DELHI • SYDNEY

METHUEN DRAMA
Bloomsbury Publishing Plc, 50 Bedford Square, London, WC1B 3DP, UK
Bloomsbury Publishing Inc, 1359 Broadway, New York, NY 10018, USA
Bloomsbury Publishing Ireland, 29 Earlsfort Terrace, Dublin 2, D02 AY28, Ireland

BLOOMSBURY, METHUEN DRAMA and the Methuen Drama logo are trademarks of Bloomsbury Publishing Plc

First published in Great Britain 2026

Copyright © Marlene Goldman, Lawrence Switzky, Alice Flaherty and contributors, 2026
Marlene Goldman, Lawrence Switzky and Alice Flaherty have asserted their right under the Copyright, Designs and Patents Act, 1988, to be identified as editors of this work.

For legal purposes the Acknowledgements on pp. xviii–xx constitute an extension of this copyright page.

Series design by Louise Dugdale
Cover image: Operating Theater © The Estate of Bernard Perlin

This work is published open access subject to a Creative Commons Attribution-NonCommercial-NoDerivatives 4.0 International licence (CC BY-NC-ND 4.0, https://creativecommons.org/licenses/by-nc-nd/4.0/). You may re-use, distribute, and reproduce this work in any medium for non-commercial purposes, provided you give attribution to the copyright holder and the publisher and provide a link to the Creative Commons licence.

No part of this publication may be used or reproduced in any way for the training, development or operation of artificial intelligence (AI) technologies, including generative AI technologies. The rights holders expressly reserve this publication from the text and data mining exception as per Article 4(3) of the Digital Single Market Directive (EU) 2019/790.

Bloomsbury Publishing Plc does not have any control over, or responsibility for, any third-party websites referred to or in this book. All internet addresses given in this book were correct at the time of going to press. The author and publisher regret any inconvenience caused if addresses have changed or sites have ceased to exist, but can accept no responsibility for any such changes.

A catalogue record for this book is available from the British Library.

A catalog record for this book is available from the Library of Congress.

ISBN: HB: 978-1-3504-6072-0
ePDF: 978-1-3504-6074-4
eBook: 978-1-3504-6073-7

Series: Performance and Science: Interdisciplinary Dialogues

Typeset by Newgen KnowledgeWorks Pvt. Ltd., Chennai, India

For product safety related questions contact productsafety@bloomsbury.com.

To find out more about our authors and books visit www.bloomsbury.com and sign up for our newsletters.

CONTENTS

ILLUSTRATIONS

CONTRIBUTORS

George Anderson was born in Boston. He was raised as a ward of the state, then spent a number of years in state custody. As an adult, he pursued continuing education in a variety of subjects, including psychology, and gained extensive experience working as a long-term companion for clients living with terminal illness. His years caring for a series of disabled academics, in particular, gave him in-depth exposure to academic life and a unique perspective on the roles patients and caregivers play.

Corinne May Botz is a photographic artist, filmmaker and educator whose books include *Milk Factory* (2025), *The Nutshell Studies of Unexplained Death* (2004) and *Haunted Houses* (2010). Her work has been widely exhibited including at The Brooklyn Museum, the Museum of Contemporary Photography, Kunstmuseum Basel, Turner Contemporary and Benrubi Gallery. Her Oscar-qualifying film *Bedside Manner* (2016) won the Grand Jury Prize at DOC NYC. Botz's work has been written about by the *New York Times*, the *New Yorker*, *Granta*, *Bookforum* and *Hyperallergic*. Botz is on the faculty of John Jay College of Criminal Justice.

Marcus Coates is a contemporary artist living in London. He exhibits internationally. He was an artist in residence at King's College Cambridge (Cambridge University), 2025–6, and a visiting fellow at Jesus College Oxford (Oxford University), 2023. His recognitions include being the first recipient of the James Lovelock Commission 2014; nominated for the fourth Plinth Commission, London, 2014; the Paul Hamyln Award, 2008; winner of the inaugural Daiwa Art Prize, 2009; and co-founder of Berwick Film and Media Arts Festival, UK, 2005. Recent publications include *UR … A Practical Guide to Unconscious*

Reasoning (2020) and *Marcus Coates*, a survey monograph (2016). He is represented by Kate MacGarry, London.

Bianca Dahl is a socio-cultural and medical anthropologist, whose research ethnographically explores the (often-unintended) social effects of global health and humanitarian responses to pandemics. Much of her work has taken place in Botswana, investigating the long-term consequences of interventions to redress the burdens of the HIV pandemic. Dahl is currently Assistant Professor of Anthropology at the University of Toronto Scarborough.

Sherry Dupuis is Professor Emerita and University Research Chair in Recreation and Leisure Studies at the University of Waterloo, Canada, the former director of the Murray Alzheimer Research and Education Program, and current Co-director of the Partnerships in Dementia Care Alliance. Her research draws on critical and relational theories and uses critical participatory action research and arts-based methodologies to promote personal transformation and social change in dementia and long-term care. She uses the arts to challenge stigma associated with dementia, expose harmful policies and practices and promote relational approaches to dementia care, including at end of life.

Alice Flaherty is a neurologist at the Massachusetts General Hospital and Associate Professor of both Neurology and Psychiatry at Harvard Medical School. She is Director of the Movement Disorders Fellowship and was the site principal investigator for the trial of the first successful genetic treatment of Parkinson's disease. While still a resident she wrote *The Massachusetts General Hospital Handbook of Neurology* (1999), which received a national award for its innovative approach and has been multiply translated. She is also the author of *The Midnight Disease* (2004), an award-winning non-fiction book about the neural basis of creativity.

Karen Fricker is Adjunct Professor of Dramatic Arts at Brock University and Editorial Director of *Intermission Magazine*. Her monograph *The Original Stage Productions of Robert Lepage: Making Theatre Global* won the Canadian Association of Theatre Research's 2021 Ann Saddlemyer Award. She is co-leader of numerous projects around equitable theatre criticism, including the free online course Youareacritic.com, and is Co-director of Circus and Its Others, an international research network exploring difference in the context of contemporary circus. She is on the core team of Staging Better Futures/Mettre en scène de meilleurs avenirs, a nationwide partnership addressing systemic inequities in theatre higher education in Canada.

Stanton B. Garner, Jr, is James Douglas Bruce Professor of English and Theatre at the University of Tennessee and is a specialist in modern drama; drama, theatre and performance theory; and the intersections of theatre and medicine. In addition to his 2023 book *Theatre and Medicine*, he has published articles on the intersections between theatre and medical technology, experimental physiology, contagion, facial reconstruction, dementia and other forms of disability, vaccination and the modern research hospital. He is also the author of *Bodied Spaces: Phenomenology and Performance in Contemporary Drama* (1994) and *Kinesthetic Spectatorship in the Theatre: Phenomenology, Cognition Movement* (2018).

Marlene Goldman is a writer, filmmaker and Professor of English at the University of Toronto. Her work spans Canadian literary studies and the medical humanities and – in addition to five scholarly books – includes film adaptations of short stories by Margaret Atwood (*Piano Lessons* (2017) and *Torching the Dusties* (2019])) and Souvankham Thammavongsa (*Mani Pedi* (2021)). She was elected Fellow of the Royal Society of Canada in 2021.

Arthur Kleinman, MD, is a renowned scholar in psychiatry, anthropology, global health and medicine in China. Educated at Stanford and a Harvard professor for fifty years, Kleinman holds multiple roles, including Professor of Global Health and Psychiatry at Harvard Medical School and Professor of Anthropology at Harvard University. He has authored six books, co-edited twenty-nine volumes and published over 350 articles. Kleinman directed Harvard's Asia Center and led several major health initiatives, including the first *World Mental Health Report*. A member of the National Academy of Medicine, he's received numerous prestigious awards and has mentored over 100 PhD students and 250 postdoctoral fellows.

Pia Kontos is a senior scientist at KITE Research Institute, University Health Network, and a professor in the Dalla Lana School of Public Health at the University of Toronto. In her research she focuses on stigma-related inequities associated with dementia and the development of theories, arts-based initiatives and policies to reduce stigma and foster relational caring in community and long-term care settings. She draws from the fields of embodiment and dementia, citizenship and human rights and uses critical qualitative, participatory and arts-based methodologies to promote more inclusive and socially just approaches to dementia care.

Matthew MacKenzie is an Indigenous playwright. A citizen of the Métis Nation of Alberta, he serves in a number of roles, including as Artistic Director of

Punctuate! Theatre, an Indigenous-led professional theatre company based in Edmonton, Alberta; as a founding member of the Pemmican Collective, which supports new Indigenous dramatic writing throughout Turtle Island; and as Assistant Professor in Dramatic Arts at Brock University. His plays include the Dora Award–winning *Bears* (2018) and *First Métis Man of Odesa* (2024), which he co-wrote with his wife, Mariya Khomutova.

Sara Masciotra-Milstein is an emerging playwright, dramaturg and researcher. She graduated from the University of Glasgow's MLitt in Playwriting and Dramaturgy. Her thesis 'Fanning New Play Development' earned her a distinction and culminated in a playwriting workshop that argued for the use of fanfiction as a means of teaching playwriting to young people. She had completed work placements with The Musical Stage Company, Playwrights Studio Scotland and Disneyland Paris. Sara's research focuses on the false binary between 'high' and 'low' art, the intersections of fandom and performance, the romanticization of Scotland and Canadian musical theatre.

Timothy McGinnis is the author of *The Dog's Letter* and other poems. He holds a Masters in Social History from Oxford and a medical degree from Harvard. He did a year of psychiatry residency before completing his surgery residency and is currently a surgical resident at the University of Chicago.

Philip McKee is a director, writer, producer and educator based in Toronto, Canada. He has directed over fifty plays and worked in the UK, Mexico, Ireland, Italy, Germany and Kenya. His artistic residencies include the Urjo Kareda Grant for Emerging Artists at Tarragon Theatre, the RBC Emerging Artist: Director Development Residency at Canadian Stage, The Tarragon Playwrights Unit, and Associate Artist at Crow's Theatre. McKee is a graduate of the Directing Program at The National Theatre School of Canada and has also completed extensive training in psychoanalysis and psychotherapy.

Deborah Ocholi was a medical student at the time of writing. She is now a first-year emergency medicine resident at McMaster University. Outside of medicine, Deborah is also a writer of poetry and prose. Her work explores the intersection of clinical practice, social justice and the arts, with a focus on fostering more inclusive and human-centred healthcare environments.

Marlis Schweitzer is Professor of Theatre and Performance Studies at York University. She is the author and editor of several books, including *When Broadway Was the Runway: Theatre, Fashion and American Culture* (2009) and *Bloody Tyrants and Little Pickles: Stage Roles of Anglo-American Girls in* *the Nineteenth Century* (2020), which is a recipient of the George Freedley Memorial Award from the Theatre Library Association. With the support of an Insight Grant from the Social Sciences and Humanities Research Council of Canada, she is undertaking a revisionist analysis of George Alexander Stevens's *Lecture on Heads* (1764) and the emergent cultures of celebrity and conspiracy that surrounded it.

Kirsten E. Shepherd is Professor of English and Theatre Studies in the Faculty of English and Tutorial Fellow at St Catherine's College, Oxford University. Her research encompasses three main areas of interest: the interaction between theatre and science; the writings of Henrik Ibsen; and the relationship between modernism and theatrical performance. Recent publications include *The Cambridge Companion to Theatre and Science* (2020), *Modern Drama: A Very Short Introduction* (2016) and *Twentieth-Century Approaches to Literature: Late Victorian into Modern* (2016, co-edited with Laura Marcus and Michele Mendelssohn).

Doris Sommer is Ira and Jewell Williams Professor of Romance Languages and Literatures and of African and African American Studies at Harvard University. She is Founding Director of 'Cultural Agents' at Harvard and an NGO to revive the civic mission of the humanities. Her academic outreach includes the 'Arts and Policy Certificate', for civil servants; and 'Learn With', a scalable pedagogy that combines literacy, arts and citizenship. Her books include *Foundational Fictions* (1991), *Proceed with Caution when Engaged by Minority Literature* (1999), *Bilingual Aesthetics* (2004) and *The Work of Art in the World: Civic Agency and Public Humanities* (2014). Sommer advocates and promotes good public school education.

Lawrence Switzky is Associate Professor of English & Drama at the University of Toronto and co-editor-in-chief of the journal *Modern Drama*.

Adele Vogelsang (nom de plume) is a registered nurse with over forty-five years of bedside experience working with inpatient populations in major Boston teaching hospitals. She recently retired from clinical practice. Adele graduated from a well-known conservatory in the Boston area. She has won international awards for her fragrance journalism.

Rachel Warr is a theatre director and dramaturg, specializing in puppetry. Her puppet work includes string marionettes, rod, glove, light, shadow puppetry and object theatre. She is based in the UK and has presented work at venues including Little Angel Puppet Theatre, The Barbican Centre and Victoria and

Albert Museum. She has also worked internationally in Europe, North America and Asia. Her interdisciplinary work includes collaborating with clinicians, as well as projects with product designers and scientists. She is a performer in residence at The Centre for Performance Science, and Artistic Director of Dotted Line Theatre.

Katherine Williams is Associate Professor of English at the University of Toronto. She is the author of the award-winning *Unfixable Forms: Disability, Performance, and the Early Modern English Theater* (2021) and has published widely on early modern drama, critical disability studies and performance. She edited Chapman, Jonson and Marston's *Eastward Ho* for *The Routledge Anthology of Early Modern Drama* (2020) and guest-edited 'Disability Performance and Global Shakespeare', a special issue of *The Shakespearean International Yearbook* (2024); with Elizabeth B. Bearden, she is co-editing *The Oxford Handbook of Disability and Literatures in English, 1500–1700*.

ACKNOWLEDGEMENTS

The spark that ignited this volume was lit in a coffee shop in Toronto, when Marlene Goldman and Alice Flaherty met for the first time and couldn't stop talking. Over the next few years, partly as an excuse to spend more time together, they developed and co-hosted a Harvard Radcliffe Institute Exploratory Symposium entitled 'Medicine as Theatre: Theatre as Medicine' in June 2021. The COVID-19 epidemic, by driving the symposium online, transformed the event unequivocally into a medical and performative spectacle. We are grateful to the Radcliffe Institute staff – Becky Withiam, Maura Madden and Sean Tath O'Donnell – for helping us to pivot gracefully online. Immense thanks also to the participants who joined us online: Geroge Anderson, Corinne Botz, Luna Dolezal, Tony Errichetti, Arthur Kleinman, Henry Llewellyn, Tim McGinnis, Philip McKee, Deborah Ocholi, Niki Cesare Schotzko, Doris Sommer, Lawrence Switzky and Katherine Williams. While listening to each other's voices, sharing images and experiences, and, on occasion, playing theatre games together, we discovered and rehearsed some of the performative elements and tactics explored in the volume.

Recognizing that the conversations and questions generated during the symposium deserved more time and space for consideration, Flaherty and Goldman determined to co-edit a volume on the subject with the aim of contributing to the emerging field of performative medicine. Neither, however, were trained in drama or performance studies, so they turned to Larry Switzky for help. Not only did Larry take up the role of co-editor, he and Goldman co-hosted a year-long 'Theatre and Medicine' Jackman Humanities Working Group at the University of Toronto in 2022–3. Thanks to Switzky's friendship, kindness in mediating disputes and brilliance, co-editing this volume has truly been an exuberant experience of serious play for all of us.

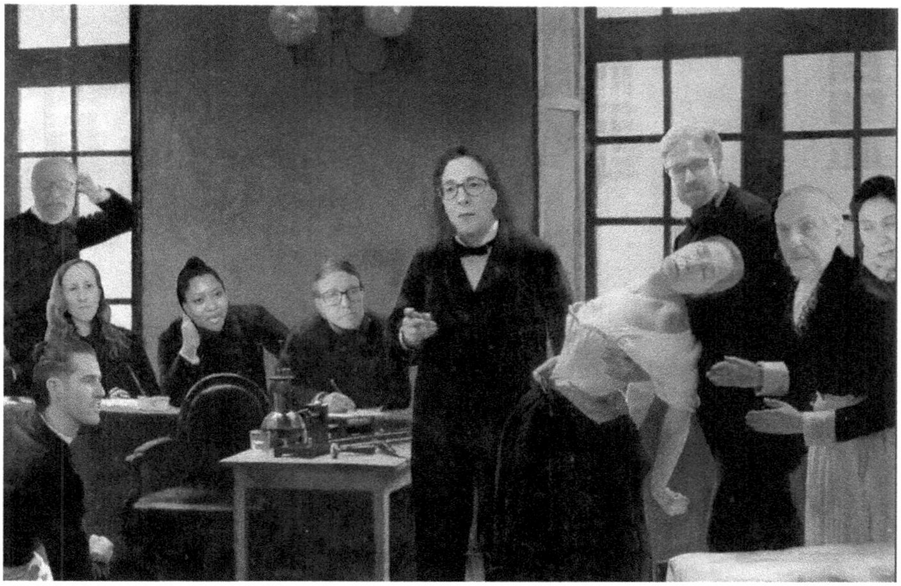

FIGURE A.1 A playful photomontage made for the 2021 Harvard Radcliffe Institute Special Seminar *Medicine as Theatre: Theatre as Medicine*. Heads of seminar participants are stuck on the bodies of the famous neurologists and hysterics in André Brouillet's 1887 painting *A Clinical Lesson at the Salpêtrière*. From left to right: George Anderson, Timothy McGinnis, Corinne Botz, Deborah Ocholi, Katherine Williams, Marlene Goldman, Alice Flaherty, Lawrence Switzky, Arthur Kleinman and Doris Sommer. Figure 13.3 shows the original painting.

Over our years working together on this project, we have relied on the Jackman Institute for the Humanities as our playground. We remain grateful to its director, Alison Keith, a visionary champion of interdisciplinary humanities, and her staff – Kimberly Yates and Monica Toffoli – for supporting us. It was also a privilege to work with the faculty at the University of Toronto and abroad who participated in the Theatre as Medicine Working Group and contributed to our evolving understanding of the spatially and temporally dynamic links between medicine and theatre: Sarah Bay-Cheng, Jill Carter, Lisa Cherniak, Xing Fan, Stan Garner, Caylen Heckel, Alex Eric Hernandez, Hartley Jafine, Pia Kontos, Andrea Most, Arthur Rose, Marlis Schweitzer, Doris Sommer and Katherine Williams. Thanks also to Caitlin Gowans, Ilana Khanin, Soykan Karayol and Walter Villanueva – graduate students at the University of Toronto who shared their insights and experience.

We are also grateful to the scholars and artists whom we sought out with questions and, in some cases, requests for interviews. Our community was enriched by the experience and expertise of Cariad Astles, Claudia Orenstein, Marina Tsaplina, Leonard Bloom, Hillel Finestone, Anne Stanwix, Alexis Milligan and

Katie Stock. We owe particular thanks to two non-academic contributors to this book – George Anderson and Adele Vogelsang. They brought us unique and diverse perspectives and gracefully collaborated with our desire to adapt their fresh views into our academic framework.

In preparing the book for the press, it has been a delight to work with our editors at Bloomsbury – Ella Wilson and Mark Dudgeon. Thanks also to Claire Weatherhead at Bloomsbury for facilitating our permissions requests. Kurt Carstensen at *Weekly World News* was also tremendously generous, saying 'yes' to an image request in less than three hours.

Words cannot do justice to the inestimable privilege of working with our in-house editor, Joel Faber, who has been ably assisted by Ben Pulver, at the University of Toronto. Faber has been integral to *Theatre as Medicine* from its inception to its completion. His scholarly discernment and writerly sensibility helped articulate and accommodate the markedly different, interdisciplinary perspectives that make up this polyphonic volume.

We hope that readers will appreciate the communal joy that went into creating the book and join us in exploring the exciting field of performative medicine.

Introduction

MARLENE GOLDMAN, LAWRENCE SWITZKY
AND ALICE FLAHERTY

A fundamental tenet of *Medicine as Theatre: Theatre as Medicine* is that the clinical encounter is performative and dynamic: patients interact with doctors and caregivers. Medical performances cannot be understood in isolation, nor does interpretation happen in only one direction. The contact that occurs between patient, doctor and caregiver makes illness an ensemble drama. The art of medicine practised by physicians and caregivers is so enmeshed with the art of being a patient that we propose viewing them together as the art of illness. Ignoring the performative aspects of doctors', patients' and caregivers' identities can cause real-world harm.

Foregrounding the art of illness helps health humanities scholars and clinicians grapple with medicine's longstanding yet undertheorized relationship to theatre. Medicine arose from healing rituals that complemented herbal remedies and surgical procedures to address the 'physical and metaphysical aspects of well-being'.[1] Scholars of both classical and early modern culture have productively charted the intersections between medicine and theatre. Perhaps because the relationship between the disciplines has changed so profoundly, scholars have paid less attention to the links between modern

[1] Chukwundu Elendu, 'The Evolution of Ancient Healing Practices: From Shamanism to Hippocratic Medicine. A Review', *Medicine* 103, no. 28 (2024): 5.

medicine and modern and contemporary drama. This oversight means that many scholars have overlooked how theatre remains grounded in the medicalized body.

As early as the fifth-century-BCE Hippocratic corpus, medical schools trained physicians in the manner of taking on a medical role: posture, gait and tone of voice were deliberate and rehearsed. Wittingly or unwittingly, patients likewise adopt scripted gestures, phrases and learn how to communicate distress. The phrase 'the art of illness' should not suggest that medical performance is deceptive or false. Instead, it emphasizes that the embodied and verbal communication between doctors and patients relies on performative elements ranging from setting, lighting and props to the doctors' and patients' costumes. Performance is never simply an act of seeming, nor is theatre merely an instrument of play-acting. The theatrical elements in the clinical encounter enhance doctor–patient–carer interactions. Properly understood, the art of illness lends such interactions emotional and therapeutic dimensions that transcend a purely biomedical framework of cure.

This book arose from the multidisciplinary friendship between the three editors: a physician, a literature professor and a professor of drama studies. We came together when organizing an exploratory seminar held at the Harvard Radcliffe Institute in 2021. Besides physicians and scholars from North America and Europe, speakers included patients and home health aides – stakeholders whose voices are rarely heard in the medical humanities. The book has expanded that roster to include interviews with a nurse, a paid companion, an Indigenous playwright, artists who directly interact with doctors, patients and the general public, as well as healthcare activists and scholars of disability studies and theatre and performance history.

To some degree, the field of performative medicine described in this volume already exists and thrives in practice: in the postures with which both doctor and patient choose to enter a room; in the modulations of voice, gesture and costume that caregivers artfully *and* compassionately employ; in the ways so many of us rehearse what we're going to say to communicate our needs effectively before entering a clinical or healing environment. Yet, because the theatrical dimensions of medicine have been neglected and sometimes even actively disavowed by medical workers who fear that they will be seen as not authentically empathetic or professional enough (see Figure I.1: *Weekly World News* headline), performative medicine has largely been a diffuse, underground endeavour.

The contributors to this volume bring into the open discussions that are already carried out quietly between colleagues or mentors and medical students or that take place in occasional training workshops for clinicians on dramatic analysis and applied theatre. In that sense, much of the work of this

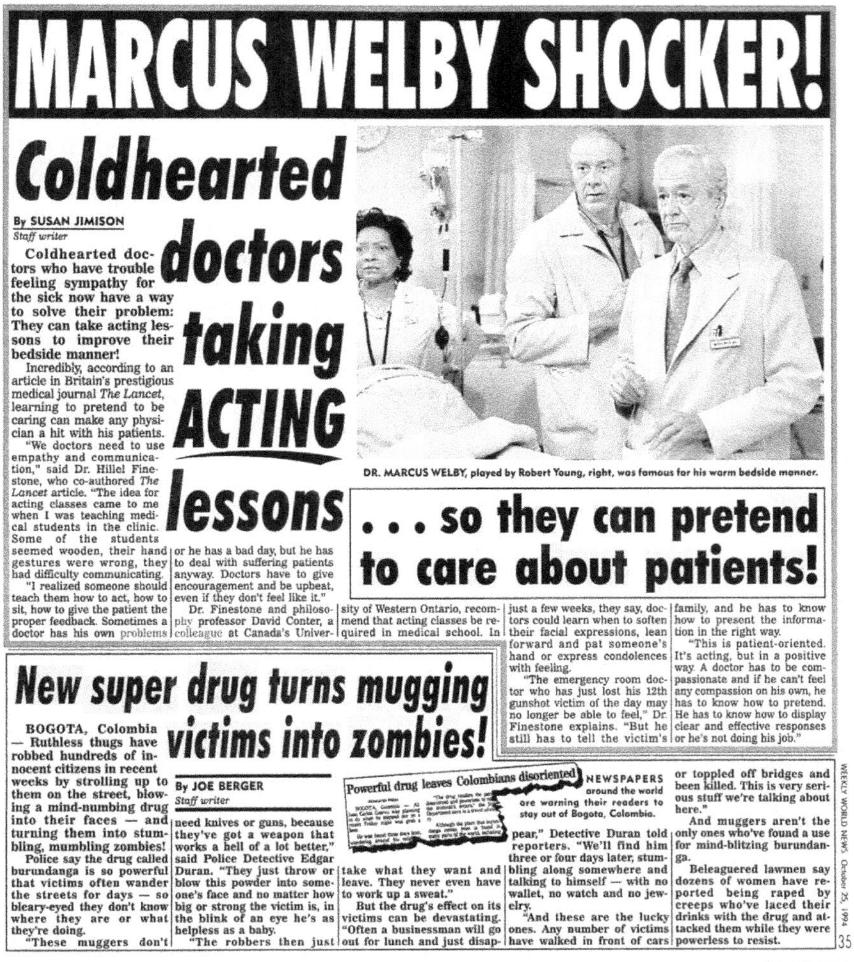

MARCUS WELBY SHOCKER!

Coldhearted doctors taking ACTING lessons

. . . so they can pretend to care about patients!

By SUSAN JIMISON
Staff writer

Coldhearted doctors who have trouble feeling sympathy for the sick now have a way to solve their problem: They can take acting lessons to improve their bedside manner!

Incredibly, according to an article in Britain's prestigious medical journal *The Lancet*, learning to pretend to be caring can make any physician a hit with his patients.

"We doctors need to use empathy and communication," said Dr. Hillel Finestone, who co-authored *The Lancet* article. "The idea for acting classes came to me when I was teaching medical students in the clinic. Some of the students seemed wooden, their hand gestures were wrong, they had difficulty communicating.

"I realized someone should teach them how to act, how to sit, how to give the patient the proper feedback. Sometimes a doctor has his own problems or he has a bad day, but he has to deal with suffering patients anyway. Doctors have to give encouragement and be upbeat, even if they don't feel like it."

Dr. Finestone and philosophy professor David Conter, a colleague at Canada's University of Western Ontario, recommend that acting classes be required in medical school. In just a few weeks, they say, doctors could learn when to soften their facial expressions, lean forward and pat someone's hand or express condolences with feeling.

"The emergency room doctor who has just lost his 12th gunshot victim of the day may no longer be able to feel," Dr. Finestone explains. "But he still has to tell the victim's family, and he has to know how to present the information in the right way.

"This is patient-oriented. It's acting, but in a positive way. A doctor has to be compassionate and if he can't feel any compassion on his own, he has to know how to pretend. He has to know how to display clear and effective responses or he's not doing his job."

DR. MARCUS WELBY, played by Robert Young, right, was famous for his warm bedside manner.

New super drug turns mugging victims into zombies!

By JOE BERGER
Staff writer

BOGOTA, Colombia — Ruthless thugs have robbed hundreds of innocent citizens in recent weeks by strolling up to them on the street, blowing a mind-numbing drug into their faces — and turning them into stumbling, mumbling zombies!

Police say the drug called burundanga is so powerful that victims often wander the streets for days — so bleary-eyed they don't know where they are or what they're doing.

"These muggers don't need knives or guns, because they've got a weapon that works a hell of a lot better," said Police Detective Edgar Duran. "They just throw or blow this powder into someone's face and no matter how big or strong the victim is, in the blink of an eye he's as helpless as a baby.

"The robbers then just take what they want and leave. They never even have to work up a sweat."

But the drug's effect on its victims can be devastating.

"Often a businessman will go out for lunch and just disappear," Detective Duran told reporters. "We'll find him three or four days later, stumbling along somewhere and talking to himself — with no wallet, no watch and no jewelry.

"And these are the lucky ones. Any number of victims have walked in front of cars or toppled off bridges and been killed. This is very serious stuff we're talking about here."

And muggers aren't the only ones who've found a use for mind-blitzing burundanga.

Beleaguered lawmen say dozens of women have reported being raped by creeps who've laced their drinks with the drug and attacked them while they were powerless to resist.

Powerful drug leaves Colombians disoriented

NEWSPAPERS around the world are warning their readers to stay out of Bogota, Colombia.

WEEKLY WORLD NEWS October 25, 1994 35

FIGURE I.1 A headline from the tabloid *Weekly World News*, 25 October 1994. Credit: Bat Boy LLC.

book is exploratory, as reflected in the significant number of interviews we feature here to uncover how and where performative medicine happens. In the early 1990s, British playwright David Hare called his method of research 'asking around': talking to the people who make up institutions about how they do their jobs, sustain relationships and envision transformation. A similar spirit has guided the acts of asking, listening and reporting that went into the creation of this book.

FROM NARRATIVE MEDICINE TO PERFORMATIVE MEDICINE

While putting this book together, we have all, at one point or another, found ourselves trying to introduce the new field of performative medicine, only to discover that our interlocutors immediately assume we're talking about narrative medicine. Their confusion is understandable. Narrative medicine, whose origins date back over twenty years, is frequently understood to encompass the entire field of medical humanities. Its first global conference in 2013, hosted by two of narrative medicine's most recognized champions, physicians Rita Charon and Brian Hurwitz, aimed to promote '*a narrative future for healthcare*'. That future has arrived: to date, narrative medicine's proponents have founded university departments and launched programmes dedicated to disseminating its theories, clinical practice and approaches to medical training.

As one of the founders of narrative medicine, sociologist Arthur Frank, observes, its method is predicated on using stories to enhance 'creativity and imagination in healthcare work'.[2] Narrative medicine proposes that literature encourages health professionals to be more compassionate healers. Reading sparks clinicians' imaginations and generates empathy for characters that can be transferred to patients. As Charon explains, narrative medicine began 'as a rigorous intellectual and clinical discipline to fortify healthcare with the capacity to skillfully receive the accounts persons give of themselves – to recognize, absorb, interpret, and be moved to action by the stories of others'.[3] The method's inaugural and ongoing aim entails teaching clinicians and trainees in healthcare the skill of close reading that entails attending to 'such narrative features as temporality, narrative situation, voice, metaphor, and mood'.[4] Its proponents' faith lies in 'an egality that emits from storytelling [which] levels even hard-bitten power asymmetries, so that members of interprofessional healthcare teams or groups of teachers and students or clinicians and patients can meet one another as equals, bent on reflexively giving and receiving, teaching and learning'.[5] While we remain grateful to narrative medicine for highlighting the manifestly fruitful relationships between the humanities and the medical arts, at times its long shadow prevents people from grasping alternative approaches, concepts and tactics.

[2] Arthur Frank, 'What Is Narrative Medicine?', review of The Principles and Practice of Narrative Medicine, by Rita Charon et al.', *Journal of Medical Humanities* 38 (2017): 339.
[3] Rita Charon et al., *The Principles and Practice of Narrative Medicine* (Oxford Academic, 2016), 1.
[4] Ibid., 157.
[5] Ibid., 5.

Performative medicine complements narrative medicine's focus on books and stories by offering an embodied analytic framework for the performative elements that directly inhere in the clinical encounters' embodied interactions. Whereas close-reading skills can be applied to the clinical situation, performance elements constitute its rebar. Rather than rely on books to spark ethical engagement, an awareness of theatre and performance allows medical practitioners to understand their largely unexamined and culturally codified performative operations. In this volume, we use performance theory to highlight the foundationally theatrical nature of the doctor–patient encounter. Exploring the intersection between medicine and theatre also corrects narrative medicine's primary emphasis on the spaces and interactions restricted to physicians, nurses and other healthcare workers. Commenting on medicine's unwavering attention to the physician, Frank argues that 'close reading becomes what Michel Foucault would call a form of care of the self … a discipline of self-formation'.[6] Ironically, the attention paid to the physician's self threatens to create a solipsistic loop that undermines the goal of levelling the hierarchy between patients and physicians.

To appreciate the difference between the two approaches, we invite readers to consider Yale drama critic Elinor Fuchs's point that a play is completely different from a narrative. As she explains, 'A play is not a flat work of literature, not a description in poetry of another world, but is itself another world passing before you in time and space. Language is only one part of this world. Those who think too exclusively in terms of language find it hard to read plays.'[7] By analysing the active roles of patients and family caregivers, our volume casts new light on the complexity of the ensemble drama of illness.

The art of illness – with its operating theatres, its costumes such as white coats and patient gowns, and its use of ritualized lines and physical gestures – lends the doctor–patient interaction emotional and therapeutic dimensions that exceed narrative medicine's practice of focusing largely on the doctor's close reading of the patient and her story or on the patient's capacity to organize their experiences through speech. These dimensions include acknowledging the process of creating and sustaining an embodied attunement to the other. This attunement, in turn, provides the foundation for intimate and compassionate dialogue and ritual gestures that shore up patients' agency and sense of personhood.

---

[6] Frank, 'What Is Narrative Medicine?', 341.

[7] Elinor Fuchs, 'EF's Visit to a Small Planet: Some Questions to Ask a Play', *Theater* 34, no. 2 (2004): 6.

THE PERFORMATIVE TURN IN HEALTH HUMANITIES

For humanists, the word 'performance' may conjure images of a costumed actor playing a character on stage. For physicians, performance refers to the implementation of a skill and the success of an activity based on a given standard. Yet doctors also wear costumes and assume different personae. As part of their training and work, they also rehearse and intone scripted lines, as, for example, when they are breaking bad news to patients. The seemingly disparate definitions of performance – playing a role and performing a skill – are in fact bound by a common denominator since all performance involves an awareness of a model or a standard and, in some cases, an audience – what performance theorists term 'consciousness of doubleness'.[8] All performance relies on mimesis or doubleness, regardless of whether 'the actor or the observer suppl[ies] the action with a comparator ... Although people typically associate performance with the theatre, performance studies scholars have applied the concept more broadly to make sense of historical, social, and cultural process'.[9]

During the late 1950s and 1960s, sociologist Erving Goffman's groundbreaking research analysed how people perform in everyday life. He observed that what appear to be improvised behaviours in social situations actually 'consists of pre-established patterns or routines'.[10] Viewed in this light, everyone is an actor, and all the world is a stage. Goffman distinguished between the 'front' of the house – the spaces reserved for the audience – and the 'back' of the house – the spaces where the actors and the production team let down their guard. In the medical context, the front of the house constitutes the public-facing spaces in the clinical setting of the doctor's office or the hospital. For performance theorists, frontstage and backstage performances are equally constructed and equally deserving of scholarly analysis.

American sociologist Talcott Parsons also began to conceptualize the performative aspects of medicine in his 1951 study *The Social System*. As Parsons recognized, becoming ill entails taking on a special social status, which he called 'the sick role'. Patients cast in the sick role are temporarily exempt from social expectations – chiefly the expectation to be economically productive – but are also subject to the normative obligation to recover swiftly under a doctor's care and rejoin the world of work. As he later observed, 'the acceptance of the role of patient ... may be said to impose a definite responsibility on the patient in working toward the common goal of the system as a whole' (267). The doctor also enacts a social role that dovetails with her professional role, taking on

[8] Richard Bauman, quoted in Marvin Carlson, 'What Is Performance?' in *The Performance Studies Reader*, ed. Henry Bial and Sara Brady (Routledge, 2016), 75.
[9] Marlene Goldman, *The Social, Aesthetic, and Medical Implications of Performing Shame: Interdisciplinary Approaches* (Routledge, 2023), 19.
[10] Erving Goffman, *The Presentation of Self in Everyday Life* (Doubleday, 1959), 61.

an altruistic duty of care while agreeing to regulate the patient's return from a 'deviant' condition of sickness on behalf of society and its institutions. Critics have subsequently contested Parson's model, particularly his seeming endorsement of a fundamental asymmetry of power between a child-like patient and a parent-like doctor, though later theorists and clinicians have been influenced by his conception of medical care in terms of the multiple and changing parts that sick people are required to play.

In the 1960s, social scientists, keen on analysing cultural performance – 'the living, embodied expression of cultural traditions and transformations', championed new theoretical approaches to performance and performativity.[11] A preference for embodied performances, as Goldman observes, became increasingly prevalent when the setting shifted from the theatre to the street protests in support of civil rights and Black Pride, second-wave feminism, Gay Pride and disability rights, which relied on theatrical elements to mount politically progressive and embodied public performances.[12] Performance studies as a scholarly discipline finds its roots in this historical era of social upheaval. Anthropologists including Milton Singer and Victor Turner – who coined the term 'social drama' – adopted and adapted 'the forms and approaches originally linked to theatrical performance into research tools'.[13] As Jon McKenzie observes, the term 'performance' became central to the newly emerging field of scientific management.[14] Within this context, 'performance' resonated with connotations of improving labourers' efficiency and productivity – connotations that were readily applicable to medicine.

In the early 1960s, philosophers and linguists were proposing a very different conception of performance that applied the concept to 'non-embodied, textual performances'.[15] Leading theorists included J. L. Austin, who emphasized that 'speech acts', or 'performative utterances', do things.[16] Drawing on Austin's insights, literary theorist Judith Butler noted that language combined with the codified and 'repeated stylization of the body' to produce gender rather than merely describe it.[17] The insights of Austin and Butler help us to understand the powerful role healthcare professionals possess since they alone have the power to name and assert the legitimacy of disease entities – and pronounce people as healthy or diseased. Just as a minister changes the identities of individuals when his speech act names them 'man and wife', a

---

[11] Jon McKenzie, *Perform or Else: From Discipline to Performance* (Routledge, 2001), 8.
[12] See Goldman, *Performing Shame*, 18–20.
[13] Ibid., 19.
[14] McKenzie, *Perform or Else*, 6–7.
[15] See Goldman, *Performing Shame*, 23–5.
[16] For an overview of speech act theory, including quotations of Austin's work, see the *Stanford Encyclopedia of Philosophy* entry on 'Speech Acts' (https://plato.stanford.edu/entries/speech-acts/).
[17] Judith Butler, *Gender Trouble* (Routledge, 1990), 33.

doctor's pronouncement of a diagnosis can likewise create a new self. Thus Atul Gawande, for example, writes about patients, after a fatal diagnosis, 'learning to play the dying role'.[18] This power, as medical historians demonstrate, has been wittingly and unwittingly abused. The power that inheres in the relationship is not actually stable, either, since patients and family caregivers can now use the internet to self-diagnose or treat, thereby intervening in the hierarchical act of medical care.

There have been attempts before now to articulate a specifically performative approach to medicine. These, however, have been diffuse and have taken the form of relatively brief essays and letters written by medical professionals that primarily address physician training. Their models have rarely been promoted or developed beyond an initial provocation owing to the authors' busy schedules. Although the underlying methods and theories of theatre that guide these approaches vary, they consistently focus on a few key features: destigmatizing acting, using theatrical concepts as frames for understanding and revising social and communicative norms, and imagining acting as a tool to generate emotional availability and empathy in adverse circumstances (e.g. exhaustion, antipathy) while preventing doctor burn-out.[19] Finestone and Conter (1994) and McManus (1994), for example, recognize that supporting patients emotionally is crucial to their physical health and endorse acting as a tool to fine-tune a doctor's expressive behaviour, which patients often attend to more closely than explicit messaging. Persaud (2005) takes the stance that acting can bring the contradictory expectations of patients – who want both emotional support and authority from carers – to conscious awareness, enabling the rescripting of roles. Case and Brauner (2010) use methods from performance studies and acting theory to move past the rote modelling and mimicry in medical communications education, instead endorsing a flexible '*empathetic imagination*' that can be a source of comfort and enjoyment for doctors and their patients.[20] Whorwell and Shanahan (2016) likewise emphasize the potential pleasures of acting in medical environments – as a way of providing reassurance in time-strapped contexts and for building confidence in doctors to 'release [their] personality' to benefit patients.[21]

[18] Atul Gawande, *Being Mortal: Medicine and What Matters in the End* (Anchor Canada, 2014), 249.

[19] Many of these essays engage in debates – sometimes in reference to each other – about the conditions under which empathy might be learned or trained and the permissibility of creating appearances of empathy. This remains a contentious issue in many fields; for a discussion of how the limits of empathy are the grounds of many legal structures, see Elaine Scarry, 'The Difficulty of Imagining Other People', in *For Love of Country?*, ed. Joshua Cohen (Penguin, 2002), 98–110.

[20] Gretchen A. Case and Daniel J. Brauner, 'The Doctor as Performer: A Proposal for Change Based on a Performance Studies Paradigm', *Academic Medicine* 85, no. 1 (2010): 159, emphasis in original.

[21] P. J. Whorwell and F. Shanahan, 'In the Performing Art of Medicine: The Doctor as Actor', *QJM: An International Journal of Medicine* 109, no. 3 (2016), 159–60. These references form a brief

Many of these essays also give voice to anxieties that bringing theatrical acting into medicine compromises authenticity. Such concerns can be addressed by noting, as medical educator Hartley Jafine does, that although we may change our personae in different circumstances our values do not change, and thus we maintain integrity across our performances.[22]

HISTORICAL CONNECTIONS BETWEEN THEATRE AND MEDICINE

Performance theorists adopt theatrical metaphors to describe social behaviours while approaching theatre per se as only one among many ways of performing. Within the ensemble dramas of illness and healing that the essays in this collection explore, however, theatre plays a pivotal role – as a repertoire of conventions, locations, materials, metaphors and relationships that can inform and enrich healthcare. For thousands of years, theatre and medicine have worked together as disciplines that 'converge on the somatic body, its capacities and vulnerabilities'.[23] As a 'complex engagement' that has often gone 'in waves rather than in steady, progressively deepening intertwinement', the invention and abundance of intersections between theatre and medicine can offer a roadmap for present and future partnerships between theatre, medical training and patient care.[24] A lightning sketch of representative instances suggests how historical collaborations between these two arts of somatic knowledge might enrich present-day practice.

In the ancient world, theatre was often part of a healing process or a means of healing in its own right. Treatment took place during, alongside and through performances. In Ancient Egypt (*c.*3000 BCE), healers arranged elaborate

---

theoretical and philosophical backbone for our inquiry. It's also important to note that there have been many instances of introducing practical and applied theatrical training into undergraduate and professional medical education as well as to enhance the skills of doctors and carers. See, for example, Katie Watson, 'Serious Play: Teaching Medical Skills with Improvisational Theatre Techniques', *Academic Medicine* 86, no. 10 (2011): 1260–5; L. Gao et al., 'The Role of 'Improv' in Health Professional Learning: A Scoping Review', *Medical Teacher* (2018), https://doi.org/10.1080/0142159X.2018.1505033; Bronte K. Johnston and Hartley Jafine, 'Applied Theatre and Drama in Undergraduate Medical Education: A Scoping Review', *McGill Journal of Medicine* 20 (2022); and three chapters in *The Routledge Companion to Health Humanities*, ed. Paul Crawford, Brian Brown and Andrea Charise (Routledge, 2020): Rick Iedema, 'Intervention Theatre'; Marina Tsaplina and Cariad Astles, 'Puppetry'; and Gretchen Case and Sydney Cheek-O'Donnell, 'Applied Theatre'.

[22] Personal conversation with Hartley Jafine, 2 June 2025.

[23] Stanton B. Garner, Jr, *Theatre & Medicine* (Methuen Drama, 2023), 4.

[24] Kirsten Shepherd-Barr, 'The Diagnostic Gaze: Nineteenth-Century Contexts for Performance and Medicine', in *Performance and the Medical Body*, ed. Alex Mermikides and Gianna Bouchard (Bloomsbury Methuen Drama, 2016), 39.

theatrical productions to 'drive away a patient's sickness'.[25] In Zhou-Dynasty China (1045–256 BCE), the songs and dances of wu-shamans warded off both 'evil spirits and epidemic diseases' and also became predecessors of Chinese opera.[26] The colossal Theatre at Epidaurus (*c.*400 BCE) is located within a sanctuary complex dedicated to Asklepios, the Greek god of medicine, and a temple to Asklepios sits next to the Theatre of Dionysus on the Acropolis in Athens. At the complex and temple where patients resided – essentially, early hospitals – performances were included in a regimen of recovery from illness alongside bathing, special diets and receiving dreams from the gods.[27] Ritual and theatre were also used to manage public health by stimulating, purifying and rebalancing the emotions, as was practised in Ayurvedic medicine in India and Traditional Chinese Medicine and as Aristotle likewise proposed in his *Poetics* (*c.*330 BCE). Hildegard of Bingen (*c.*1098–1179 CE), a German Benedictine nun and composer, as well as a medical practitioner and author of treatises on medicinal herbs and treatments, regarded musical performances and sung sacred drama as 'a kind of regulator, a therapeutic agent of the first order'.[28]

In the fifteenth and sixteenth centuries, theatre and medicine borrowed techniques from each other for producing and disseminating knowledge about the body and its hidden interiors. Humoral medicine, derived from the ancient Greek physician Hippocrates (*c.*460–370 BCE) and popularized by the philosopher Galen (130–200 CE), explained human character in terms of the imbalance of four internal fluids, or humours, that governed the human body. Shakespeare and contemporary playwrights used humoral theory to 'visualize and externalize inner processes' and to provide a gallery of instantly recognizable types with an excess of one humour – the brooding and suspicious melancholic, the short-tempered choleric – that could be set into dramatic conflict.[29] Demonstrations in anatomy theatres, which originated in the same period, imitated theatrical performances, while 'dissection took its place alongside the Shakespearean monologue, as an alternate stage for the testing of the limits and pathologies of the human'.[30]

Theatrical and medical modernity in the late nineteenth century participated in a similar series of exchanges. Realism in the theatre emerged out of developments in experimental physiology and an 'ideology of the visible' that cast

---

[25] Sade Musa, 'Historic Abundance', in *Artists Remaking Medicine: The Practice of Imagination and the Power to Create a Better Healthcare Future*, ed. Emily F. Peters (Procedure Press, 2023), 19.

[26] Xiaohuan Zhou, 'Nuo Altar Theatre on a Liminal/Liminoid Continuum: Reflections on the Shamanic Origins of Chinese Theatre', *TDR: The Drama Review* 63, no. 2 (Summer 2019): 59.

[27] Karelisa V. Hartigan, *Performance and Cure: Drama and Healing in Ancient Greece and Contemporary America* (Duckworth, 2009), 29–30.

[28] Heinrich Schipperges, *Hildegard of Bingen: Healing and the Nature of the Cosmos* (M. Wiener, 1997), 86.

[29] Amy Kenny, *Humoral Wombs on the Shakespearean Stage* (Palgrave, 2019), 3.

[30] Jane Taylor, 'Newes from the Dead: An Unnatural Moment in the History of Natural Philosophy', in *Shakespeare's Things*, ed. Brett Gamboa and Lawrence Switzky (Routledge, 2020), 208.

audiences in the position of doctors, rendering diagnoses of physiological and social ills based on observable symptoms.[31] During the same period, doctors learned from the theatre the symbolic value of a costume change: they traded black formal dress for white coats, still potent emblems of medical authority, to emphasize the cleanliness of clinics after discoveries about the value of antiseptics and hygiene to prevent infection.[32]

Medicine and theatre have also converged in 'medical spectacles', performance genres in which clinical knowledge joins forces with showmanship to educate non-specialist publics, display non-normative bodies and advertise medical services and drugs.[33] Travelling medicine shows in rural North America after the Civil War sold patent cures between entertainments like restaged battles between Native Americans and settlers and magic tricks. Freak shows throughout the nineteenth and early twentieth centuries put non-standard bodies on display as titillating exhibitions of pathology, authenticated by 'respected medical doctors' who documented 'their examinations in language at once clinical and reverent'.[34]

Lecture-performances likewise merged medicine and theatre and frequently took place within scientific institutions. Neurologist Jean-Martin Charcot's highly theatrical public demonstrations at the Paris hospital La Salpêtrière in the 1870s and 1880s presented mostly female patients coached and hypnotized by neurologists to perform in 'hysteria shows': simulations of symptoms, poses and even sometimes short scenes, all in a darkened auditorium with footlights and a limelight.[35] Spectators similarly paid entry fees to medical asylums throughout Europe to watch productions put on by the inmates. Although earlier medical spectacles gained a reputation for being manipulative and exploitative, theatre that draws from these genres has been an important vehicle for spreading news about medical discoveries and instigating policy debates and social change. Throughout the 1930s in the United States, for example, a spectacular genre of theatrical performance called Living Newspapers staged stories about current events and controversial social issues, including healthcare reform. Activists and theatre-makers have acknowledged the spectacular singularity of disabled

---

[31] Stanton B. Garner, Jr, 'Is There a Doctor in the House? Medicine and the Making of Modern Drama', *Modern Drama* 51, no. 3 (2008): 311–28.

[32] Mark S. Hochberg, 'The Doctor's White Coat: A Historical Perspective', *AMA Journal of Ethics* 9, no. 4 (2007): 310–14.

[33] Alex Mermikides and Gianna Bouchard, 'Introduction', in *Performance and the Medical Body*, ed. Mermikides and Bouchard, 4.

[34] Rosemarie Garland-Thomson, Introduction, *Freakery: Cultural Spectacles of the Extraordinary Body* (New York University Press, 1996), 10.

[35] Elaine Showalter, *Hystories: Hysterical Epidemics and Modern Media* (Columbia University Press, 1997), 34; Matthew Wilson Smith, *The Nervous Stage: Nineteenth-Century Neuroscience and the Birth of Modern Theatre* (Oxford University Press, 2017), 139.

bodies for their unique creative capacities and as tools that build access and inclusion for physical and cognitive difference.[36] Indigenous performers have likewise reclaimed the medicine shows that appropriated and misunderstood their traditions, instead making medicine through theatre 'by reconnecting through ceremony, through the act of remembering, through rebuilding community, and by negotiating solidarities across communities'.[37]

While the art of medicine and the art of theatre have frequently been allied or complementary, they have also, at times, been fiercely critical of each other. Medical drama since the Renaissance has generally scourged doctors as self-absorbed and obsessive, fixated on incomprehensible Latinate terms and pet theories at the expense of their suffering patients. Even in the realist drama of the late nineteenth and early twentieth centuries, when doctors were largely portrayed on stage primarily not as buffoons but rather as earnest and well-meaning healers, playwrights still rendered them as ineffective in the face of complex lives and systems, as 'expert diagnosticians but inept curers'.[38] From the perspective of medicine, credentialed and licensed professionals have long dismissed the theatricality of so-called mountebanks and 'quacks', medical operators who gaudily advertised their wares in the marketplace and offered dubious placebos and cure-alls in place of legitimate knowledge and experience. According to historian Roy Porter, the outcry against quacks came to a head in the early eighteenth century as the need to compete for patients' business in a crowded and confusing field escalated.[39] Informed by the long history of the intersection of theatre and medicine, a suspicion of theatricality in medicine continues to the present day: the clinician's refusal of duplicitous practitioners and malingering patients, and theatre's rebuke of monomaniacal and ego-driven comedy doctors. This suspicion, however, is only a small part of a much longer and ampler story – one that this collection attempts to tell anew, with participation from both sides.

A PERFORMATIVE THEORY OF ILLNESS

As we move from cultural history to consider the lived experiences of modern patients, caregivers and doctors, it might first be helpful to elaborate on what we mean by a performance theory of illness. To a great extent, in this section of

---

[36] See, for example, Petra Kuppers's discussion of 'disability as spectacle' in *Theatre & Disability*, especially pp. 13–17, and Katherine Williams's chapter on how disability knowledge can reshape theatre and medicine in this volume.

[37] Yvette Nolan, *Medicine Shows: Indigenous Performance Culture* (Playwrights Canada Press, 2015), 3. See also the interview with Matthew MacKenzie on 'good medicine' in this volume.

[38] Kirsten Shepherd-Barr, *Science on Stage: From Doctor Faustus to Copenhagen* (Princeton University Press, 2006), 157.

[39] Roy Porter, *Quacks: Fakers and Charlatans in English Medicine* (Tempus, 2000), 30.

the introduction, we are foregrounding physician and co-editor Alice Flaherty's approach and experiences. Interpreting clinical encounters as an ensemble performance goes beyond being a fertile turn for medical humanists: it can also help real-world people get and give care. A patient who can movingly communicate her suffering to doctors will more often get the treatment she needs. Medical roles are inherently performative: if a sick person does not act the way caregivers expect sick people to act, they may not get care. Likewise, if a clinician does not play doctor well, their patients won't take their meds.

For many readers of this volume, the theatricality of medicine will already be obvious, but the general public often finds the idea disturbing. Most sick people and caregivers associate words like 'theatrical' with artifice and use 'performative' to mean the opposite of real or authentic, as in virtue signalling. The popularity in medical schools of narrative medicine – of drawing parallels between the art of medicine to the art of literature – may reflect physicians' desire to avoid being associated with theatre's reputation as a low, deceptive art form. That reputation, however, paradoxically lies in theatre's persuasive power and its closeness to real life. Patients, caregivers and doctors can beneficially harness that power and immediacy.

Most doctors are willing to talk about their 'performance' because performance metrics seem distant from the theatre's artful associations and confer a quantitative gloss. In educating doctors and patients about the theatrical aspects of medicine, it may help, initially, to use more neutral terms: 'gesturally communicating kindness' is less tied to artifice than 'acting kind'. Given the varied definitions of performance, as noted above, it is useful to distinguish between performances that communicate and performances that complete a task – though a single performance can do both. When a nurse puts her hand on a patient's hand, she may simultaneously communicate goodwill and assess the patient's temperature. But the two types of performance are still fundamentally different. We argue that doctors need to overcome their reluctance and accept the long-standing connection between theatre and medicine. Accepting that connection can allow doctors to reflect on and, potentially, enhance their performances.

Doctors' attitudes are beginning to change, in part because of the introduction into medical education in the late 1970s and 1980s of actors trained to mimic illness behaviour. These actors are known as standardized patients because they give similar performances each time. Medical schools' reliance on standardized patients is making new generations of doctors more open to the importance of their words and gestures. Yet medical professors still often tell students, 'Don't act! The patient can always tell.'[40] Because medical educators

[40]For more on this, see the conversation between Timothy McGinnis and Arthur Kleinman in this volume, and Corinne Botz's essay on her work *Bedside Manner* (2016).

and the general public valorize empathy as honest and as inherently leading to compassionate action, some young doctors strive to feel the patient's pain in the hope that doing so will create sympathetic expressions and helping acts. Empathy, though invisible to patients, can be vivid enough that carers trust their own emotion and discount patients' reports that do not fit the carer's experience. Empathy can make carers act in ways that relieve their own pain, not the patient's. Affect theorist Doris Sommer notes empathy can mimic imperialistic tendencies to assume that we can know and master another person's experience.[41]

When doctors step away back from their subjective experience to focus on their performance of helpful actions, they tend to frame that performance as a one-man show that they practise in front of a passive patient audience. This solipsistic model ignores the importance of teamwork: in the operating theatre, for example, the surgeon is just one member of a highly skilled troupe.[42] The art of illness as it is lived and practised is an ensemble drama that depends on patients, doctors, nurses and home caregivers, with walk-on roles for insurance adjusters, priests and pharma reps. When patients, doctors and a whole network of caregiver 'co-actors' recognize their interdependence, they can make better healing performances.

Patients' attitudes are changing too. The patients' rights movement has begun to empower sick people to act in ways that will enhance their care. There are, of course, challenges facing patients and caregivers alike. Both are dragged onto the medical stage without knowing they should have learned their lines. By contrast, medical students get explicit training in bedside manner, and even practising doctors conduct serious illness conversations by using palliative care scripts. This asymmetry in training how to 'play sick' (the way that clinicians learn to 'play doctor') leads patients to find ad hoc examples. They must model their patient manner on what they have seen or heard from families and friends, on social media or on TV doctor shows.

The medical humanities can help guide societies to be more mindful and deliberate about empowering patients and family caregivers to act. Although patients may learn after the fact how to tell their stories, storytelling doesn't always help during the immersive, multi-sensory, moment-to-moment present in which suffering happens, care gets negotiated, and bodies, with all their expressive tools, physically change each other. Appreciating the potential of performative medicine, medical humanists can expand their scope to

---

[41] See Doris Sommer, 'Attitude, Its Rhetoric', in *The Turn to Ethics*, ed. Marjorie Garber, Beatrice Hanssen and Rebecca Walkowitz (Routledge, 2000), 201–20.

[42] For more on the ensemble drama of medicine, see the chapters in this volume by Alice Flaherty and Rachel Warr.

empower their students to learn an embodied communication of suffering and compassion.

MAPPING *MEDICINE AS THEATRE: THEATRE AS MEDICINE*

The essays in this volume scrutinize what it means to play doctor and to assume the sick role, directly examining the effects of gender, race, class, sexual orientation, disability and age on patient–caregiver interactions. By expanding scholarly knowledge and interdisciplinary conversation, shedding new light on medical and patient education and rewriting the scripts for embodied interactions between patients and physicians, the volume will benefit scholars, practitioners, caregivers and patients.

The book is structured in five main parts, which correspond to the chiasmus in the title of *Medicine as Theatre/Theatre as Medicine*. The first three parts focus on the performative aspects of three kinds of participants within the ensemble drama of illness: the doctor, the patient and the caregiver; the final two parts then explore how theatrical performance in the past and present has abetted, interrogated and worked to transform medical care by modelling performative medicine.

PART ONE: FASHIONING THE DOCTOR'S CHARACTER

Part One's contributors underscore the basic premise of performative medicine: physicians, patients and caregivers are *embodied* actors, who collaborate in a specific setting (a clinic, hospital or at home), and who work with (and, at times, without) scripts and props as part of their daily performance. This part features three contributors who, in very different ways, challenge contemporary North American medical schools' overly rigid standardized approach to teaching doctors how to perform. The problem is not standardization per se; it is when adherence to a set procedure prevents innovation and the inclusion of diverse health professionals. Equally critical, overreliance on a standardized procedure can undermine attunement to the patient as a person and potentials for healing collaborations. Works in this part also consider how medical programmes can address these limitations by embracing insights generated by the performative arts.

In Chapter 1, Dr Tim McGinnis, who recently completed his surgical residency at the University of Chicago, interviews Arthur Kleinman, Professor of Medical Anthropology and Psychiatry at Harvard Medical School, who conceived of the concept of 'the illness narrative'. According to Kleinman, in the medical context 'performance' and 'theatre' ideally entail that actors – in this case, physicians – infuse their role with felt emotion and respond to patients authentically and in the moment, as opposed to mechanically playing a scripted part. Anything that interposes itself between doctor and patient and impedes this type of humane connection, which he terms 'presence', undermines medical performance. Even ostensible gains in diagnostic testing, pharmacology, along with broader structural changes in the healthcare system, in Kleinman's view, can inadvertently undermine the primary doctor–patient dyadic connection, thereby degrading 'the humanity that should be at the core of medicine'.

In Chapter 2, Dr Deborah Ocholi, a recent medical graduate, reflects on her training in her personal essay 'Medical Training and Character Development: The Hidden Curriculum in Learning to Act'. Recalling Kleinman's concerns about medical schools' reductive, mechanistic approach, Ocholi explains that her education aimed to mould students into a unitary, standardized prototype as if there were only one socially approved type of doctor. Although North American medical schools purport to support diversity, Ocholi regularly witnessed students with diverse backgrounds encountering interpersonal and structural barriers that had a negative impact on the formation of their 'physician character'. Drawing on her recent medical training, Ocholi argues that everyone caught up in the ensemble drama of illness stands to benefit ethically and therapeutically from conceiving of themselves as actors who have the power to both fashion and adopt a particular persona.

The final contribution to Part One, Chapter 3's interview with UK puppeteer, dramaturg and medical educator Rachel Warr, 'Puppetry and Medical Performance', offers a deep dive into what the art of puppetry, in particular, can teach medical residents. Surgical residents working with Warr, for example, learn about their shared reliance on teamwork, on the human hand and on the skilful manipulation of knots and thread.

Taken together, the chapters in Part One highlight a common thread that runs through the entire volume: the recognition that doctor's, patient's and caregivers' roles are implicitly and, at times, explicitly scripted. By reflecting on these scripts, everyone involved in the collaborative drama of illness is afforded an opportunity to refine their performance and, where appropriate, to revise unhelpful or worse, iatrogenic roles. Relying on theatre, which is essentially a collaborative art, to shed light on experiences of illness and healing has the added benefit of correcting for medicine's overemphasis on the doctor's role. This traditional overemphasis typically elides the agency and insight afforded by patients and caregivers.

PART TWO: PATIENTS AND THE ART OF ILLNESS

As the title of Part Two suggests, Chapters 4–6 explore patients' agency. The essays in this part demonstrate that both doctors' and patients' agency is challenged by experiences of chronic illness and intractable suffering.

In Chapter 4, 'Performing the Art of Illness: How Patients Can Ail Well and Caregivers Can Help', neurologist Dr Alice Flaherty outlines how patients can 'learn to play sick well'. To receive appropriate aid from others, Flaherty argues that ailing individuals need to do more than communicate their symptoms; they must learn how to 'act sick' – how to grimace, groan and gesture – so as to clearly convey their distress. Although playing sick well is not easy when one is ill, Flaherty insists that we can recover or cope better with our condition if we consciously plan our words, gestures and actions.

In Chapter 5, 'The Ensemble Arts of Healing and Learning: Forum Theatre and Pre-Texts', Doris Sommer likewise addresses how theatre can empower patients. Her approach differs from Flaherty's because it imagines moving beyond the clinical context. To empower patients, Sommer relies on Forum Theatre, a community-based improvisatory art created in the early 1970s by Brazilian theatre artist August Boal. Rather than putting the onus on individuals to learn to play sick well, Forum Theatre brings community members together to stage and enquire into local public health problems. For example, in January 2018, Sommer together with eighty local participants used techniques from Forum Theatre in Lima, Peru, to analyse and develop solutions to obstacles to much-needed tuberculosis treatment. In Boal's model, health-related problems that are generated structurally can only be addressed by a community acting together.

In Chapter 6, 'Rehearsing Failure: What Theatre Can Teach Medicine About Being Present', anthropologist Bianca Dahl and theatre director Philip McKee rely on personal experience to address the challenges presented by patients' suffering and chronic pain to aesthetic and biomedical narratives, both of which are predicated on an implicit dramaturgy of resolution and closure. Rather than view these challenges as anomalies that can be dismissed, they argue instead for centring experiences that defy conventional plotting and instead rely on co-presence and shared susceptibility. As a corollary, they affirm the value of acting that represent living within limits, the inescapability of suffering and the risk and experience of failure.

As Part Two's contributors attest, healing does not occur merely because like a magician pulling a rabbit out of his hat, doctors come up with a diagnosis. At times, healing requires the support of one's co-actors and community. The attunement needed to initiate and sustain healing also requires that patients and doctors recognize their agency and limits as actors.

PART THREE: CAREGIVERS

Part Three (Chapters 7–9) considers often elided yet essential players in the ensemble drama of illness. As the interviews in this part demonstrate, depending on the illness, its duration and its trajectory, patients and doctors share the stage with a host of actors ranging from specialists to home-care aids to performance artists. Health humanities approaches that focus exclusively on the doctor–patient dyad convey the erroneous impression that the drama of illness is a two-hander, consisting of a doctor, who observes, and a patient, who is observed. By allocating this part to caregivers, we aim to correct this impression and challenge the implicit hierarchy it maintains.

Chapter 7, 'Nursing Tactics: Voice, Touch, Scent', features an interview with Adele Vogelsang, a former in-patient nurse in Boston, Massachusetts. Reflecting on skills honed over forty-five years of nursing patients on neuroscience and oncology wards, Vogelsang outlines how she purposefully appealed to her patients' senses. By relying on embodied, performative skills, she enhanced both her rapport with patients and their comfort and healing.

Chapter 8, 'What Part of the Stage Are You Standing On?', extends the volume's exploration of diverse approaches to caregiving by offering an interview with George Anderson, a mixed-race home caregiver whose clients were primarily white, well-educated, wealthy 'mean old men'. Having spent his youth and most of his adulthood in the US prison system, Anderson was able to assist his privileged clients in resolving past inter- and intrapersonal conflicts. As someone who had never occupied the limelight, he was well positioned to accept their essential vulnerability and helplessness which, for them, was only apparent when faced with death.

Chapter 9, 'I Like to Act Vicariously on Behalf of People', offers a very different perspective on the caregiving role by tracing performance artist Marcus Coates's intimate and imaginative work with psychiatric patients. In Coates's interview, he focuses on two of his recent performances – 'The Trip', a series of disc audio recordings generated with patients at St John's Hospice in London, and *The Directors* (2022), five short films that collaboratively present the experience of psychosis. According to Coates, performance artists can meaningfully contribute to caregiving and healing by highlighting the value of the imagination and tailoring performances that are 'pragmatic, purposeful, and enabling'.

As the interviews in this part attest, caregivers' performative tactics include engaging in open-ended dialogue, rituals and a range of compassionate gestures. These embodied practices underscore that at every moment of illness, no matter how devastating or mortifying, we remain open to the possibility of healing.

PART FOUR: THE PASTS OF PERFORMATIVE MEDICINE

Performative medicine long predates the current moment, and its uses today are conditioned by engagements between medicine and theatre from the past (many of which persist in the present). Because an anti-theatrical bias has long been present in medical practice, which often denies its performative dimensions, theatre and drama history provide an important window into historical instances of performance-based approaches to healthcare. Part Four (Chapters 10–12) investigates how late nineteenth- and twentieth-century theatre, in particular, engaged with medical approaches to the human body, as well as public health and society's understanding of the normal versus the pathological. Building on insights from works in Bloomsbury's series on science and performance such as *Performance and the Medical Body*, our volume offers a diachronic account of medical performance, ranging from the fascinating intersections between medical performance and narrative in the modern period – a period associated with the 'bipolarization' of the human body at the turn of the twentieth century, and the increasing understanding of the human body as revealed by biomedical science – to the present.

Chapter 10 presents our interview with theatre scholar Stanton B. Garner, Jr, 'Medical Influences on Modern Theatre and Theatrical Influences on Modern Medicine'. Garner's pioneering work laid the foundation for analysing the profoundly intimate yet undertheorized relationship between medical and theatrical representations of the human body. During the interview, Garner reflects on his early, seminal insight that how a society explains bodies medically influences how it presents them theatrically. He goes on to consider how disability studies usefully complicates biomedicine's totalizing conceptions of the body. A reprint of Garner's ground-breaking essay, 'Is There a Doctor in the House? Medicine and the Making of Modern Drama' (2008), follows the interview.

In Chapter 11, '"250,000 Unnecessary Deaths": Theatricalizing the National Healthcare Debate in Broadway's *Medicine Show* (1940)', theatre historian Kirsten E. Shepherd offers a detailed analysis of medicine and healthcare on stage in the mid-twentieth-century United States. Shepherd's essay focuses on the highly innovative and imaginative Living Newspaper *Medicine Show* (1940) – a powerful collaborative drama that eschewed medicine's traditional, limited focus on the individual by embracing exuberant theatricality and presenting a snapshot conveying the current state and stakes of American healthcare. As Shepherd demonstrates, *Medicine Show* was openly critical of both the American Medical Association's refusal to support national healthcare and the ideological biases of realist drama that only accepted visible evidence of structural flaws. The fact that Americans continue to face the same problem in healthcare makes *Medicine Show* all the more relevant to contemporary scholars.

In Chapter 12, 'Performance and Medical Education: Bridging the Gap Between Public and Private Phrenology', Marlis Schweitzer and Sara Masciotra-Milstein's essay traces how friendships and, in some cases, intimate relationships between medical professionals and theatre artists shaped the development and dissemination of phrenology, the wildly popular nineteenth-century 'science of the mind'. As the authors demonstrate, supporters of phrenology were coached in theatrical techniques that profoundly contributed to phrenology's rapid uptake in Britain and North America, many of which anticipate the populist strategies of celebrity doctors on social media and television today.

Throughout these chapters, the theatrical past offers a way of understanding the past of performative medicine. It also provides models for and warnings about performative medicine in the present. Theatre is a technology for concentrating and directing attention; studying previous medical theatres illuminates shifting patterns of attention in ensemble acts of care – what we see, what we don't see (or don't want to see) and what we can only see while acting together.

PART FIVE: PERFORMATIVE MEDICINE IN CONTEMPORARY THEATRE AND DRAMA

Theatre today offers a wealth of forms and strategies for exploring the applications and efficacy of performative medicine: from activist and interventionist theatre that brings communities together with artists to give voice to collective problems to applied theatre that represents and addresses pressing social issues to multimedia theatre that incorporates live performance alongside film and photographs. The essays in this part continue the volume's exploration of the ways that interrelationship structures both theatre and medicine using contemporary theatre to highlight new perspectives on the clinical encounter. Combining contributions from scholars and artists, the interviews and essays presented here draw on media studies, age studies, disability studies and Indigenous dramaturgy.

In Chapter 13, 'Bedside Manner', Corinne Botz offers an autoethnographic analysis of her film *Bedside Manner*, which traces the use of Standardized Patients in medical education. Botz's behind-the-scenes focus on novice doctors as they interact with people – some of whom are actors – who assume the role of patients for clinical exams highlights the performative facets of medicine and portrays doctors navigating vulnerability, self-reflection, shame and failure.

In Chapter 14, 'Theatre for Social Change in the Dementia Context: A Conversation Between Two Activist Academics', Sherry Dupuis and Pia Kontos describe their co-written production *Cracked: New Light on Dementia*. As they demonstrate, in contrast to a scholarly article or a book, their research-based play created a world featuring an array of compelling characters living with dementia, along with their families and caregivers. Their immersive, dramatic, embodied scholarship functioned as research and rhetoric, reaching a broad, intergenerational audience, and powerfully conveyed the challenges of the impact of dementia and the challenges and benefits of long-term care facilities.

In Chapter 15, 'Beyond the Cost of Care: Connection, Disability and Embodied Reciprocity in Martyna Majok's *Cost of Living*', Katherine Williams likewise focuses on caregiving, as portrayed in Martyna Majok's Pulitzer Prize–winning play *The Cost of Living*, by considering how lived experiences of 'disability knowledge' can simultaneously influence contemporary healthcare and the production of commercial theatre. As Williams demonstrates, Majok's script benefitted from input from disabled performers about theatre and embodiment. As Williams attests, disabled actors served as co-authors who both inscribed and portrayed alternative temporalities and models of reciprocal care that challenge capitalist concerns with cost and efficiency.

In Chapter 16, 'Knots That I Can't Seem to Easily Undo', playwright Matthew MacKenzie, a citizen of the Metis nation of Alberta, converses with Karen Fricker and Lawrence Switzky about what constitutes 'good medicine' in the context of playwriting and theatre. During their wide-ranging discussion of creativity, caregiving, sickness and grief, Mackenzie and his friends identify important differences between theatre that serves individual interests and art that heals by witnessing and offering meaning to the entire community.

Considered together, the essays and interviews in this part demonstrate the variety and inventiveness of recent theatrical approaches to performative medicine while offering directions for further research. Theatre is, as contributor Stanton B. Garner, Jr, reminds us, 'the medium that looks back. To give voice on stage to someone with an illness is to bring into an objectifying field of vision a perspective and agency that can never be contained by anyone's gaze'.[43] Much as no single actor guides the art of illness, this volume, while containing many voices, is not intended to be exhaustive. Instead, *Medicine as Theatre: Theatre as Medicine* is an invitation to further research and conversation addressed to everyone involved in medicine and the medical humanities – to look back at, and perform with, the many other actors who promote, accompany and witness the event of medical care.

[43]Stanton B. Garner, Jr, 'Medical Influences on Modern Theatre and Theatrical Influences on Modern Medicine', interview in this volume.

REFERENCES

Butler, Judith. *Gender Trouble*. Routledge, 1990.

Carlson, Marvin. 'What Is Performance?' In *The Performance Studies Reader*, edited by Henry Bial and Sara Brady. Routledge, 2016.

Case, Gretchen A., and Daniel J. Brauner. 'The Doctor as Performer: A Proposal for Change Based on a Performance Studies Paradigm'. *Academic Medicine* 85, no. 1 (2010): 159–63.

Charon, Rita, Sayantani DasGupta, Nellie Hermann, Craig Irvine, Eric R. Marcus, Edgar Rivera Colsn, Danielle Spencer and Maura Spiegel. *The Principles and Practice of Narrative Medicine*. Oxford Academic, 2017.

Elendu, Chukwundu. 'The Evolution of Ancient Healing Practices: From Shamanism to Hippocratic Medicine. A Review'. *Medicine* 103, no. 28 (2024): 1–17.

Finestone, Hillel M., and David B. Conter. 'Acting in Medical Practice'. *The Lancet* 344 (1994): 801–2.

Frank, Arthur W. 'What Is Narrative Medicine?" Review of The Principles and Practice of Narrative Medicine, by Rita Charon et al.' *Journal of Medicinal Humanities* 38 (2017): 339–43.

Fuchs, Elinor. 'EF's Visit to a Small Planet: Some Questions to Ask a Play'. *Theater* 34, no. 2 (2004): 5–9.

Garland-Thomson, Rosemarie, ed. *Freakery: Cultural Spectacles of the Extraordinary Body*. New York University Press, 1996.

Garner, Stanton B., Jr. 'Is There a Doctor in the House? Medicine and the Making of Modern Drama'. *Modern Drama* 51, no. 3 (2008): 311–28.

Garner, Stanton B., Jr. *Theatre & Medicine*. Methuen Drama, 2023.

Gawande, Atul. *Being Mortal: Medicine and What Matters in the End*. Anchor Canada, 2017.

Goffman, Erving. *The Presentation of Self in Everyday Life*. Doubleday, 1959.

Goldman, Marlene. *The Social, Aesthetic, and Medical Implications of Performing Shame: Interdisciplinary Approaches*. Routledge, 2023.

Hare, David. *Asking Around: Background to the David Hare Trilogy*. Faber and Faber, 2003.

Hartigan, Karelisa V. *Performance and Cure: Drama and Healing in Ancient Greece and Contemporary America*. Duckworth, 2009.

Hochberg, Mark S. 'The Doctor's White Coat: A Historical Perspective'. *AMA Journal of Ethics* 9, no. 4 (2007): 310–14.

Kenny, Amy. *Humoral Wombs on the Shakespearean Stage*. Palgrave, 2019.

Kuppers, Petra. *Theatre & Disability*. Palgrave, 2017.

McKenzie, Jon. *Perform or Else: From Discipline to Performance*. Routledge, 2001.

McManus, Chris. 'Department of Theatrical Medicine?' *The Lancet* 344 (1994): 767.

Mermikides, Alex, and Gianna Bouchard, eds. *Performance and the Medical Body*. Bloomsbury Methuen Drama, 2016.

Musa, Sade. 'Historic Abundance'. In *Artists Remaking Medicine: The Practice of Imagination and the Power to Create a Better Healthcare Future*, edited by Emily F. Peters. Procedure Press, 2023.

Nolan, Yvette. *Medicine Shows: Indigenous Performance Culture*. Playwrights Canada Press, 2015.

Parsons, Talcott. 'The Sick Role and the Role of the Physician Reconsidered'. *Health and Society* 53, no. 3 (Summer 1975): 257–78.

Persaud, R. 'The Drama of Being a Doctor'. *Postgraduate Medical Journal* 81, no. 955 (2005): 276–7.
Porter, Roy. *Quacks: Fakers and Charlatans in English Medicine*. Tempus, 2000.
Schipperges, Heinrich. *Hildegard of Bingen: Healing and the Nature of the Cosmos*. M. Wiener, 1997.
Shepherd-Barr, Kirsten. *Science on Stage: From Doctor Faustus to Copenhagen*. Princeton University Press, 2006.
Shepherd-Barr, Kirsten. 'The Diagnostic Gaze: Nineteenth-Century Contexts for Performance and Medicine'. In *Performance and the Medical Body*, edited by Alex Mermikides and Gianna Bouchard. Bloomsbury Methuen Drama, 2016.
Showalter, Elaine. *Hystories: Hysterical Epidemics and Modern Media*. Columbia University Press, 1997.
Smith, Matthew Wilson. *The Nervous Stage: Nineteenth-Century Neuroscience and the Birth of Modern Theatre*. Oxford University Press, 2017.
Taylor, Jane. 'Newes from the Dead: An Unnatural Moment in the History of Natural Philosophy'. In *Shakespeare's Things*, edited by Brett Gamboa and Lawrence Switzky. Routledge, 2020.
Whorwell, P. J., and F. Shanahan. 'In the Performing Art of Medicine: The Doctor as Actor'. *QJM: An International Journal of Medicine* 109, no. 3 (2016): 159–60.
Zhou, Xiaohuan. 'Nuo Altar Theatre on a Liminal/Liminoid Continuum: Reflections on the Shamanic Origins of Chinese Theatre'. *TDR: The Drama Review* 63, no. 2 (Summer 2019): 57–77.

PART ONE

Fashioning the Doctor's Character

The analogies that have been proposed for medical education can tell us a lot about how the doctor–patient relationship has been imagined. In the past, medical educators drew comparisons between training doctors and airplane pilots, owing to the dangers – for patients and passengers – associated with 'flying' with novices. Just as one now expects that a pilot would have practised using simulations before being charged with the lives of actual humans, medical educators have similarly argued that doctors could benefit from training with simulated patients and artificial models before testing their newly acquired skills on vulnerable patients.[1] Other educators have turned to performance athletes for the lessons they offered doctors in perseverance, hard work, practice and precision.[2] Still others have looked to literature and the analogy of doctors as close readers to train doctors to become sympathetic close readers and creative writers.[3]

Despite this array of generative analogies, in fact, a broad array of actors and agendas participate in effective healing. The pervasive focus on lone doctors and isolated patients elides what is our key contention: that medicine is an ensemble, performative art. The need to expand the focus beyond the traditional doctor–patient dyad is borne out by the fact that physicians increasingly

[1] H. Barrows, *Simulated Patient (Programme Patients): The Development and Use of a New Technology in Medical Education* (Charles C. Thomas, 1971), 9.
[2] Atul Gawande, *Better* (Henry Holt, 2007), 4.
[3] Rita Charon, Sayantani DasGupta, Nellie Hermann, Craig Irvine, Eric R. Marcus, Edgar Rivera Colsn, Danielle Spencer and Maura Spiegel, *The Principles and Practices of Narrative Medicine* (Oxford University Press, 2016).

work in teams within hospital systems comprised of hundreds of people as well as robots and AI.[4] Where clinicians offer verbal and embodied performances for an intimate audience, they may well be akin to the acts of close-up magicians that solicit spectators' participation in sustaining illusions.[5] Properly understood, however, even this type of intimate performance is 'not provided by one person and passively witnessed by another'; instead, it too is an ensemble art, 'a process of engagement, a two-way street'.[6]

Medicine's collaborative, embodied 'process of engagement' is vividly conveyed by a friend's recent experience. While visiting a remote medieval village in Spain, a woman fell dreadfully ill. When the elderly doctor arrived at her pension, they were forced to communicate in gestures since his English was as limited as her Spanish. Initially, the doctor removed a yellow pad from his briefcase and wrote a single sentence in English: 'Don't worry, we will recognize her.' She assumed he wanted to assure her that he would be able to diagnose her illness. In her mind, his use of the pronoun 'we' made them a team. The words 'recognize' and 'her', which personified the illness, promised heroically that together they would 'recognize' the malady. After penning this sentence, he silently gestured for her to lift her shirt. Sitting beside her on the hotel bed, he proceeded to listen to her lungs with his stethoscope and to examine her throat with a tongue depressor. After this protracted moment of intimate, physical connection, he wrote a prescription. Their virtually wordless ensemble performance, which relied on ritual gestures and props to enhance the intimate connection – what Arthur Kleinman refers to as 'presence' – between the pair was, in her view, healing in and of itself.

The role of the doctor calls for technical expertise working in concert with a distinctive set of character skills including curiosity, compassion and empathy. As one might imagine, the stakes and complexity of medical performances make training doctors an urgent and essential task and the topic of heated debates. Although in the Greco-Roman era the training and practice of medicine and theatre were linked, medicine's relationship to the arts and its openness to insights from the humanities has waxed and waned over time, often correlated to the proximity of medical training to humanist academic subjects such as religion and philosophy. The development of the modern medical school – the model we have largely inherited – was revolutionized by famous physicians, notably William Osler (1849–1919). The instructional model that Osler put

[4] Anna Colivicchi, 'Doctors Increasingly Using AI and Seeing Benefits, Finds GMC Report', *Pulse*, February 6, 2025, www.pulsetoday.co.uk/news/technology/doctors-increasingly-using-ai-and-seeing-benefits-finds-gmc-report/. Accessed 25 March 2025.

[5] Roger Kneebone, 'The Art of Medicine: Performing Magic, Performing Medicine', *The Lancet* 389 (January 14, 2017): 148–9.

[6] Ibid., 148.

into effect at the newly formed Johns Hopkins Medical School, where he was professor and head of medicine, 'revolutionized medical teaching in the art and science of diagnosis and patient care':

> There were three aspects to the clinic. There was a live-in resident staff with graded experience: from the new graduate to more senior residents of several years' experience. Instruction in methods of history taking and physical diagnosis was emphasized to a degree not seen since [Pierre] Louis. Medical students became actual members of the patient care team, taking histories, doing physicals, doing the laboratory work, and making rounds with the residents and faculty. Thus evolved the medical clerkship, which was extended to surgery, obstetrics and gynaecology. This clerkship did for the clinical students what laboratory work did for the scientists.[7]

Osler's model is credited for developing a more rigorous curriculum, for adding new subjects and for transforming the medical student from a passive observer into an active participant. More than this, though, by insisting that residents live at the hospital Osler established an implicit, embodied connection between medical students and patients. For the first time, both groups lived in the same place and ate the same food. It's also worth observing that by integrating medical students into patients' care teams, Osler was implicitly realizing Aristotle's strategy for creating an ethical character through virtuous action made habitual.

We touch briefly on the history of medical education here to emphasize that embodied collaboration, co-presence and 'building a character' are already baked into modern medical training, so that the ingredients for a performative approach to medicine are fundamental to how medical education takes place – even if doctors are reticent to say so. The contributors in this section share an overriding concern with medical schools' reliance on an overly rigid adherence to standardized approaches to medical education at the expense of in-the-moment responsiveness and collaboration. It is not enough, they contend, for the medical student and, by extension, the doctor, to constitute the sole 'active participant'. It is time for patients and caregivers to share this role.

The interviews and essays in this section underscore the stakes involved in contemporary medical education and raise key questions: If training students to rehearse standard physical and verbal scripts aims to encourage creativity and interdependence, does the so-called hidden curriculum work against the mutuality, improvisation and whole-body presence doctors know they need to

---

[7] H. K. Walker, 'The Origins of the History and Physical Examination', in *Clinical Methods: The History, Physical, and Laboratory Examinations*, 3rd edition, ed. H. K. Walker, W. D. Hall and J. W. Hurst (Butterworths, 1990), www.ncbi.nlm.nih.gov/books/NBK458/.

embrace to respond effectively to patients?[8] And what of the damage to doctors, who are forced to disguise and deny their own inner emotional richness in the name of objectivity and what Jodi Halpern calls the regime of 'detached concern'?[9] The task here, and one that theatre can help with, is to find forms of emotional expression that are authentic without straining the doctor or the patient. Emotional training is needed to this end. As Raj Persaud writes in 'The Drama of Being a Doctor', 'physicians need to learn certain emotional control and manipulation techniques with which actors would be familiar, to best cope with the psychological demands of patients'.[10] This is not dissembling; it is using real emotions effectively to communicate, to feel together and to work together.

The contributions in Part One, beginning with Dr Timothy McGinnis's interview with Arthur Kleinman, carefully examine the benefits and limitations of medical schools' emphasis on constraining rather than generative modes of standardization. A world-renowned psychiatrist and anthropologist, Kleinman played a pioneering role in founding narrative medicine and formulating the concept of 'illness narratives'. Throughout his career, he remained enormously attuned to the role of theatricality and ritual in medicine. In Kleinman's view, medical schools should rely less on standardization and simulation and more on teaching doctors to become active and compassionate witnesses. He wants medical schools to prepare future doctors to enter different examining rooms and respond to each distinct patient authentically. Dr Deborah Ocholi's essay likewise challenges the standardized model of the ideal physician. She takes Kleinman's suggestion further by calling for medical schools to allow students to reflect on how the institution actively moulds their character and to choose what facets of their repertoire to retain or change. Drawing on the analogy of the 'virtuous actor' from Aristotle's *Ethics*, she suggests that people become habituated to good practices by doing them. An interview with puppeteer Rachel Warr, who teaches medical students, demonstrates how medical training can be enhanced by working with artists whose craft demands warming up and collaboration – an approach that corrects the view that the individual physician rather than the entire healthcare team is responsible for the success or failure of a given medical performance.

---

8 The 'hidden curriculum' is defined as a set of influences that function at the level of the organizational structure and culture that affect learning. It refers to the unwritten, unofficial and often unintended lessons, values and perspectives that are communicated to the learners (see R. Mackin, S. Baptiste, A. Niec and A. J. Kam, 'The Hidden Curriculum: A Good Thing?', *Cureus* 11, no. 12 (2019): e6305, https://doi.org/10.7759/cureus.6305).

9 Jodi Halpern, *From Detached Concern to Empathy: Humanizing Medical Practice* (Oxford Academic, 2015).

10 Raj Persaud, 'The Drama of Being a Doctor', *Postgrad Medical Journal* 81, no. 955 (May 2005): 276, https://doi.org/10.1136/pgmj.2004.023796.

Taken together, the chapters that follow advance a vision for what characterizes the performance of the doctor: presence, character and teamwork. They also argue, implicitly and explicitly, for the insights and training that theatre and performance studies bring to the development of those qualities in the training and practice of medicine.

REFERENCES

Barrows, H. *Simulated Patient (Programme Patients): The Development and Use of a New Technology in Medical Education*. Charles C. Thomas, 1971.

Charon, Rita, Sayantani DasGupta, Nellie Hermann, Craig Irvine, Eric R. Marcus, Edgar Rivera Colsn, Danielle Spencer and Maura Spiegel. *The Principles and Practices of Narrative Medicine*. Oxford University Press, 2016.

Colivicchi, Anna. 'Doctors Increasingly Using AI and Seeing Benefits, Finds GMC Report'. *Pulse*, 6 February 2025. www.pulsetoday.co.uk/news/technology/doctors-increasingly-using-ai-and-seeing-benefits-finds-gmc-report/. Accessed 25 March 2025.

Gawande, Atul. *Better*. Henry Holt, 2007.

Halpern, Jodi. *From Detached Concern to Empathy: Humanizing Medical Practice*. Oxford Academic, 2015.

Kneebone, Roger. 'The Art of Medicine: Performing Magic, Performing Medicine'. *The Lancet* 389 (14 January 2017): 148–9.

Mackin, R., S. Baptiste, A. Niec and A. J. Kam. 'The Hidden Curriculum: A Good Thing?' *Cureus* 11, no. 12 (2019): e6305. https://doi.org/10.7759/cureus.6305.

Persaud, Raj. 'The Drama of Being a Doctor'. *Postgrad Medical Journal* 81, no. 955 (May 2005): 276–7. https://doi.org/10.1136/pgmj.2004.023796.

Walker, H. K. 'The Origins of the History and Physical Examination'. In *Clinical Methods: The History, Physical, and Laboratory Examinations*, 3rd edition, edited by H. K. Walker, W. D. Hall and J. W. Hurst. Butterworths, 1990. www.ncbi.nlm.nih.gov/books/NBK458/.

1

Authenticity, ritual and medical performance

A CONVERSATION BETWEEN TIMOTHY MCGINNIS AND ARTHUR KLEINMAN

Arthur Kleinman and Tim McGinnis met at the Radcliffe symposium in 2021; their interview took place the following year, in March 2022. Although generations apart – Kleinman is in his eighties and McGinnis in his thirties – both physicians share a deep interest in medical anthropology and the social, performative roles of doctors and patients.

Kleinman is a distinguished psychiatrist and medical anthropologist whose career has fused clinical practice with influential scholarship in cross-cultural healthcare. He chaired both Harvard's Department of Anthropology and Harvard Medical School's Department of Social Medicine. Renowned for his foundational work on how illness is experienced and interpreted across social contexts, Kleinman's research foregrounds the roles patients, families and physicians inhabit within medical encounters. A leading figure in the medical humanities, Kleinman was one of the pioneers of narrative medicine. Since then, he has pushed the field beyond the absorption of patient stories toward an understanding of care as an embodied social performance. Currently, he advocates for a dynamic, performative medicine that acknowledges medicine's ritualistic, communal and relational dimensions.

McGinnis, a graduate of Princeton and a Rhodes scholar, completed his MPhil at Oxford where he studied anthropology and social history. His field work took him to Sierra Leone and the Democratic Republic of the Congo.

While pursuing his medical degree at Harvard, he took time off to teach anthropology at Deep Springs College, studied poetry with Jorie Graham and took courses in scriptwriting. He did a year of psychiatry residency before completing his surgery residency and is currently a surgeon in Chicago.

Kleinman's and McGinnis's collective experience spans decades of medical humanities and global health. Kleinman, who wrote the seminal book *The Illness Narratives* (1988), offers a foundational understanding of medical humanities and narrative medicine. McGinnis brings to the conversation contemporary knowledge of medical training, theatre acting and screenwriting, and has worked directly with standardized patients.

In the following discussion of the relationship between medicine and theatre they make three key observations. First, whether on stage or at the patient's bedside, the goal is to infuse performance with genuine emotion, attunement and responsiveness. Second, witnessing is likewise central to both domains. Finally, rituals support performative medicine by giving meaning to suffering, fostering hope and enacting healing that is not just biological but social and cultural. Efficiency-focused institutional routines can threaten efforts to make medicine more humane: clinical algorithms can shrink illness narratives to checklists or treat 'presence' as a billing code. Theatre invites medicine to re-enact these rituals as meaningful, embodied performances of genuine human connection.

I. PERFORMANCE

Timothy McGinnis (TM): As for so many who've studied both anthropology and medicine, my path has been shaped by your work at the intersection of psychiatric practice and anthropological analysis. When I moved from studying acting into studying anthropology and now medicine, it struck me that each discipline emphasizes an alert attunement to the other, whether it's a partner on the stage or a patient in the hospital bed or an interlocutor in the field. In each space, this attunement must also inform action – 'performance'. Having contributed so richly to diverse fields, how do you think about this relationship between attention and performance? What do you make of the guiding simile of this book, 'medicine as theatre, theatre as medicine'?

Arthur Kleinman (AK): In both anthropology and psychiatry, the idea of performance looms large. In medical anthropology, at least for two decades, there's been an emphasis on performative studies concerning personal experiences of illness and of care. In psychiatry, much of the concern with psychotherapy turns on performative acts in the anthropological sense: language that functions as a social action. There is the charismatic influence of the therapist, based in establishing trust, their responsibility for supporting, persuading and caring for the patient. Reciprocally, there is also the patient's engaged performance in accepting therapeutic interventions, including psychotherapeutic insights into parts of the self that feel unbearable. These are only a few of the performative functions in basic therapy. Hence, the leap to theatre, for me, seems logical.

I don't have any difficulty with thinking in that way, with one important reservation. I've come to believe that authenticity is a crucial aspect of the human experience of care, and I refer to it in my own work with the term presence. Presence, for me, represents that fullness of our being-in-the-world that is on vivid display when we respond deeply to the persons who matter most to us with liveliness, passion and realness of purpose. I'm referring, in particular, to the presence of the caregiver and the care recipient. As long as theatre is understood to involve players who are reaching for a kind of authenticity – infusing the role with felt emotion, and being open and immersed in the moment rather than mechanically playing a part – in their own performances, then I think the model of theatre is a good model for medicine. To the extent that theatre is seen in a more cynical vein as simply playing a standardized role, I am less inclined to believe that it is a useful way of getting at what really matters in medicine.

TM: I was struck by this mechanistic view of role-play when I arrived at medical school as well, and it often showed up, to me, as a misunderstanding of how inhabiting a role – acting it out, so to speak – can enable a vivid form of communication. For example, when we were first introduced to the classic task of a physician, 'eliciting the history of present illness', our seasoned instructor stressed what was, to her, a crucial element of a bedside manner. 'Don't act!' she implored us, 'your patients will know the difference'. We then proceeded to learn scripts to characterize pain, acronyms to help guide us through 'delivering bad news', and choreographed movements to help ease patients through the physical exam. We were evaluated on the quality of our eye contact, pensive pauses and the timing of washing our hands. The irony of getting positive feedback for the authenticity of our rehearsed bedside manner was not lost on us.

It was amusing and a touch disorienting to have 'acting' associated with a cheapening of relationships, when we had just been instructed to imitate, practise and riff on a repertoire of defined behaviours – perhaps the closest we came in medical school to theatrical rehearsal. I'm curious, do you locate the disconnect between clinicians and patients in this space of practised behaviour? Or what, in your view, are the factors that diminish doctors' and patients' abilities to experience an authentic connection?

AK: In my somewhat biased view, the great problem of medicine today has been that three things conspire to reduce the humanity of the doctor–patient encounter and care. Namely, the institutional structures, the governmental procedural requirements and the big business aspect of care networks (even so-called non-profit hospitals).

The danger of modelling illness and care on theatre – knowing that every innovative, powerful idea has negative consequences as well as opportunities – the danger of theatrical performance as a heuristic is that you don't want an emphasis on theatre to mean that people accept mechanically playing a role. I don't think that is what good theatre is about, anyway.

TM: Agreed. With a bit of experience as an actor and as a clinician now, I certainly feel the reps we had as students to practise the skills of a clinical encounter have given me a greater degree of space for emotional attention with patients. In that sense, the 'good theatre' of rehearsing the role enables a capacity to do both a 'clinical task' and to show up with and for a patient. But I imagine that practising and finding one's own clinical personae could be alienating for some while empowering for others. And if not alienating, a bedside manner can readily tilt in the direction of rote information gathering and pat gestures at empathy – the very 'acting' our instructor dreaded.

Even if you were not thinking about theatre at the time, your work in *The Illness Narratives* (1988) has proved enduringly influential for so many of us in its ability to blend a discrete skill or framework with an emphasis on learning from the specific meaning of a patient's experience of illness. Here, I'm thinking of the simple but powerful act of setting out with a goal of learning what's meaningful for a patient, whether aided by an analytical grid as the book suggested or simply with a set of questions. Though we might hope this fundamental form of relating would naturally occur in a medical encounter, by no means was the twentieth century defined by allopathic medicine's interest in patients' personal, familial, or cultural meanings. Particularly with the turn to concepts of performativity and theatre, I wonder how you relate to 'illness narratives' now. Do they help move us toward authenticity?

AK: That's an important question. As I've evolved and grown, as I've perfected my own clinical act – or, at least tried to chip away at the imperfections – I've come to think that the illness narrative, including the way it's told, and staged, and listened to, is important as an opening, as a way into conversation. But I now think the illness narrative should be the start of something, not some 'ah-ha' sense of structured insight to deploy.

For example, when I wrote *The Illness Narratives*, much of the work came from my own experience of intensely witnessing people's illness, the challenges and rewards of people opening up and sharing. I was writing from the place of that shared moment. When I later travelled as a visiting professor to medical schools across the country, I frequently had a very disheartening experience.

I would accompany the clinical team on rounds, and invariably one of the residents or medical students would point to the chart or in the electronic medical record, and say 'Here's the patient's illness narrative, their explanatory model!' Right there on their checklist.

It was as if they'd discovered an artefact, like they'd found a piece of pottery or something that had materialized in the patient's condition akin to the patient's blood pressure. But it wasn't my understanding of what 'the explanatory model' was or was 'for'. I'd written the book in the mode of anthropological study, with the view that the way you listen to an illness narrative was a conversation, a way to open a conversation and relationship. But I discovered that it was incorporated into the belly of the beast in medical settings as a conversation stopper.

There was an active shift then – in the late 1980s and 1990s – of encouraging trainees and clinicians to add a new emphasis. Clinicians got to ask someone 'What do you think is wrong with you? How do you think it works? What do you fear about it?' and then put it in the chart. But then that was it. The doctors had done their thing. It was done with the best of intentions, yet I felt this lingering sense of having produced something that contributed to the very impoverishment of care I had sought to reverse. I'd given doctors the sense that they could have a humanistic encounter just by getting the illness narrative down in the chart, almost like a frozen section in the pathology lab.

Having seen how my work was put into practice, I became very sceptical about how illness narratives were being used in medicine. I had provided bureaucracies with the perfect tool to say 'We do inquire about these things, and we take an interest in patients' lives. Here it is, you can read it.' And I felt that this was no substitute for the meaning-informed conversations I wanted doctors and patients to be having.

Watching 'explanatory model' become a check-box in the medical record helped me realize that the practice – the *how* of eliciting and sharing illness narratives, the *how* clinician and patient responded to sharing the illness narratives – was just as important as the content of the narrative per se. For me, this *how* gets at authentic witnessing. When you go to a theatre and watch a play, you give it your utmost attention, you get utterly caught up in the theatre itself – this type of witnessing is just as important as the play's narrative. I think this is what the ancient Greek playwrights had in mind when they argued that tragedy was catharsis. You get so caught up in it that you release some kind of passion within you, in your lived engagement between the presence of the actors and your presence. With this type of engagement in mind, thinking of medicine from the perspective of theatre can be refreshingly insightful and potentially effective.

II. RECIPROCAL PRESENCE

TM: When I think of 'witnessing' as an elevated, distinct act of value, I tend to think of the likes of James Baldwin and trenchant voices speaking from the very edge of truths we ought to face as a society. It's curious to think about that kind of witnessing alongside the witnessing of a play, where the relationship of engagement can make an audience member far more than a passive spectator. As clinicians, we observe and participate in some of the most intense moments of patients' lives, yet physicians can also be the most removed from the chronic suffering and care that exists outside the moments of diagnosis and intervention. Can you say more about the role of the witness in these spaces?

AK: Witnessing begins with acknowledgement of the patient (and family and friends) as full human beings deserving to be treated as ethical subjects with respect, with affirmation of the seriousness of their condition, and commitment to accompanying them on their journeys of care. But it is deeper than that flat statement would make it seem. Witnessing means feeling something akin to awe before the unfolding of a singular human experience – a drama. It means 'hearing the tone' in the therapeutic relationship like the story in Zhuangze of the lute player in ancient China who gave up playing after the close friend he played for died. When asked why he stopped playing the lute, he replied that only his friend could 'hear the tone'. I take that to mean that there is a critical awareness as well as a caring presence in moral-emotional relationships. Another way of thinking of witnessing is that it opens up a moral-emotional space of reciprocity where compassion is drawn out of the caregiver by the raw, unfiltered experience of the patient's suffering. Where, strange as it may seem, the patient responds by self-witnessing their own inner world and outer life of injury and repair. The patient–doctor relationship is more reciprocal than we usually recognize. It is an exchange of feeling and value along with practical action.

Thinking about theatre and how its power arises in the witnessing of the performance, and applying that insight to a clinician's potentially equally powerful and transformative regard for a patient could be very instructive. In the same vein, just as a theatre critic can become a professional at witnessing plays, so can any physician become more practised in the art of witnessing their patients' experiences of illness. It requires not only a kind of passion for the affirmation of and acknowledgement of the patient as a human being, it also involves a kind of critical attention.

Conceiving of the connection between medicine and theatre in this way, while reflecting on this volume, helps me rethink my aspiration with *The Illness Narratives*: as a means of encouraging an ongoing practice of refining a form of attention that clinicians could bring to the work of learning how to shape a patient or family's course of treatment and care. Listening to theatre professors and critics discuss plays and their potential application to care reminded me of how a clinician brings a critical sensibility to enquiring about the patient's context and inner life and their potential value in creating quality care. Evidence of my development of this perspective over the course of my career can be seen more fully in my later books, *What Really Matters* (2006) and *The Soul of Care* (2019).

I don't know how residents in psychiatry are trained today, but when I was a resident – with a further specialization in consultation-liaison psychiatry, where we are supposed to help other areas of medicine understand their patients' psychological and social needs – no one taught me how to explain anything to a patient. No one ever taught me how to interpret what the patient said, except in the most crude fashion. When I was in your position as a young resident, we were told: 'Listen to the patient. She is telling you the diagnosis.'

My feeling is that phrase epitomizes the worst way you can listen to a patient. What clinical teachers typically mean by that instruction is that we just need to pick out the signs and symptoms of disease from a person's story, that all this stuff about experiencing illness is clinically worthless. No one told us 'You should really attend to your patient's experience of illness, because then you'll make a connection with the patient, then you'll see where you can truly have your effect.' I think you can use a model of the theatre – particularly a model that puts the onus on the spectator's responsibility as a witness – to get at that. I am not knowledgeable enough about theatre studies to name a particular model, though in literary studies there is the formerly influential 'reader response' theory. In the Chinese tradition that I have participated in for over half a century, there is the crucial idea that you project your emotions and values onto landscape paintings, where your messiness gets ordered and made clearer by the stylized effects of the portrayal of a lone scholar wandering amongst crags, pines and mist in a Confucian ritual-like process of recentering the self by projecting it outwardly into a preformed world of value and action.

This type of attentive and immersive witnessing is crucial in the context of chronic disease where the benefit of medicine comes from tinkering, making attentive changes where a small improvement in functionality can make the difference between a modicum of wellbeing and an agonizing situation. For some people, with asthma for example, if you're able to reduce a person's shortness of breath by 10 per cent, that can be the difference between a person who is able to do what they want to do in a day and someone who is housebound. In a society with widespread chronic disease, aging and the demands of end-of-life care, this type of beneficial tinkering is much more likely to come out of an authentic relationship grounded in the presence of the practitioner eliciting the presence of the patient and the family to foreground what matters most in the experience of illness and wellness.

TM: With the breadth of disciplines that emerge in medicine, from psychiatry to surgery, it seems even competing emphases on the role of listening pose a challenge to curricular design that might strive to emphasize this goal of witnessing. Prior to all that differentiation though, they do try to get us all to think of ourselves as 'physicians' first, perhaps more core than any identity as a reconstructive urologist or neuro-ophthalmologist. That's certainly where my earlier clinical instructor stepped in during week one of orientation, encouraging us not to act; the didactic series was even called 'TDP: The Developing Physician'.

Along the way, I thought there were missed opportunities to lean into the theatre of it, times when the 'don't act' sentiment impeded what could have been more conscientious moments of learning with and from techniques of acting. That said, even if medicine could stand to grow more nuanced, attentive and present in drawing lessons from the theatre, do you see any detriments to drawing the two closer together?

AK: There are aspects of the way theatre has, in a sense, been cannibalized by medical educators. I don't like simulated patients as teaching tools, perhaps from having had bad experiences with the exercise. Simulated patients don't give you the sense of awe, the engagement with the real, that arises from being with a patient or from being with someone who is living out their serious problem. Simulated patients tend to be much more articulate than most patients initially are in their illness. It takes time for a person to learn, to create, or discover, their illness narrative. Creating that genuine articulation of suffering arises in the troubled course of living with illness in the process of domesticating the fear, habituating to the 'wild' experience of threat and giving it a name. In becoming patients, people learn how to talk about illness. That helps attenuate its threat to our everyday reality. The 'reality' of the story orders the wild mysteriousness of the life experience, reducing anxiety, and thus itself becomes a treatment.

As clinicians working with patients, we create a safe distance by putting the illness in symbolic space. This is an old idea in social and cultural anthropology, and in medical anthropology in particular. As developed by the influential anthropologist Victor Turner, especially in his book *The Forest of Symbols* (1970), healing rituals are interpreted to work on several levels simultaneously: physical, interpersonal, cultural. One level is the symptom as physical experience. Another level is the symptom and treatment as a community or social engagement. While the third level establishes the symptom and diagnosis as cultural metaphors. Those metaphors like 'pain in the neck' are symbolically manipulated in healing rituals so that a new state is legitimized in the symbolic space: the state of renewed health and accomplished healing on the cultural plane. The healing ritual is deemed successful in this symbolic space as the patient and the diagnosis as symbolic forms, cultural symbols, move from suffering to healing. The ritual legitimates healing in the symbolic space no matter what happens physically and socially. For example, a patient with chronic asthma comes to an emergency room where they have been a number of times before because of shortness of breath unrelieved by a bronchial-dilating inhaler, and even before the medical intervention has begun, their just being in the waiting room legitimates a transformation from the frightening uncertainty of breathlessness to the expectation of therapeutic success, and voila, the shortness of breath is 'mysteriously' reduced and the patient already feels partially or fully healed while waiting for the steroids and other medications to be administered. I have seen this happen, not just with patients, but in my own experience as an asthmatic. Here, the symbolic ritual of moving from the threatened domestic space to the formal clinical space legitimates a cultural transformation that becomes experienced in the body, so that the symbolic ritual actually has a physiological effect.

When I have watched simulated patients work with medical students, the simulated patients are already way beyond the narrative forms of someone learning their illness. They are not simulating the singularity of a particular illness or a particular patient. The actor often simulates a patterned disease process, or clinical scenarios that can be challenging to the clinician in order to teach pattern recognition. But I myself have not observed them go beyond pattern recognition and get at the existential uncertainty and fear at the outset of a serious illness and the relief in its clinical transformation to a named condition. Nor, in my admittedly limited experience, do the actors resonate with the experience of being healed – that emotional and moral energy of transformation on the cultural-personal level.

This limitation in the employment of actors as patients is present not just in acute conditions but with chronic illnesses, which absorb like a great sponge the meanings of their local worlds. In my work, I have tried to get students and doctors to begin by seeing things through the patients' eyes, not just from the biomedical perspective. Of course, the biomedical understanding of the disease and treatment is critical, but all too frequently it intervenes before the clinician understands who the patient is and what their needs and resources are. The classic outcome is doctor-centred care rather than patient-centred care, which today, thank goodness, is widely taken to be the essence of quality care.

TM: That's interesting – I haven't thought about how early versus later stages of illness narrative show up in our standardized patient encounters. A lot of our OSCEs (Observed Structured Clinical Encounters) hinged on a 'first' moment of some kind: diagnosing a new illness, sharing a cancer diagnosis, learning how to do a physical exam. Few of them were geared towards the chronic or later stages of a condition, although we did have opportunities to practise some behavioural health techniques regarding addiction. The emphasis was often less on the content so much as on the form of the interaction. For example, in some scenarios actors were not supposed to reveal crucial information (such as a history of abuse) unless the trainee came across as appropriately empathetic at other moments.

Despite these richer or even overwhelming scenarios, plenty of the OSCE's did emphasize time management in such a way that we could feel the rhythms of the ideal clinic or inpatient workflow shaping our interactions. And the end, we would stop for feedback from the actors. They often focused on what we could do better to be more caring or curious. But sometimes the actors would offer glimpses into how they (and we all) as patients shape our behaviours to signal to clinicians what it is we think we need.

Our curriculum could have done more to emphasize this performative feature of the clinical relationship, somewhat in line with how, in *The Empathy Exams*, Leslie Jamison describes becoming more effective at communicating in her own health visits after working as a standardized patient.

III. RECENTRING THE PATIENT

TM: Arthur, while you and I have been elaborating how clinicians enact forms of presence and witness, how do you think about the performance from the patient's point of view?

AK: Patients must perform their symptoms for a clinician who often fails to perceive or respect the patient's illness experience. With clear aetiologies of pain – a broken bone, a mass, an inflammatory state – much of our clinical training involves an attempt to 'see through' experience and context to discern and address the cause. But that model breaks down when we encounter the limits of diagnosis, and when we mistake our diagnostic abilities as exhaustive of human experience. The chronic pain patient, the patient with chronic fatigue syndrome, the Long COVID patient, suffers whether we can 'detect' a cause or not. The helpful theatre of the therapeutic encounter can break down in this context, especially with the forms of training we have today, the strain of mediating care through an electronic medical record, and the time pressures of 'efficient' care.

If you think of the chronic conditions I listed above, they are diagnoses of exclusion. The very definition of the disease is predicated on exhausting our diagnostic tools of measurement and imaging, leaving physician and patient with the demoralizing sense of failure. Patients arrive at the point of diagnosis after those tools have failed, and often clinicians will talk about this disconnect in terms of the patients themselves *failing*, as in, for example, the phrase 'they've failed treatment' – rather than saying 'the treatment has failed the patient'. The common error of the physician entails assuming a position of disbelief, acting in ways that don't acknowledge or affirm the actual experiences of the patient.

Much of my career has involved working with patients with chronic pain and chronic fatigue syndromes. Perhaps there are a few exceptions, but nearly every patient I have encountered has come to see me after having had miserable experiences with doctors and even family members – because they feel that, not only is their pain not understood, it isn't believed. Forced to endure protracted testing and ineffectual therapies, many of the patients find themselves having to perform or exaggerate their symptoms to receive the medical attention they feel they deserve. Faced with that classic threadbare pain scale, which asks a chronic pain patient 'how would you rate your pain on a scale of one to ten?' a patient might well be driven to say 'thirteen'.

This kind of exaggerated communication may make some clinicians even more sceptical, widening the gap even further between patient and clinician. To me, this iconic disjuncture in performance arises from a clinician's failure to attend authentically to a patient, whether from consciously or unconsciously biased dismissal or from some other source causing an inability to appreciate the suffering. Or, because, as I have previously suggested, the patient's experience of the *illness* (symptoms, functional impairment, coping methods, self and family care) is systematically disregarded and replaced by reductionistic pattern recognition of the underlying *disease* pathology only. The latter is the fault of biomedical education itself becoming the thief of clinical evidence and the practical sense of how to live a life.

TM: Thinking of chronic pain syndromes and how theatre helps us attend to what matters, I have been wondering about the role of belief in medical care. Our training rests on an underlying conviction in the objectivity of our tools and technologies to get at unit of bodily fact. Medical training doesn't often teach the anthropologist's or medical historian's awareness that these technologies are helping create forms of perception.

By way of contrast, in the theatre we all show up agreeing to believe in a different mode of reality – if only for a moment. Depending on the kind of play or show, that different reality could be fantasy, historical realism, theatre of the absurd, a twenty-four-hour show of endurance, or something else. But in some way, from actors to audience, we share a willingness to play with reality, at times to profound effect on our lives' meaning and how we go about our day afterwards. How, if at all, does something similar arise in medicine?

AK: It is best if the patient and physician come together with the hope or belief that the experience of illness can change for the better. Such is the traditionally legitimated emotional and moral quality of the patient–doctor relationship in our culture and others, that that transformation can routinely occur. But I don't know if physicians are trained any more to create this belief, which I suppose is akin to how theatre fosters a belief in an imagined world. We're trained to use the technology, to really hunt for a diagnosis, with the great truism that the right diagnosis enables the right or best treatment. And we are trained to directly convey our critically minded reading of the 'evidence', no matter if it strips the patient and family of hope. But this can rush past the social or moral commitment to shifting the treatment narrative that endows the symptoms with meaning and, by extension, transforms the patient's experience of them, at least as they 'feel' those symptoms, even if it doesn't affect disease outcome. And yet, often this approach does make a difference.

All illnesses, whether they frustrate medical diagnosis like a chronic pain syndrome or whether they're as seemingly clear cut as hypothyroidism, coronary artery disease, or colon cancer, can be amplified or dampened. I think the role of the physician should be to dampen the illness experience of pain and suffering, to tune it down.

TM: I have seen and certainly made mistakes when attempting to dampen an aspect of illness. The most common one seems to be when an expert, like a burn surgeon, tells a patient their wounds 'look great' or that their pain is 'normal'. From a physiologic point of view, the wound may be healing robustly with reassuring signs that the skin will regain integrity. But the attempt to reassure can carry with it a powerfully alienating disregard for the presence of pain, fear and disfiguring scars. While that kind of mistake can easily arise from overfamiliarity and losing touch with the particularity of individual's suffering, I wonder if there are moments among the repetitions in medicine that can help us reorient to the person at hand. Do you see any medical rituals, so to speak, that might draw on the energies of theatre that can forge – or undermine – the connection between patients and clinicians?

AK: The physical exam is a great example of this type of ritualistic gesture. We've all but lost the value of the laying on of hands. We teach the physical exam, but its teaching and application on a regular basis is all but perfunctory. When I join internal medicine residents on rounds, it's easy to see how cursory the physical exam has become. A brief moment of the stethoscope, with little honest attempt to listen. Doctors know they've got all this other technology, if a patient has a heart problem, where the diagnostic information is clinically far more important to the treatment than the sound of the murmur through a stethoscope. You can get an echocardiogram to figure out the degree of mitral valve stenosis or the wall motion of the heart. In the scenario of a primary care physician discovering the murmur for the first time, that's an essential moment of moving a patient towards a helpful diagnosis. But once the patient is well down the path of chronic management, the murmur nearly becomes a curiosity. With our scans, tests and the like, the physical exam is often less important as a means of data acquisition.

This misses the primary value of the physical exam, the shared physicality of touch, of being with the patient. The exam has always been rooted in that objectifying effort of gathering physical information. But it is also crucial for gathering knowledge of the patient's suffering and demonstrating that we have shared it for a moment. We live with and via our bodies, and the physical exam uses the intimacy of touch and proximity as a bridge to the social and psychological intimacy of care. It can communicate 'I am with you in this! I am here in this [emotional and moral as well as] physical space with you! You are not alone!' It is an essential part of the performance's ability to effect therapeutic change. We don't teach it like we used to. The huge gains in pharmacology and diagnostic tests along with the larger structural changes in the systems of care seem to have degraded the humanity that should be at the core of medicine.

TM: To that point, it seems like our medical lexicon based on billing codes has captured the term 'care' without including, or having a way to include, the intimacy you describe. The codes turn 'care', and the time spent furnishing it, into a payment metric rather than a human action or practice. Does theatre enliven this in any way? How can the medical humanities contribute to the moment?

AK: The medical humanities might entice a young physician like you, or an anthropologist-physician like me, and they might help us in our practice. We might be able to model and advocate for a richer physical exam informed by an awareness of theatre. Nonetheless, maybe you've found me on a bad day, but I don't think the medical humanities have enough power to resist or overcome the more inhuman structural issues in medicine – our failures at the level of political economy. Where institutional efficiency has come to substitute for quality care in our healthcare system dominated by big business and government regulation.

My generation failed yours when we allowed the economists to capture the terminology of medicine and boil it down to cost effectiveness. When we gave into and prioritized legal, bureaucratic and financial value as opposed to the overriding value of care. The medical humanities, which are cut off from the finances and regulatory power of this gargantuan neoliberal health system, simply do not have the scale of influence to challenge what's happening in medicine, the degradation of the human. That is what is visible today in both patient dissatisfaction as well as physician burnout.

This is the challenge for your generation, restoring and attending to all the things that matter: the attention, the being with the patient, really learning from and with patients in suffering. Using the term 'care' to mean something about the quality of a relationship rather than the speed of obtaining a test result or providing a prescription. And I do think change is possible. The fact that I haven't seen this kind of change too often doesn't matter – what matters is that people continue to work on bringing this change about. Paul Farmer, my former student, then colleague, then boss, who died unexpectedly in 2022, possessed a remarkable ability to combine moral commitment and clinical effectiveness. He never wavered in his moral commitment to the poor, and, somehow, he did get many practices and many systems to change in such a way as to improve social and health inequality via accompaniment (meaning, being with the patient with presence over the entire course of illness and treatment) as a model of human care. I do not discount that some kind of moral reform can take place in the practice of medicine. There is promise. We can, we must, get it right.

2

Medical training and character development: The hidden curriculum in learning to act

DEBORAH OCHOLI

I am sitting at my dining table editing a medical school application essay, as I have done for mentees sporadically since my own admission in 2020. As I work through the essay, I smile fondly – she's done it well, I think, better than I did on my first draft. There is a cliché among medical school applicants, one so well known that they are often reminded to avoid it throughout the application process: 'I want to help people.' While this is a genuine declaration for most, over time it seems to have lost meaning to admission committees. The challenge, instead, is to describe how the applicant plans to utilize medicine to help people, without quite using those words. This is where the performance begins. Medical school hopefuls with earnest intentions begin to learn the 'right' way to communicate, how to present who they are in a palatable form, in hopes of achieving what for many is a lifelong dream.

Supporting med school hopefuls through the application cycle offers me an opportunity to reminisce about my own path to medicine. I recall preparing for interviews in front of my mirror with my new suit on, practising everything from the way that I would introduce myself to the sequence and content of my answers, reminding myself to smile, to be 'bubbly' (but not annoyingly so).

Most importantly, I reminded myself not to ramble, meaning my tendency to repeat myself when attempting to illustrate a concept. While preparing with medical student mentors, I learned that this habit of mine would not be well received during interviews, so I focused my attention on quelling this trait. Weeks of rehearsal later, I walked into my first interview and put on the most important show of my life.

I started medical school armed with knowledge of the realities of being a person of colour in medical education. I promised myself that I would hold onto my authentic self, even in the face of pressures to change aspects of my identity. Armed with this resolve, I believed that I was already a few steps ahead in challenging what I would later learn was called the hidden curriculum – the implicit norms, values and lessons that are transmitted to students through role-modelling, interactions and institutional culture.

In this chapter, I propose that a major, overlooked feature of the hidden curriculum is the shaping of the physician as a character. For the purposes of this discussion, 'character' refers both to the role of the physician and to the collection of virtues that comprise an individual's identity. Much as a director choosing an actor for their unique set of skills and working with them towards the final depiction of their character, medical institutions choose their students for their unique traits and guide them along the path of maturation into their final form as practising physicians. In what follows, I draw on models from my background in screenwriting and philosophy to explore how pressures to conform can insidiously mould diverse medical learners into the same outmoded prototype of a physician. I use my own experience as a medical learner to illustrate this process and propose an approach to character development that addresses this aspect of the hidden curriculum. Ultimately, I advocate for a self-conscious approach that takes into consideration both the character and cultural background of the individual learner and the institutional demands to self-fashion a more holistic, content and effective physician-character.

I. THE HIDDEN CURRICULUM AND DIVERSITY IN MEDICINE

The hidden curriculum

Professor of Medical Education F. W. Hafferty distinguishes three dimensions in medical learning, which he names the formal curriculum, the informal curriculum and the hidden curriculum.[1] While the formal curriculum is the official

[1] Frederic W. Hafferty, 'Beyond Curriculum Reform: Confronting Medicine's Hidden Curriculum', *Academic Medicine* 73, no. 4 (1998): 403–7, https://doi.org/10.1097/00001888-199804000-00013.

content that is explicitly taught, the informal curriculum is concerned with the interpersonal interactions between student and staff where teaching occurs. The hidden curriculum, on the other hand, exists within the structural and cultural practices in medicine. This method of socialization of medical students has since been described extensively, with factors such as rules, culture and structures within an organization identified as significant drivers of the process. I learned about the hidden curriculum in medical school, put on guard against the potentially biased information and practices that often oppose the content of formal instruction, conveyed tacitly through interpersonal interactions between medical learners and instructors. Sessions that aimed to attenuate the negative effects of the hidden curriculum were often focused on maintaining student empathy in the face of patient mistreatment. My view of the process was straightforward: when you observe your preceptor mistreating patients, this teaches you to mistreat patients. Therefore, the antidote to this threat, I thought, would be to purposefully retain empathy for my patients throughout my training. I believed that if I could just hold on to my ability to relate to others and to value their experiences then maybe I would not fall victim to the so-called hidden curriculum.

Although the literature supports the idea that the hidden curriculum is a systemic issue, my initial understanding of it, based on how it was taught, aligns more accurately with what Hafferty describes as the informal curriculum. Incorrectly labelling the informal curriculum as the hidden curriculum is not just of semantic concern. Practically, it might mean that we have only been focusing on two of the three dimensions in medical learning – the formal and informal curricula – leaving the true hidden curriculum, the structural and cultural factors that shape medical education and the characters of medical students, unaddressed. Hafferty proposes priority areas to address within the hidden curriculum, including policy development, evaluation, resource allocation and institutional terminology. He argues that 'medical training is, at root, a process of moral enculturation' and that medical schools function as 'moral communities' (a socially integrated group with shared values, norms and beliefs).[2] It is only by understanding this aspect of the hidden curriculum that medical reform might be possible. Only, we do understand the hidden curriculum: we define it, we research it, and then we address the informal curriculum instead.

As I began my journey through medical education, I continuously drew on my previous experiences working with diverse populations to maintain my capacity to display empathy. Despite my avid participation in tutorial discussions around the social determinants of health and my ongoing passion for patient advocacy, I felt my patience wearing thin, especially with patients who repeated

[2] Ibid., 406.

themselves often or did not answer questions directly. I was careful to remain polite and professional, but I sensed the distance grow. I no longer identified easily with people who shared the same traits that I struggled with myself, such as repetitiveness. I could identify contributors to this decline, such as exhaustion, self-protection and competing demands on my time. Overall, I feared that some part of me was changing, not because I had picked up unpleasant habits from observing preceptors, but from structural constraints on my time and the fear of receiving negative evaluations due to supposedly undesirable traits previously identified by my instructors.

I cared deeply for my patients and had been forewarned about the existence of a hidden curriculum which might undo what I most valued in myself as a physician. It wasn't enough. By neglecting structural problems while futilely attempting to change the behaviours that result, we are attempting to treat the symptoms without eradicating their cause. We overlook how the treatment of medical learners and the structure of medical education work insidiously to mould learners into a standardized prototype of 'the physician', perpetuating a one-dimensional approach to patient care.

Diversity in medical education

Medical educators and researchers often blame the drop in empathy that medical learners experience over the course of their training on fatigue and negative role-modelling. However, I also found my empathy flagging due to a less tangible cause.

During a tutorial on health inequities, my group found ourselves discussing the social determinants of health and ways to address the financial barriers that play a role in health inequity in Canada. Our group of students was often left-leaning in discussions such as these, and brought up the concept of 'taxing the rich'. The attending, unimpressed, retorted, 'Physicians *are* the rich in Canada, and we get taxed plenty. You only feel this way because you are not practising yet. Ten years down the line, we'll see how you feel.' Although parts of this statement were grounded in fact, and their opinion on this complex topic was just as valid as mine, this example is significant for a few reasons. First, this comment assumed a supposedly unavoidable change in my political views. As a first-generation immigrant who grew up with financial insecurity, I appreciated that my socio-economic status would change because of the nature of the career I chose to pursue. But the attending's statement presumed that with that change, rather than maintain my integrity, my political values would realign to match the upper middle class. However, if my opinion on financial privilege is expected to change once I acquire wealth myself, then what is the relevance of seeking prospective physicians who come from lower socio-economic backgrounds?

Furthermore, I received feedback that my inputs were 'too political', and my instructors criticized me for rambling, suggesting that I rehearse my points ahead of time to avoid this habit. Given that most participation was discussion based, it was virtually impossible to prepare all of my responses ahead of time. Additionally, many of the discussions in this particular tutorial required combining lived experience with knowledge gained from readings and lectures. Topics were often political in nature, and I frequently drew from my experience working in the non-profit sector. So, I resorted to speaking less frequently in discussions. When this alone improved my evaluation, I realized that my perspective was not welcome. As Hafferty notes, 'Tools of evaluation ... are not simply instruments of assessment. They also are vehicles for conveying what is and is not important within the organization.'[3] My ideas and background were not important if my perspective did not align with that of the instructor, and especially if I could not get my point across without repeating myself. I have come to recognize that my repetitions were not unstructured 'rambling', but a reflection of my life experiences – whether from listening to the preacher's sermon every Sunday growing up or during my education in literature and poetry, I learned that repetition can be an effective tool to communicate. A pattern of similar negative feedback throughout pre-clerkship and clerkship made medical school feel like a constant uphill climb, however, and I would find myself suppressing not only my voice but my personality just to make it through one tutorial, one call shift, or a whole clinical rotation with my academic standing intact.

Ironically, this powerful suppressive effect is a broader counter-current running directly against institutional efforts to attract diverse voices into medicine. Recognition of the social determinants that contribute to health inequity in society has led medical schools to focus on diversifying the medical student population. Admissions staff in Canada, where I received my medical training, rely on multiple strategies to increase learner diversity with the goal of improving health equity.[4] This push to diversify the medical field is necessary and laudable, because the ability of a diverse student to bring their authentic selves into patient interactions and the learning environment is critical. While we often think of race when we think of diversity, it also encompasses other facets of identity, such as socio-economic status, visible and invisible disability and religious diversity, to name only a few. Minority patients have better experiences and outcomes with physicians who look like them, which may have less to do with physical

[3] Ibid., 405.

[4] Nelson Saddler et al., 'Taking Initiative in Addressing Diversity in Medicine', *Canadian Journal of Science, Mathematics and Technology Education* 21 (2021): 309–20; Tisha R. Joy, 'Strategies for Enhancing Equity, Diversity, and Inclusion in Medical School Admissions: A Canadian Medical School's Journey', *Frontiers in Public Health*, Jun. 24, 2022, 879173.

resemblance and more to do with shared identity.[5] Beyond physical sameness, a shared identity drives connection that contributes to the success of patient interactions. Additionally, diversity in medical education increases comfort amongst medical students when caring for diverse patient populations.[6] However, despite successful efforts at diversifying the matriculating medical classes, students with diverse backgrounds continue to report facing both interpersonal and structural discrimination based on their race, gender, sexual orientation and disability. This is worrisome since students in unfavourable learning environment experience higher burnout rates, declining mental health status, decreased levels of empathy and higher rates of attrition.[7] For diverse students, survival may depend on their ability to downplay or hide aspects of their identity to match the implicit cultural expectations in their learning environment, just as I did.

I found solace in commiserating with other students with diverse backgrounds. We would exchange tales of interactions with educators and trade jokes at the absurdity of our experiences. A bilingual student was mocked by their educator for mispronouncing a word that had no bearing on their understanding of the content of the lecture. A neuro-divergent student was repeatedly criticized for their lack of neurotypical traits; as a result, they feared that at their core, they did not have what it takes to become a physician. A racist educator was reported to the administration repeatedly, but due to bureaucratic procedures, administrators were unable to intervene; their students of colour continued to nod and smile in response to microaggressions and blatantly racist remarks. These examples are not meant to reflect on a single institution, as mistreatment is a shared experience among diverse medical learners. Instead, they highlight how the structure of medical education in general has not been adjusted to accommodate people who were previously underrepresented or considered unsuitable for admission.

Early on in my medical training, as I observed myself shrink out of fear of negative feedback, I was convinced that the problem was at the level of the instructors. Perhaps if they received better training, I mused – such as trauma-informed, inclusivity training – they would not cause such harm to their students. Although some part of this may ring true, as time passed and I waded deeper into medical education, I wondered if the harms were less tied to

---

[5] Ibid.

[6] Joy, 'Strategies for Enhancing Equity, Diversity, and Inclusion'.

[7] Liselotte N. Dyrbye, Daniel Satele and Colin P. West, 'Association of Characteristics of the Learning Environment and US Medical Student Burnout, Empathy, and Career Regret + Invited Commentary + Supplemental Content', *JAMA Network Open* 4, no. 8 (2021): 2119110; Liselotte N. Dyrbye et al., 'Race, Ethnicity, and Medical Student Well-Being in the United States', *Archives of Internal Medicine* 167, no. 19 (2007): 2103–9; Mytien Nguyen et al., 'Letters Association of Mistreatment and Discrimination with Medical School Attrition', *JAMA Pediatrics* 176, no. 9 (2022): 935–7.

instructors and more to the system which employed them. It was not simply disapproval that I feared, but the power they had to impact my career. Not only were my instructors solely responsible for deciding if I passed the course, they were also afforded the freedom to write comments on the final rubric that would be shared with residency programmes that I applied to in the future. Therefore, a pass was not enough: I needed to ensure that comments such as 'too political' or 'lacks concision' did not make it onto my application file. One day, while discussing our tutorial with a classmate who did not belong to an underrepresented identity group, I shared my ongoing struggle. She squinted at me, seemingly confused when I told her that I felt my rambling was interfering with my ability to communicate. 'I love your contributions in tutorial', she replied. 'Yeah, you ramble sometimes, but you always make sure that your point is clear. I have no trouble understanding you.' This validation matched the positive feedback I received from patients in the clinical setting – who sometimes *needed* to hear points repeated to digest the complex medical information – about my communication skills. This was validating, but I continued to lose points on communication in my tutorials. So who was correct? Was I an effective communicator or not? One thing was clear, however: my classmates and my patients were not the ones who would complete my final evaluation.

Initially, I viewed pressures to change as indicators that I was doing something wrong. Later, I became defensive, viewing the pressure to change my habits as inherently negative. Neither approach I adopted – I am wrong/they are wrong – allowed me to reconcile basic contradictions. Was it wrong that I practised concise communication to pass interviews or get through the OSCE (a timed exam), or was this a necessary form of code switching? Is concision an inherent marker of a good communicator, or is good communication the ability to get your point across to a variety of audiences, having the patience to answer questions and clarify where needed? How often does a patient receive seemingly clear and concise instructions from their physician, after all, only to return a few weeks later with inadequate compliance simply due to misunderstanding or misremembering the instructions? I looked for answers and models within medical education and the medical training literature, but without much success. To reconcile the contradiction, I found it helpful not to think of myself as a monolithic person, but instead, as a potentially malleable performer in a drama.

II. CHARACTER ARC AND ETHICS IN MEDICAL EDUCATION

Character development in medical education

During a visiting clerkship elective where I travelled to a different province to complete a clinical rotation, I was placed in a clinic where I quickly developed a cadence with my attending. Every time we entered a room to see a new patient, we would perform the same routine. She would introduce me as her medical student, at which the patient would smile politely. She would point out how I travelled from another province to be there, and almost every patient would respond 'Oh! That's a lovely place', or something similar; then she would say, 'Yes, she's come a long way just to see you', and we would all laugh. I would smile widely as she asked if it was okay if I joined the interaction (most patients said yes), and then we would begin. We did this more than thirty times a day for two weeks, and it never got old. Each time we entered a room, we were putting on a routine that was new to each patient and allowed us to build rapport quickly. Even when we were running behind, or we were exhausted, the performance continued.

In a traditional clinical interaction, the physician and the patient are characters embodied by individuals whose life experiences have brought them to this point. As Hafferty and Franks point out, this means that 'medical training is not just learning about becoming a physician, it involves learning how to cease to be a layperson. Medical training is not just about acquisition of new knowledge and skills, it is about the acquisition of a physician identity and character'.[8] If the physician is a role that we embody, then the acquisition of a physician identity and character must occur throughout the process of training and beyond. Instructors transmit the physician-character with its values and culture to medical learners in both explicit and tacit ways throughout medical education. However, these pedagogical processes are often in conflict with each other. Medical students are faced with the difficult task of reconciling the repeated contrasts between explicit and implicit lessons. When faced with this challenge, people adopt one of several strategies to resolve the conflict, including adopting implicit values with justifications that appease their discomfort, rejecting traditional values in favour of cynicism, or, less commonly, maintaining their original values in the face of the conflict.

As I came to see medical education as character development, the discipline of film studies provided a valuable analytical tool for understanding these conflict resolution strategies. Screenwriter Anthony Mullins theorizes an approach called arc analysis, an exploration of a character's external and internal worlds, which are interrelated.[9] For the character of a medical learner, the external world would include their role as a student and caregiver, as well as any interpersonal or situational conflicts that arise. Their internal world would consist of their values, hopes, motivations and other entities that form their identity.

---

[8] Frederic W. Hafferty and Ronald Franks, 'The Hidden Curriculum, Ethics Teaching, and the Structure of Medical Education', *Academic Medicine* 69, no. 11 (1995): 865.

[9] Anthony Mullins, *Beyond the Hero's Journey: Crafting Powerful and Original Character Arcs for the Screen* (Oldcastle Books, 2022).

Their character arc in the story which unfolds is determined by the interaction of external events, with the pressure they exert on the individual, and the character's inner choice. External events, whether positive or negative, create conflict between the external and internal worlds, forcing the character to make an internal choice to resolve this conflict. Two types of characters emerge, change characters and constant characters: a change character responds to conflict by making unfamiliar choices, while a constant character meets challenges by a consistent application of their values. Over time, a change character's internal world will adapt to align with the actions and choices they make. Alternatively, the internal world of a constant character remains the same over time as they continue to make choices that align with their original value system, encountering whatever consequences this approach to conflict might bring.

When applied to medical education, arc analysis indicates that the final form of the physician's identity relies on internal choices made throughout the process of medical education (and beyond). A 'change' physician-character is one who adopts the implicit lessons taught during medical training, and a 'constant' physician-character is one who stands firm in their value system. However, my experience also illustrated a third option, neglected by arc analysis, in which cynical physician-characters adopt new behaviours without adopting the beliefs which ought to underpin them – leading to dissatisfaction and a simmering internal contradiction.

The change in identity that can occur over time for a medical student was illustrated by a cross-sectional study of the hidden curriculum across the stages of medical training. Early on, medical students viewed emotional neutralization negatively, but students who were further along in their training viewed emotional neutralization as a 'necessary coping mechanism for daily life as a physician'.[10] Faculty within the study saw this change as a rite of passage on the journey to becoming an 'effective physician'.[11] Setting aside the contested value of emotional neutralization and its utility in clinical practice, I want to emphasize what the study reveals about the process of value adaptation in medical education. As medical students perform traits deemed more desirable, their inner beliefs, values and desires tend to change in accordance with those performances. Attempting to resolve external world conflict through choices that are misaligned with internal world values results in an altered identity – and we are not often aware that this internal change is occurring.[12]

---

[10] Asif Doja et al., 'The Hidden and Informal Curriculum across the Continuum of Training: A Cross-Sectional Qualitative Study', *Medical Teacher* 38, no. 4 (2016): 415.
[11] Ibid.
[12] Alexandra Kilian, Victor Do and Lyn K. Sonnenberg, 'All of Residency's a Stage: Fostering Authenticity and Individuality Among Learners', *Medical Science Educator* 33, no. 1 (2023): 243–45.

Given that diverse medical students often feel pressure to hide or alter aspects of their identity, they are at risk of losing some of the unique attributes that medical schools recruited them for in the first place. These are displaced in favour of new behaviours and values which resemble the monolithic type of how a physician looks, sounds and thinks, with potentially significant effects for patients. For instance, consider the fact that appearance is an important part of the psychiatric evaluation. If a Black student repeatedly receives unprofessionalism complaints based on their hair and are forced to adapt to more 'agreeable' hairstyles, how might their assessment of a Black patient's appearance change? Furthermore, if their classmates bear witness to these unprofessionalism complaints, how might this shape their understanding of what a dishevelled appearance looks like? Alternatively, picture a student who uses a wheelchair and who must attend a tutorial on the second floor with no ramps or elevators close by. If this student spends the next four years adapting to buildings that are not created for them, expected to arrive at the same time as their able-bodied classmates, how, then, can they be expected to empathize with their patient who is repeatedly late or misses appointments due to mobility issues? However, if this student witnesses their institution actively making changes to accommodate them, they learn that their experience is just as valuable as the rest of their colleagues, and perhaps, in the future, might be more likely to consider the barriers that are impacting their disabled patient.

Inclusion and proactive accommodation are not merely features which might improve the experience of medical training, but essential steps to return agency over their own 'arc' to students. By enabling medical students to more consciously shape the dramatic character of the physician, medical schools will garner a much more diverse cast of physician-characters and will, I believe, themselves become much more diverse.

Virtue ethics and character development

With my background in creative writing, I often found myself making connections between the practice of medicine and the art of literature. By the time I became a senior medical student, I had been grappling with this concept of character formation in medicine, so during a clerkship elective in biomedical ethics, I undertook the intimidating task of reading through Aristotle's *Nicomachean Ethics*. I wanted to understand how virtue ethics, which discusses character development, could be integrated into medical education – but I had an ulterior motive as well. I hoped to prove how our institutions were failing medical learners and in turn, failing patients. After repeated attempts to make my bias align with the interpretation of the literature, however, I was forced to reassess my position. In understanding that the problem was not as simple as I initially believed, I also realized that I had become the cynical character, resenting the behaviours I had adopted for safety and the institution (medical education) I belonged to. My silence was the external response as I attempted to stay constant to my initial values, but in the absence of an intentional choice, the conflict between my external and internal worlds was never resolved.

A few days into my clerkship elective, we had a patient who repeatedly asked the same questions about her symptoms, even as we reassured her repeatedly there was nothing to be concerned about. As I felt my own irritation begin to appear, I noted how patient my attending was, taking time to address the patient's concerns with no signs of irritation. Later, I said to her, 'You're so patient with your patients. I'm not sure if you always feel it or just portray it, but it's admirable.' She paused to consider how much of her behaviour was acting and how much was genuine, then shrugged and said, 'It comes down to listening to your patients. Even when you're running behind or stressed, even when you don't feel it, people want to feel that satisfaction, and they deserve it.' It struck me, listening to her, that she made a choice to listen to her patients – a choice that put the patient above both personal needs and institutional values.

The concept of choice as a driving force in character development is reflected in both humanities and medical literature. Mullins sees choice as crucial to Western storytelling, for example, located 'at the heart of understanding both character and story. Choice makes the intangible internal world of the character tangible as they try to impose their will on the external world'.[13] But when is a choice made due to an intellectual decision and when is it simply a matter of habit? Jack Coulehan and Peter Williams argue that tacit learning pertains to action, which makes it more powerful than explicit learning, which is concerned with words.[14] This aligns with Aristotle's distinction in the *Nicomachean Ethics* between intellectual virtue, which is taught, and moral virtue, which comes by habit and ultimately defines character.[15] In their exploration of ethics and the hidden curriculum, Hafferty and Franks highlight the difference between teaching ethics as a variety of concepts that can be applied in clinical settings (autonomy, beneficence, non-maleficence, justice) versus teaching ethics as permanent values that are integrated within the learner's identity. They argue that ethical principles must be integrated into the identity of the physician, echoing Aristotle's conclusion that character cannot be separated from the person.[16] The screenwriter's insight about the formation of dramatic character applies to ethical character as well: external pressures on the person shape the internal character.[17]

---

[13] Mullins, *Beyond the Hero's Journey*, 237.
[14] Jack Coulehan and Peter C. Williams, 'Vanquishing Virtue: The Impact of Medical Education', *Academic Medicine* 76, no. 6 (2001): 598–605.
[15] Aristotle, *Nicomachean Ethics*, i.1.
[16] Hafferty and Franks, 'The Hidden Curriculum', 862; Aristotle, *Nicomachean Ethics*, ii.1.
[17] A good example from medical education comes from the finding that the tolerance of unprofessional behaviour, not only the existence of the behaviour, has effects on students' own personal code of ethics (Doja et al., 'The Hidden and Informal Curriculum', 415).

Applied to medical education, the type of physician a learner becomes will be determined by the choices and actions they continuously make during training and beyond. Healthcare interactions are gruelling repeated performances which blend 'character' in both dramatic and ethical senses, where full-fledged characters emerge and interact, to create something worthy of their efforts. If a learner consistently acts in accordance with their original value system – as a constant character would – they may be better protected against the changes in identity brought on by the hidden curriculum. Indeed, having persistent dedication to personal ideals and values can be a protective factor against the harms of the hidden curriculum.[18] The challenge, then, is to uphold one's core principles as a learner while facing conflicts in the learning environment which communicate implicitly that those core principles are unwelcome.

In the *Nicomachean Ethics* Aristotle terms the third type of character, someone stuck half-way between the constant character and the change character, as 'incontinent'.[19] This is an individual who knows what not to do, yet gives in to this action to relieve pain. Although Aristotle's use of this term focuses on self-indulgence, an equivalent character in medical training is the learner who attempts to hold on to their core values but feels forced to adopt behaviours that will attenuate pain – for example, someone who remains quiet to pass a course at the expense of sharing useful lived experience with colleagues. A character who behaves in this way does not resolve the conflict between their internal and external worlds. They neither change nor remain constant, instead becoming stalled in unresolved conflict which risks their becoming cynical about medical values, positive and negative alike.

In my own misguided attempt to avoid internal change while giving in to actions that allowed for survival, I embodied the stalled character. I have come to understand that the stalled character may be the worst arc that a diverse learner can live out, as it is of no benefit to diverse patients and the individual's own conflict is not resolved. I began to wonder how many diverse leaners are finding themselves stalled, burnt out, portraying a role they have no connection to.

III. APPLYING ARC ANALYSIS AND VIRTUE ETHICS TO THE HIDDEN CURRICULUM

In retrospect, I had entered medical school assuming that the optimal character arc would be the constant character. I had no idea that to remain constant would run directly against the goals of medical education, as Hafferty

[18] See Coulehan and Williams, 'Vanquishing Virtue', 601.
[19] Aristotle, *Nicomachean Ethics*, v.9.

and Franks emphasize: '[students] are not *supposed* to exit from the training process unaltered – at least as far as the culture of medicine is concerned'.[20] Some scholars regard the hidden curriculum as a valuable method of socialization, one which cannot be discarded. They argue that the focus of critique or analysis should be less on the existence of the hidden curriculum, and more on the content of the socialization that occurs.[21] This position is a valuable addition to the discussion. Take the earlier example of emotional neutralization, for instance: without further exploration, it is difficult to claim that this change in perspective is inherently negative or harmful to patient care. Since so much of clinical medicine is learned through practice, we must leave room for the possibility that just as there are harmful aspects of the hidden curriculum, there may be necessary changes that learners must undergo through tacit socialization to practise clinical medicine successfully.

The contemplative approach: From Aristotle to Grey's Anatomy

As I came to recognize the complexity of character formation, including my own, I had to acknowledge the possible utility of the hidden curriculum. In this final section I want to turn to the popular medical drama *Grey's Anatomy* to illustrate the role of the hidden curriculum in driving positive change characters. Setting aside the often unrealistic dramatic aspects of the show and focusing solely on the journey of the characters as surgical residents, the original cast of characters portrays a useful combination of arcs. Alex Karev, the arrogant and competitive resident, clashes frequently with clinicians and patients until he slowly adopts values which lead to his success as an empathetic – albeit direct – paediatric surgeon. This is an example of a change character whose adoption of values taught by his environment made him a more effective physician. Alternatively, Izzy Stevens, the ever-empathetic resident, is arguably a constant character. While her empathy was helpful in certain patient presentations, her ongoing inability to compartmentalize led to over-involvement with her patients and, inevitably, a dramatic burnout.

Literature has highlighted the significance of reflective practice in combating negative effects of the hidden curriculum.[22] This is a key point in Aristotle's virtue ethics, as well. He argues that for an individual to pursue human flourishing for the self and the other, they must adopt a contemplative life and make choices that lead to the formation of good character, regardless of consequence.

---

[20] Hafferty and Franks, 'The Hidden Curriculum', 865.

[21] See, for example, Hafferty and Franks, 'The Hidden Curriculum'; Maria Athina Martimianakis et al., 'Humanism, the Hidden Curriculum, and Educational Reform: A Scoping Review and Thematic Analysis', *Academic Medicine* 90, no. 11 (Suppl.) (2015): S5–S13.

[22] See Martimianakis et al., 'Humanism, the Hidden Curriculum, and Educational Reform'.

Living this kind of contemplative life during medical training would invest learners with both agency and responsibility to engage in continual introspection and intentionality in choices that align with the type of physician one wants to become. The *Grey's Anatomy* character who best reflects the contemplative approach is its protagonist Meredith Grey. Most episodes of the show are framed with her voiceovers, which include active reflection on the external events occurring, acknowledgement of the conflict at hand, and attempts to reconcile internal values through choice. At times, this process requires change on her part, and at other times, it requires her to stand firm in her core values. Ultimately this leads to the formation of a character who emerges as a leader among her peers and a strong advocate for her patients.

It is worth acknowledging that throughout my undergraduate medical journey there have been many sessions on the importance of reflective practice, and plenty of encouragement to adopt tools such as journaling. However, a more radical approach is needed. As early as the first week of medical school, students should be alert to the complexity of character formation and their role in this process. They should outline the type of physician they want to be and the aspects of their identity that will shape their role. Students' application essays could form the basis of this reflective exercise, where they would have already made declarations of values and intent in efforts to be admitted. As they progress in their studies, it would be important to return repeatedly to their formation, reflect on the conflicts they are experiencing and the choices they have made, and assess whether their internal and external worlds are aligned. It should be expected that some of the specific traits they deemed important may change, but this intentional practice would help empower each individual to make contemplative choices about their own character arc.

Understanding that we are all playing a role in our healthcare interactions, and that character is defined by action not thought, can empower medical students to act not as we feel but as the type of physician we want to be. Throughout medical school, we learn and are tested on showing empathy through body language, word choice, etc., so that in the face of competing priorities when one feels their patience wearing thin, we can put our years of rehearsal to use, as our audience deserves.

It was through embracing the contemplative approach that I was able to enjoy medicine again. However, I remained aware that the responsibility to shape my physician identity does not belong to me alone.

CONCLUSION

The stakes are high on the road to becoming a physician. As part of the informal and hidden curriculum, medical students – especially diverse learners – are painfully aware that how they are perceived can have direct impacts on their evaluations, their residency match and their ultimate goal of becoming a physician. When students consider these consequences and recognize that their identity expression is in contrast with implicit culture, it is understandable why many choose the relative safety of acculturation.

The personal virtues of learners that have been shown to protect against identity attacks, but it is important to register that systemic changes can be protective as well.[23] The rules, structures and culture of an organization are highly influential elements of the hidden curriculum.[24] An example of structural change that would support contemplative character development would be protected time or recurring small group sessions where students are meant to work on their character formation document. In order to make this an effective intervention, however, these sessions should not be haphazardly added to the students' already demanding schedule, which would only worsen stress and promote disdain for the process. Rather, this would need to intentionally be paired with a corresponding restriction in duty hours. Attempts to change the hidden curriculum often target individual behaviour and sometimes target institutions, but rarely address the greater structural foundation of medical practice and education.[25] The focus on increasing diversity in medical education by attracting a diverse student body is one example of an attempt to challenge the discriminatory foundations within medicine. While this necessary bottom-up approach has proven successful in improving medical school diversity, casting is only the first step in the long journey towards the full production. Admission diversity alone cannot achieve true health equity unless we also address the implicit standards that threaten to extinguish the intended benefits of a diverse medical workforce.

The formation of good character is a shared responsibility between medical learners, their teachers and the institution that trains them. Institutions must interrogate how their policies, employee training and management, may be contributing to the ongoing perpetuation of the hidden curriculum. Practically, this may look like conducting focus groups (or undertaking other forms of data collection) to pinpoint which policies, rubric items, structural elements, etc., are creating internal conflict for students. Based on this data, medical schools can then revisit the intention behind these highlighted items, explicitly outlining which traits are truly necessary to physician and patient flourishing, and which rules are unexamined remnants of an original medical culture. For example, who decides what passes for effective communication? Which aspects of

---

[23] See Coulehan and Williams, 'Vanquishing Virtue'.

[24] Yaser Sarikhani, Payam Shojaei, Mohammad Rafiee and Sajad Delavari, 'Analyzing the Interaction of Main Components of Hidden Curriculum in Medical Education Using Interpretive Structural Modeling Method', *BMC Medical Education* 20 (2020): 176.

[25] See Martimianakis et al., 'Humanism, the Hidden Curriculum, and Educational Reform'.

what we define as 'professionalism' truly impact clinical practice and which are more cultural? How can our physical and academic learning environments be adjusted to better reflect the needs of our student population? This will be gruelling work, but by undertaking it we can create learning environments in which students are not pressured to choose between safety and identity.

REFERENCES

Aristotle. *Nicomachean Ethics*. Translated by W. D. Ross. Global Grey, 1925.

Coulehan, Jack, and Peter C. Williams. 'Vanquishing Virtue: The Impact of Medical Education'. *Academic Medicine* 76, no. 6 (2001): 598–605. https://doi.org/10.1097/00001888-200106000-00008.

Doja, Asif, M. Dylan Bould, Chantalle Clarkin, Kaylee Eady, Stephanie Sutherland and Hilary Writer. 'The Hidden and Informal Curriculum across the Continuum of Training: A Cross-Sectional Qualitative Study'. *Medical Teacher* 38, no. 4 (2016): 410–18. https://doi.org/10.3109/0142159X.2015.1073241.

Dyrbye, Liselotte N., Daniel Satele and Colin P. West. 'Association of Characteristics of the Learning Environment and US Medical Student Burnout, Empathy, and Career Regret + Invited Commentary + Supplemental Content'. *JAMA Network Open* 4, no. 8 (2021): 2119110. https://doi.org/10.1001/jamanetworkopen.2021.19110.

Dyrbye, Liselotte N., Matthew R. Thomas, Anne Eacker, William Harper, F. Stanford Massie, Jr, David V. Power, Mashele Huschka, Paul J. Novotny, Jeff A. Sloan and Tait D. Shanafelt. 'Race, Ethnicity, and Medical Student Well-Being in the United States'. *Archives of Internal Medicine* 167, no. 19 (2007): 2103–9. https://doi.org/10.1001/archinte.167.19.2103.

Hafferty, Frederic W. 'Beyond Curriculum Reform: Confronting Medicine's Hidden Curriculum'. *Academic Medicine* 73, no. 4 (1998): 403–7. https://doi.org/10.1097/00001888-199804000-00013.

Hafferty, Frederic W., and Ronald Franks. 'The Hidden Curriculum, Ethics Teaching, and the Structure of Medical Education'. *Academic Medicine* 69, no. 11 (1995): 861–71. https://doi.org/10.1097/00001888-199411000-00001.

Kilian, Alexandra, Victor Do and Lyn K. Sonnenberg. 'All of Residency's a Stage: Fostering Authenticity and Individuality Among Learners'. *Medical Science Educator* 33, no. 1 (2023): 243–45. https://doi.org/10.1007/S40670-022-01700-Z/METRICS.

Martimianakis, Maria Athina, Barret Michalec, Justin Lam, Carrie Cartmill, Janelle S. Taylor and Frederic W. Hafferty. 'Humanism, the Hidden Curriculum, and Educational Reform: A Scoping Review and Thematic Analysis'. *Academic Medicine* 90, no. 11 (Suppl.) (2015): S5–S13. https://doi.org/10.1097/ACM.0000000000000894.

Mullins, Anthony. *Beyond the Hero's Journey: Crafting Powerful and Original Character Arcs for the Screen*. Oldcastle Books, 2022.

Nguyen, Mytien, Sarwat I. Chaudhry, Mayur M. Desai, Candice Chen, William A. McDade, Tonya L. Fancher and Dowin Boatright. 'Letters Association of Mistreatment and Discrimination with Medical School Attrition'. *JAMA Pediatrics* 176, no. 9 (2022): 935–7. https://doi.org/10.1001/jamapediatrics.2022.1637.

Saddler, Nelson, Seana Adams, Lisa A. Robinson and Ike Okafor. 'Taking Initiative in Addressing Diversity in Medicine'. *Canadian Journal of Science, Mathematics and Technology Education* 21 (2021): 309–20. https://doi.org/10.1007/s42330-021-00154-6.

Sarikhani, Yaser, Payam Shojaei, Mohammad Rafiee and Sajad Delavari. 'Analyzing the Interaction of Main Components of Hidden Curriculum in Medical Education Using Interpretive Structural Modeling Method'. *BMC Medical Education* 20 (2020): 176. https://doi.org/10.1186/s12909-020-02094-5.

Joy, Tisha R. 'Strategies for Enhancing Equity, Diversity, and Inclusion in Medical School Admissions: A Canadian Medical School's Journey'. *Frontiers in Public Health* (2022): 879173. https://doi.org/10.3389/fpubh.2022.879173.

3

Puppetry and medical performance

AN INTERVIEW WITH RACHEL WARR

Rachel Warr is a puppetry director and dramaturg. She has collaborated with medical professionals for over a decade, focusing on surgery, medical education and public engagement; in this interview she particularly references her long-standing collaborator Roger Kneebone, Professor of Surgical Education and Engagement Science at Imperial College London, and Co-director of the Centre for Performance Science in the UK. Clinicians initially wonder what a seemingly minor theatrical genre – the 'children's' art of puppetry – can teach them about the serious work of operating in a medical theatre. Incredulity quickly gives way to respect when the juxtaposition of puppetry and surgery opens a space for valuable and life-sustaining insights. Puppetry's emphases, for example, on warming up, collaborating on the collective endeavour, honouring the centrality of the hand and practising active listening can offer solutions to serious and often elided challenges that surgeons encounter in the operating theatre. Clinicians come to appreciate that the consulting and operating room constitutes a theatre of sorts. As Warr explains, 'patients as well as doctors can benefit if they see the consultation as a sort of performance', in which both parties engage in a carefully structured semi-improvised exchange. Warr's work in medical education demonstrates how stagecraft can help ensure the audience (i.e. the patient) receives the intended message, and, equally critical, that the healthcare professional is 'actively listening'.

I. THINKING ACROSS THEATRES

What does the title of our volume, Medicine as Theatre: Theatre as Medicine, *bring to mind?*

Rachel Warr (RW): When I first met with a group of medical professionals to share our working practices, it didn't take us long to realize we were using similar terminology. Most obviously the term theatre/theater – it's an operating 'theatre' after all, and for good reason. In the 1800s, operations were often performed in front of audiences: students and the public. Much has changed in medicine since then, of course, but even so, the modern operating room is still like a theatre space – many of the clinicians I've met acknowledge that. It's quite usual for a modern operation to include a group of students watching, as part of how medical students train. Also, if a patient is awake, under local rather than general anaesthetic, then the patient is both a player in the proceedings and an audience to it.

A theatre is a space where people come together at a designated time to take on specified roles and enact a rehearsed sequence in concert with one another, sometimes having to improvise if the circumstances force some deviation from the planned choreography. This definition of theatre applies just as much to the operating theatre as it does to my work in the performing arts. Both have a set of procedures that support those carrying out their roles. I've heard surgeons describe getting into scrubs and scrubbing up as the time where they focus their mind on the task ahead – 'getting into the zone'. Of course, scrubbing up is about cleanliness, but it also enables a mental shift, in the same way as for performers as they get into costume and prepare to go on stage. I think it's a bit like an air lock between two worlds or states of being, a place of mental transition, a transformation in focus and role, aided by a change in clothing and a ritualized physical action.

Other parallels include managing nerves before and during, and dealing with the big comedown after the event to adjust back into the everyday world. I've heard performers from the arts and members of surgical teams speak about these challenges in exactly the same way.

Some years ago, I had an appointment with my family doctor and he asked me, 'What do you do for a living?'

'I'm a theatre director', I said.

He responded, 'Oh, you work in a hospital.' I had to clarify that I work in the performing arts, with puppetry. As a clinician the word 'theatre' automatically led him to think of a hospital.

How do people react when you explain that you work with puppets? What kinds of assumptions do they make?

RW: When you say the word 'puppet', everybody has a different image in their head. There are many types of puppetry: shadow puppets, rod puppets, string marionettes and so on. Each type requires different skills. There is a widespread perception in the contemporary Western world that puppetry is just for children. It's a bit frustrating; I sometimes have to work at shifting that assumption. There's lots of contemporary work for older audiences. Historically and globally puppets are more associated with the adult world, or the whole community. Puppets have an innate ability to address grown-up themes, and are particularly good at themes of the sacred and the disruptive.

When and how did you first get involved in work with clinicians?

RW: I've been working with Professor Roger Kneebone now for over twelve years (I've worked with other medical practitioners, too, but mostly with Roger.) The work I've been involved in is broader than training medical students: there is also cross-discipline research and writing academic papers, and public engagement events that demystify the operating theatre. We've also held outreach events for the next generation, highlighting how medical skills are not just about academic knowledge but also hands-on craft skills and performance skills.

My collaboration with Professor Kneebone began when a mutual friend named Prue Cooper, who is a potter, invited me to a talk at The Art Workers' Guild in London. Before the talk, we were chatting and I mentioned that years before I'd presented work at a theatre festival organized by an engineering college. The engineering faculty had identified that the skills you learn doing drama echo the skills you need in civil engineering: project management, scheduling, teamwork, managing people with diverse skills, turning a concept into a physical entity, structural awareness, narrative and communication – all sorts of stuff. The students had courses in drama as part of their engineering degree. I mentioned this, and Prue said, 'Oh, you need to meet Roger.' He was also at the event, so Prue introduced us.

Roger is very outward looking. He has a genuine curiosity and is interested in looking at things from different perspectives. Looking outward helps you look inward anew. We started collaborating by a simple sharing of our practices, and we started to identify connections. It grew from there. We are still finding new parallels to explore. Roger works with other creative practitioners, too, not just me.

What types of medical learners have you worked with and where have you worked?

RW: I've worked with students training to become family doctors, clinicians in the final stages of becoming consultants, mid-career medical staff, as well as teenagers considering a career in medicine.

I've worked with a variety of different hospitals in London as well as institutions such as the Wellcome Trust and the Science Museum. At the moment, I am puppeteer in residence at the Centre for Performance Science, co-led by the Imperial College and the Royal College of Music, which investigates notions of performance across different disciplines, including medicine.

What forms has your work taken?

RW: Discussions, demonstrations, simulations and practical sessions. It is always interesting getting clinicians to have a go at puppeteering, with some guidance. It's an embodied way of learning. Watching someone puppeteer for the first time can expose their aptitude for leadership, coordination and listening.

II. PARALLELS BETWEEN THEATRE AND MEDICINE

You're challenging some of the basic tenets of medical culture. How do people react? Are the medical students and surgeons open to your ideas or do they get stonewalled?

RW: I am not trying to tell someone how to do their job, nor force them to be excited by puppetry. If I frame it as merely sharing my way of working and inviting others to use it to reflect on their own work through a different perspective, then people open up. Some people are beguiled by a puppet, others can be wary of them. Sometimes I have to give people a moment to express these reactions before we can get into a discussion.

People can be sceptical at the start, but that changes fairly quickly, partly because the parallels are so strong. And credit to Professor Kneebone, he does much to prepare participants to think in new ways.

One of the strengths of drawing parallels between surgery and puppetry rather than, say, surgery and acting, is that puppetry is more externalized. In medicine, it's not really about you – the clinician – it's about the patient. Likewise, in puppetry, it's not about the puppeteer, it's about the puppet. The puppet is seen by the audience rather than the puppeteer. Even if the puppeteer is visible to the audience, it is the puppet they are looking at. Having said that, during a demonstration of puppetry an observer can see straightaway that there is expertise in seeming to bring a puppet to life. There can be sensitivities about language. There can be a horror or distaste from clinicians at the idea of 'pretending', which is so often associated with fakery. For some doctors, even the word 'performing' can be challenging as it has connotations of 'pretending'.

What kind of connection do medical students tend to make beyond the basic analogy that expertise lies in your hands in both professions?

RW: Expertise in our hands is a way in, yes. How objects are handled effectively between team members is important to both disciplines, for surgeons particularly during an operation. There are other parallels which are more resonant and these soon dominate the discussion, although it depends on what type of clinician is present.

The parallels for family doctors are about reframing the consultation process as small scale semi-improvised performance, where doctor and patient make sense of a narrative together through active listening.

For surgeons it's the way both disciplines work as a team, including working in close physical proximity, the way the team needs to position itself in the space and the stress positions we sometimes have to hold at length. There are parallels in the hierarchy of a surgical and puppetry team, and parallels in how they need to communicate. With eyes focused on the patient or puppet's body the team communicates through shared movement and rhythm rather than eye contact. The skills required by open surgery are particularly aligned with multi-person table-top puppetry. Skills for laparoscopic or keyhole surgery are akin to long rod puppetry, having to sense and control movement at the end of a rod with a trigger mechanism. We both experience the same kinds of physical strain in our wrists, arms, shoulders and neck. We've looked also at knots and thread management in medical suture from the view of handling string marionettes. Dealing with notions of failure, burn out, nerves – these topics sometimes come up too.

The parallels for technicians, who oversee animatronic dummies used by some hospitals for simulation, are how these complicated devices can be afforded a degree of human authenticity when they represent a patient during a simulation.

Let's follow up on that last statement – do you consider dummies used for simulations as 'puppets'?

RW: They are representations of the human form, and everybody has to invest in the idea that they are alive to some degree for a simulation to be effective. Professor Kneebone doesn't work with animatronic dummies in simulation but I've collaborated with a couple of hospitals that do.

At one hospital I was told about a simulation where the animatronic dummy started malfunctioning. The students being assessed were responding to its malfunction, a continually winking eye, and understandably mistook it as a symptom of the patient and part of the role play. In conversation with the trainers afterward, it was acknowledged that the complex animatronics are often a hindrance to the simulation – not just because of malfunctions, but also because while using dummies is an attempt at high-level realism in fact it often leads to the opposite. The dummies feel uncanny and alien. Enabling participants to *feel* immersed in the simulation comes from suggesting essential visual triggers rather than attempting full realism, and also from how the instructor frames the experience and the way participants are led into the narrative. The dummies in isolation don't do that. Something becomes a puppet because of the puppeteer/storyteller's skill. The transformation comes from the puppeteer. You need an awareness of how to make a dummy appear to have meaningful life in a situation, otherwise it is just a dead object and not really serving the purpose.

Another group I worked with voiced a very different concern. At their Christmas party, some of these dummies were dressed up and wheeled out in jest. Their question to me was, how can they then come back and respect the dummies as a patient in a simulation after that? There was a sort of boundary that had been crossed. I was asked to come and talk to them about how to treat their dummies as I would a puppet.

Beyond the parallels you've mentioned so far, what are other puppetry skills that can specifically benefit surgeons?

RW: A physical warm-up is an example. In my work it is common practice to warm up before performing, particularly focusing on hands, arms, shoulders, neck, back. At the start of a rehearsal I instigate a warm-up using exercises according to what kind of puppetry we're doing. When I've shown some simple hand warm-up exercises to surgeons they found it novel. That is not part of medical practice at all. When I first heard this I was shocked. I've met surgeons who say that they get a cramp in their hands during an operation. I know surgeons who've had to give up because of strained hand muscles and can't rely on a steady hand anymore. They're heartbroken that they've had to abandon the work they love. Warming up might have helped protect against that.

Warming up does a lot of things: it prepares your muscles for the task; it increases your range of dexterity; and it can help protect against strain. Equally important, it enables you to get into the right frame of mind and put mind and body in sync. It needn't take long – a couple of minutes could be built into the routine of scrubbing up. Once you become aware of the benefits of warming up, you can also think about warming down, which can help support you emotionally in dealing with the stress and high stakes of surgery, especially when things haven't gone as smoothly as you'd hoped.

III. USING THEATRE TO OPEN DIFFICULT CONVERSATIONS ABOUT MEDICINE

What problems in medicine and medical education, in the UK or more generally, has your collaboration with healthcare professionals exposed?

RW: I'm not an expert on medical education, I only have a basic overarching sense of it. But from my limited perspective it seems to me that while we share many parallels in the skills we require, the pedagogy of our training is completely different. In puppetry we train in puppeteering a puppet but also in working as a team, and that's transferable to any team. In medicine one trains in a specialism, but not as a team across roles. There is hands-on training as a junior in a hospital, learning your specialism in situ, but I don't think there is focused training on how to work effectively as a team. Effective team work and good leadership can make a big difference to an outcome. Also, I think puppetry and medicine have very different responses to the notion of failure. This is also related to teamwork.

Can you say more about those different perspectives on failure? How does puppetry offer an alternative to medical culture, which views failure as an individual and highly litigious issue?

RW: I think performers on stage or in rehearsal tend to see failure as part of the process, to be alert to it, to see it approaching and to work together to respond to it collectively. We have the good fortune to be able to use mistakes as a useful tool in a rehearsal process. And we have feedback. In my work feedback is part of every stage of the process, coming from all directions, in a structured way, from auditions to rehearsals to shows to post production.

I don't think feedback is embedded in that way in medical training or medical practice. My personal view is that that is to everyone's detriment. Feedback is best done in a supportive structure, not just top down, and with an understanding that it is about shared aims and not personal ones. If your response to failure is to cover up or shield yourself by blaming others, then failure becomes something to fear, and harder to pre-empt or manage well.

Doesn't failure in medicine inspire such fear because the stakes are higher in the operating theatre?

RW: Well, yes of course. While performing on stage can feel high stakes, emotionally exposing and physically exhausting, of course lives aren't at stake.

Although, some years ago, I brought a few puppeteers along to meet some surgeons for a discussion, and the puppeteers all voiced the sentiment that 'the stakes are much higher in medicine'. But the surgeons said, 'Well no, not really.' They explained that many operations aren't life or death – many are routine, and they carry out the same operation many times in the week. They described their training a bit like an apprenticeship, an equivalent of a rehearsal, in the sense that every single operation is an opportunity to improve your skill. This was spoken with no disrespect to the patient – of course they are the most important consideration. I think we sometimes like to turn the role of surgeon into a superhero, which maybe isn't very nuanced or helpful, and maybe adds personal pressure and takes away from surgery being a team endeavour.

How do you help healthcare professions to elicit and acknowledge feedback?

RW: Giving and receiving feedback is difficult if it isn't supported and embedded in the way of working. I led a session for students in their last term of training to be general practitioners (family doctors). Lack of feedback or poorly given feedback seemed to have led a large number of them to feel like they were failing. In the session we looked at making feedback constructive, given appropriately, not just top down, in an open manner.

In the early days of this work, I remember getting medical students in threes or fours to collaboratively puppeteer a single table-top rod puppet, to watch and give feedback on the puppet's movement with the aim of improving its accuracy. They all struggled with how to give feedback. 'No that's not right, make it do this', is not an effective way of enabling someone to change the action of the puppet. Giving feedback in this context is about understanding the mechanics of what isn't working well, putting yourself in the position of the other person in order to understand their challenges, communicating the issue clearly and without recrimination, and having a suggestion of how to resolve it while also involving that person in finding a solution that is achievable from their position.

Some years back, Roger and I designed a public engagement activity to demystify the operating theatre, a group exercise echoing the way a surgical team functions under pressure. It was interesting hearing the audience reflect back on their roles in the exercise, both those participating and those watching. What was more surprising and interesting to me happened afterwards. The medical professionals in attendance started asking questions about their own experiences in the operating theatre. Hearing members of the public give an embodied response to an abstract exercise made the professionals open up and self-evaluate their own feelings, in particular about individual versus team dynamics, notions of success and failure and facing pressure.

IV. HOW TO BRING A PUPPET TO LIFE

How do you bring a puppet to life?

RW: Well, depends on what type of puppet: shadow, string, rod, glove puppets each require different approaches. All, though, require the puppeteer to do something contradictory, to make a connection with the puppet (physical and psychological) in order to lend the puppet life and intention, while at the same time keeping some distance (physical and psychological) so that the puppet appears autonomous. You have to hold this dual contradictory state.

Bringing a puppet to life has to start from somewhere, and that's often from a sense of breath. Everything that has life has breath, even if it is an inanimate object given impetus from a force, such as a ball being thrown. As an audience we see the breath and the impetus it conveys, and we read its intention or trajectory. In terms of puppetry, breath is impetus for intention and action, as much as lung capacity.

I once showed a nurse a breathing exercise from puppetry, mimicking breath movement in an object, and she said, 'It's just like when you need to give manual ventilation to a patient.'

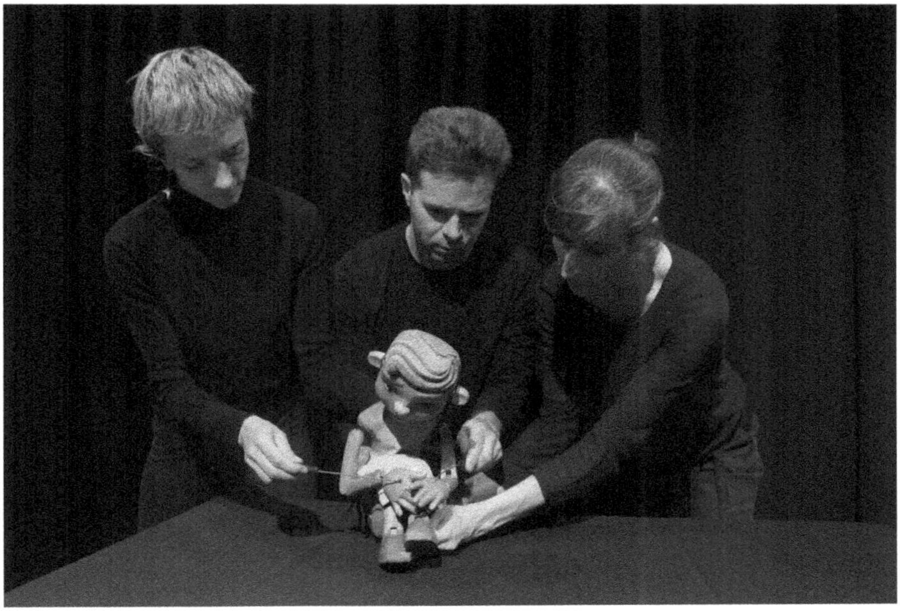

FIGURE 3.1 Three puppeteers working collaboratively to bring a puppet to life. Their physical positions, gaze, team structure and methods of team communication is a parallel to that of a surgical team. Puppeteers (L–R): Edie Edmundson, Gilbert Taylor, Rachel Warr; puppet made by Jan Zalud; photographer: Tom Crame.

How can the kind of breath and intention you're talking about in the puppeteer's work be extended to the coordinated action of an entire medical team?

RW: Clinicians need to hold that contradictory state too: they need to have both a connection with and a distance from their patient. They need to engage with and genuinely care about their patient to respond to the patient's medical needs, but at the same time they need some distance to carry out medical procedures on the patient, such as cutting with a scalpel.

A patient's breathing is an important guide for clinicians. Clinicians read a patient's rhythm and tone of breathing, and it can inform what action they take. In an operating theatre, a patient's breathing is monitored and is often audible to the operating team through the monitor. It's a guiding soundtrack to the operating team's decisions and actions. If the heart rate changes or the anaesthetist is concerned about the breathing of the patient, then the actions and pace of the surgical team may change.

There's this fascinating thing that happens in a theatre performance. An engaged audience will start to breathe in keeping with the pace and flow of the performance. The audience's breathing is in a sort of dialogue with the performance. It's also like that with surgeons and puppeteers: they breathe and move in response to the patient's breath or puppet's breath, not copying it but in dialogue with it. Of course I know that a puppet isn't actually breathing, and that the illusion of breath comes from the puppeteers, but the puppet's breath isn't a copy of the puppeteer's breath – it has its own rhythm, connected to the movements and ideas it is being made to express. The puppeteer responds to the rhythm and intention the puppet requires.

When a single puppet is being puppeteered by a team, they work collectively by reading the rhythm and pace of the puppet's breath. They are all looking at the puppet, not at each other, so the puppet's breath is their point of connection. Sometimes they don't all have a good view of the puppet, so they are also reading each other's movements in order to work in sync. Surgical teams function in a similar way. Both teams have their eyes focused on the body they are supporting or the tools they are using, not on one another. So they are not communicating through facial cues but through breath, rhythm and movement. When I first saw an operating team working together it looked so familiar, it was just like a puppetry team in the positions they were standing in and their gaze. I could have taken a photo of one team and transposed it on onto the other.

There's a similar hierarchy in both these teams. Generally, the puppeteer working the head of the puppet takes the lead while each of the other puppeteers has specific responsibilities, which echoes the roles in a surgical team, from the lead surgeon to the scrub nurse.

Puppet theatre can help medical professionals replace a myopic focus on their individual performance with an awareness of making the best of the team. Teamwork and leadership are not separate things. In puppetry, leadership and hierarchy need a degree of flexibility. Sometimes we are not led by our thoughts, our head. If we slip or fall, our body tries to regain balance – we have automatic responses. So the lead puppeteer, working the head of the puppet, has to know when to lead and when to relinquish to another team member so that they can lead the movement at the appropriate moment. Leadership involves giving space for others to employ their expertise when required, and resuming leadership to keep the action coherently flowing action.

In puppetry, it's clear when the team is not working well because the puppet's movement is clunky, uncoordinated, either from the team not listening to the puppet or each other, or from an individual trying to lead by force. The puppet is an embodied visual indication of whether the team is working well.

You've given us a great sense of the insights that emerge from the collaboration between surgeons and puppeteers in an operating theatre. Does puppetry also relate to the more intimate consultations between doctors and patients in the clinic?

RW: As a theatre director in the performing arts, I am always thinking about how I communicate information, what affect will it have on my audience, what message will they take away. I'm thinking about where I direct the audience's attention: what do I want them to look at and see on the stage, and what journey I am taking them on, emotionally or philosophically? Of course it is up the audience to interpret and make sense of something from their perspective. It's a two-way process. This is akin to the consulting process between doctor and patient. A medical consultation is not just a casual passing conversation. It is a structured sequence that enables the exchange of intimacy and information. It is a kind of performance (I use that term with care).

Both doctor and patient are playing designated roles, probably both have rehearsed what they're going to say in some way, and both misinterpretation and confusion could lead to serious problems. Perhaps patients as well as doctors can benefit if they see the consultation as a sort of performance. Performing is about presenting a focused version of yourself in heightened circumstances – minimizing the parts of you that could be a hindrance in that moment in order to carry out some purpose.

If a patient doesn't feel listened to and loses confidence in the doctor's skill based on how the consultation has been handled, or comes away confused about the course of action they have been directed to take, then the consultation has not achieved its purpose. Relatively simple things like how a doctor inhabits and uses the space, eye contact, body language, directing the patient's focus, the narrative arc of the information exchanged – all these things can change the encounter.

These are all skills that can be learnt, skills which are at the core of the performing arts. It is not misdirection or subterfuge or 'acting' or 'pretense'. It is managing focus, active listening, understanding how to use space, voice and body to communicate. What I mean by 'active listening' is not just listening with your ears but reading all aspects of the communication, the physicality, the pauses, the unsaid. Listening with all your faculties, while being aware of how your own responses are being perceived, demonstrating that you are listening.

An awareness of performance skills can help in the consulting room. Are there specific skills from puppetry that can also help?

RW: In puppetry we specialize in how to handle objects. We really look at how the object looks and moves, its emotional resonance. We explore what we can make that object do. We push at the limitations of the object in our hand, trying to make the most of what our hand or body can make it do. Doctors don't need to do this exactly, but how they handle and use objects, such as medical instruments, is important. There is handling an instrument well, with ease and expertise, for the work they need to accomplish, and there is also handling it in a way that inspires confidence and ease in the patient. These aren't always the same thing, and it can affect how relaxed or tense a patient is about being examined.

A puppeteer gets an audience to look at a puppet rather than at them. In some performances, if a puppeteer is also playing a character alongside the puppet, then the puppeteer is getting the audience to repeatedly switch their focus between the puppet and puppeteer. This direction of focus can also be an invaluable skill during a medical consultation. It can help ensure engagement and clear flow of information to the patient.

PART TWO

Patients and the Art of Illness

The essays in this section invite readers to reconceive the agency of patients as in the ensemble drama of illness. For some doctors and patients, conceiving of patients as agential is virtually inconceivable. In Margaret Edson's play *W;t* (1993), one of the most celebrated modern medical dramas, the protagonist, Vivian Bearing, is a fifty-year-old English professor diagnosed with stage four ovarian cancer and abruptly ushered from the kingdom of the well to the kingdom of the sick.[1] The play is set entirely within the hospital after Vivian – once a formidable researcher and scholar of the seventeenth-century poet John Donne – consents to undergo eight brutal rounds of chemotherapy as part of a highly aggressive, experimental research project.

To reclaim a sense of personhood and agency during the dehumanizing and ultimately ineffective medical treatment, Vivian repeatedly breaks the fourth wall, speaking directly to the audience. When the entire medical team makes their weekly rounds for educational purposes – an event known as 'Grand Rounds' – for example, she reflects ironically on the fact that once she played the part of the powerful, intimidating professor: 'Once I did the teaching, now I am taught. This is much easier. I just hold still and look cancerous. It requires less acting every time.'[2] Her comment can be taken to mean that as her cancer progresses, she no longer has to act *as if* she is cancerous, but it also suggests that as a patient she is increasingly losing an agential role.

---

1 Susan Sontag, *Illness as Metaphor* (Farrar, Straus and Giroux, 1978), 3.
2 Margaret Edson, *W;t* (Nick Hern Books, 1995), 22.

Becoming a patient involves undergoing a process of effacement and objectification. After surviving eight treatments, breaking the record, Vivian boasts that 'I have become something of a celebrity'; both her doctor and his research fellow are 'delighted'.[3] Their elation springs not from her heroism, she observes, but from the 'celebrity status' which they too will accrue 'upon the appearance of the journal article they will no doubt write about me'.[4] Ultimately, however, she admits: 'But I flatter myself. The article will not be about me, it will be about my ovaries. It will be about my peritoneal cavity, which, despite their best intentions, is now crawling with cancer. What we have come to think of as *me* is, in fact, just the specimen jar.'[5]

Whether you imagine yourself or a fictional protagonist being the one thrust into the kingdom of the sick, the basic question remains the same: Is there any way to affirm the role of the patient, to avoid reducing her to a specimen while the doctor takes on celebrity as the central, heroic performer? Put differently, what exactly are the implications when we refer to illness as an ensemble drama? How can patients imagine and enact a role for themselves alongside and in collaboration with other actors?

To help us imagine how healthcare professions might act differently, we draw on the insights of performance artist and puppeteer Marina Heron Tsaplina, whose work makes 'visible a unique artistic practice that can bring articulate bodies into being'.[6] As a puppeteer living with a disability (diabetes), Tsaplina brings 'puppetry work related to illness, disability and health to the forefront of artistic practice-as-research, disability studies and the medical/health humanities'.[7] At the heart of her work, she maintains that 'the art of animating a puppet trains a deep embodied listening that gives voice and form to material and immaterial presences through the imagination'.[8] Training in this art, she insists, can also transform patients' understanding of their illness.[9] By teaching people 'to perceive materials both physically and poetically, puppetry allows silenced bodies and histories to speak'.[10] Rather than fixate on a single actor or monologue, she finds and empowers diverse 'actors' who do not usually get to speak

---

[3] Ibid., 34.

[4] Ibid.

[5] Ibid.

[6] Marina Heron Tsaplina, 'Bodies Speaking: Embodiment, Illness and the Poetic Materiality of Puppetry/Object Practice', *Journal of Applied Arts and Health* 11, nos 1&2 (2020): 85–102, https://doi.org/10.1386/jaah_00020_1.

[7] Ibid., 85.

[8] Ibid.

[9] In a particularly fascinating development of her work, following a key moment in 2013, Tsaplina's 'artistic research became about the blurry lines between how my experience with "this diabetes" was at once ... my own body speaking, and the body of "diabetes" speaking, and the conversations that took place to and through one another' ('Bodies Speaking', 90).

[10] Ibid., 85.

in the clinical encounter: the patient (who claims the right to speak because they know their own body), the body and even the illness itself as an actor.

Perspectives attentive to 'silenced bodies and histories' are crucial because they convey the stakes of the contributions in Part Two of our volume, the seemingly intractable challenge of perceiving the patient as performer. How can we reconceive of the sick role, traditionally associated with passivity born of pain and suffering, to allow patients to act collaboratively with doctors and elicit their respect and compassion? Just as Part One challenged us to move beyond a focus on the individual doctor to embrace the collaborative, 'ensemble' nature of illness and care, the essays in this section also ask how we can move beyond conceiving of the singular patient to encompass the patient and her community. These chapters trace the process of finding one's voice, or creating the conditions for someone else or, in some cases, a group of people to speak.

In addition to reconceiving of illness as truly an ensemble that includes the patient, doctor, illness and the community, we must also consider what other scripts can be written or rewritten. How can we empower patients, doctors and members of the community concerned with public health not only as performers but as dramaturges, with the aim of creating a better play? Equally critical, how can we move beyond the curative script to deal honestly and empathetically with patients who 'fail' to get better – who must negotiate new limitations, pain and suffering without any clear sense of closure or resolution? How can patients make use of the conventions and instruments of theatre to communicate their experiences and live fuller, authentic lives?

Dr Alice Flaherty's essay is keenly attentive to how patients seek care by performing well for themselves and others. As her essay asserts, patients can learn to rely on costume, voice, role-play, props, self-scripting and an improvisatory invitation – the foundational 'as-if' – that allows one to explore different versions of the self, while exploring outcomes of proposed drugs and procedures. When patients learn subtle codes of communication traditionally reserved for medical professionals, as Flaherty's essay reveals, they can deploy verbal and non-verbal, embodied gestures that convey pain and suffering to elicit optimal care. According to Doris Sommer's essay, taking a more active role might also require broadening the biomedical focus on the isolated patient, bringing an advocate, or narrating and responding to the challenge instigated by illness as a communal rather than individual problem. The resilience and situational inventiveness of 'patients' offering up their psychological blocks in Forum Theatre, in Sommer's view, empowers patients and entire communities. In other words, it is not just that patients are not passive; they may be the engines of effective medical performances far more than anyone recognizes. Finally, as Bianca Dahl and Philip McKee's essay emphasizes, playing an active role might also necessitate revising one's life script and revising the belief that a biomedical, curative plot ends with the restoration of health. For doctors and patients alike, it can be a shock to realize that medicine cannot always pull people through. Nevertheless, revising outdated, hierarchical scripts can offer its own form of relief.

As the contributions in this section demonstrate, clinging to outmoded scripts and roles obscures alternative, collaborative approaches to living with illness, pain and suffering right in front of us, waiting to be recognized.

REFERENCES

Edson, Margaret. *W;t*. Nick Hern Books, 1995.

Sontag, Susan. *Illness as Metaphor*. Farrar, Straus and Giroux, 1978.

Tsaplina, Marina Heron. 'Bodies Speaking: Embodiment, Illness and the Poetic Materiality of Puppetry/Object Practice'. *Journal of Applied Arts and Health* 11, nos 1&2 (2020): 85–102. https://doi.org/10.1386/jaah_00020_1.

4

Performing the art of illness: How patients can ail well and caregivers can help

ALICE FLAHERTY

> I have always been myself, even when I was ill, only now I seem myself. That's the important thing. I have remembered how to seem.
>
> (Alan Bennett, *The Madness of King George III*)

Over the course of my life I have been, by turns and simultaneously, a doctor, a patient and a family caregiver. The intersection of these roles has helped me see that the art of medicine, practised by doctors in a top-down way on patients, is only part of a two-way 'art of illness'. In performing the art of illness together, sick people actively interact with a range of caregivers – at home as well as in medical settings – in ways that go far beyond acquiescing to doctors' orders. When illness constrains what patients and their family carers are able to do, it naturally weakens their sense of agency. In this essay, I argue that patients and family benefit from learning how to exercise that agency, however constrained, as actors in the drama of illness. The benefit includes not only receiving optimal medical treatment, but participating in the kind of sustained, compassionate care that, even when a cure proves unattainable, everyone deserves.

Recognizing moments when agency can and must be exercised in tandem with other carers is crucial to the mutual drama of treatment.

As we enact life's dramas, whether a first date or a doctor's visit, we all rely both on pre-rehearsed scripts and improvisation. Historian of science Andrew Pickering tells us that much of what we learn formally in school is 'representational knowledge' – phenomena that are transparent or can be made so and therefore are available to be mastered.[1] But knowledge that arises through a 'performative epistemology', as he calls it, can't be known in advance of that performance because it emerges relationally. Patient and caregiver roles by definition require interaction with each other: you can be sick and die alone, but you cannot be a patient without engaging with a caregiver. A surgeon's or an invalid's performance, like all human performances, is two processes at once: it is a set of actions that change the physical world, and it communicates the performer's character and intentions to others.[2] Describing medicine and illness as performative – a word recently used to refer to insincere posturing – reclaims the term's older meaning: a role determined and signalled by the repeated performance of socially prescribed behaviours.[3] If you don't act like a patient, caregivers won't treat you like a patient, and vice versa. Like my fellow contributors to this book, I argue that the health humanities can incorporate performance practices far more than they currently do. Building a critical mass of people who appreciate the performative art of illness can change the perspective of a far larger population of patients and family caregivers, helping them recognize and gain a measure of control over their roles.

In what follows, I offer tips for how to think about medicine as an ensemble art. I also include a range of specific anecdotes which, I hope, will evoke the context-specific, granular and changing conditions in which a medical performance arises. Any doctor, carer, or patient needs to wield both scripts and performative adaptability to communicate effectively during the complex event of illness.

In Section One, I examine how the art of illness includes both demands on and opportunities for sick people. I begin by exploring how sick people learn to enact, or sometimes dodge, their culture's expectations of how patients should behave. Making these challenges explicit can help patients learn illness behaviour that is both truthful and effective. In Section Two, I turn to family caregivers' struggle to perform the demands of an art whose daily, repetitive tasks bear less resemblance to modern, plot-driven dramas than to the older genre of religious devotional ritual. The mutual care that underlies family life means that patients and caregivers often swap or fuse roles. In Section Three,

---

[1] Andrew Pickering, *The Cybernetic Brain: Sketches of Another Future* (University of Chicago Press, 2010), 13.

[2] Erving Goffman, *The Presentation of Self in Everyday Life* (Doubleday, 1956).

[3] Judith Butler, *Gender Trouble* (Routledge, 1999).

I show how patients and caregivers who consciously enact their roles can create meaningful and healing human bonds.

Just as there is an implicit contract between patients and paid healthcare providers, and between patients and family caregivers, there is also an implicit contract between medical writers and their readers. When doctors like me write scientific papers, we list conflicts of interest so that readers can learn about our biases and whether to trust our opinions. Although I have no pharmaceutical industry ties, a word about my 'character' might be helpful. I didn't go to medical school because of an empathic desire to help others; I studied medicine to uncover the brain's role in controlling volition – and also because I hated doctors. I thought knowledge of medicine would enable me to treat myself and my family and keep other doctors far away. My training did not go as planned. To my surprise, learning how to help people taught me the joy of it. To my dismay, my dream of avoiding doctors lasted only half-way through my neurology residency. During my first few years as a doctor, my family and I dealt with a series of unfortunate events including a fulminant autoimmune disease, a hospital stay for psychosis and three emergency surgeries. I consoled myself with the hope that these experiences would make me a better doctor. Instead, I became absorbed by learning to play the complex and more universal roles of becoming a patient and a family caregiver. I began to compile tips I learned from other patients and their families, and to reflect seriously on what it takes to practise the art of illness. The tips I outline below are not rules to follow unswervingly, but they illuminate ways in which patients and carers have more options than they may know. By the end of this chapter, I hope to show that learning to act sick and caring are both essential and ethical activities.

I. ACTING SICK

Imagine you have the worst headache of your life and go to the emergency room for help. You try to stay calm, for fear the doctors will think you are a whiner. The triage doctor notes that 'Patient complains of eleven out of ten pain but shows no distress, photophobia, or phonophobia; he asks for hydromorphine and reports that weaker opiates never work.' For clinicians, every aspect of that sentence characterizes a very familiar type: a drug-seeking patient, not a migraineur. Now imagine an alternative scenario in which you don't rate your pain off the scale or ask specifically for opiates. Instead, you describe your pain's real-world consequences ('I've been in bed for two days') and ask for earplugs and dimmed lights. If you adopt this second approach, your clinician will be more likely to adequately treat your pain. Your headache is a biochemical event visible only through its effects on your behaviour, and, as the different outcomes of these scenarios indicate, the behaviours you choose powerfully influence your caregivers' reciprocal performance.

Because diseases are involuntary, biochemical conditions, it is unfair for caregivers to expect very sick people to act 'appropriately'. Disease thrusts us into the patient role without preparation, and the mind-warping disorientation of pain can make it hard for us as patients to act in ways we normally never would. We also may feel unable to do things we know would help us, such as physical therapy, and we may long for the ideal caregiver who cares for us without our having to lift a finger. Yet patients often have more agency than they or their caregivers believe. In the end, patients do far better when they work together with caregivers rather than when being worked on by them. Recognizing the agency of all members of an ensemble of care transforms the one-way art of medicine into the truly collaborative art of illness.

Acting sick versus being sick

Before exploring how patients and caregivers act in illness ensembles, we need to understand what drives people to care strongly about the distinction between acting sick and being sick. For many contemporary humanists, the sick role may seem a neutral term that describes how sick people interact with other members of society. Most healthcare providers see the sick role more negatively, limiting patients' freedom and draining resources from others. Sociologist Talcott Parsons codified this attitude in his 1951 definition of the sick role as a socially undesirable state that benefits patients at the expense of society.[4] (His analysis overlooked many things, including emotional rewards that caregivers can get from their work, and economic growth from healthcare jobs and products.) Parsons highlighted the common belief that caregivers need to police the boundaries of illness, to exclude as cheaters people who play the sick role without actually being sick.[5]

Modern medicine draws the line between acting sick and being sick by defining disease and its symptoms as involuntary. By definition, medical conditions limit patients' ability to act – their agency – and are distinct from what sociologists call illness behaviours – voluntary actions, such as hiding a rash under long sleeves.[6] The aphorism 'You can't choose your symptoms, but you can choose how you respond to them' sums up the way that the realm of modern medicine is defined by a fault line. On one side are involuntary symptoms that are not the patient's fault. On the other side are voluntary acts that are open to praise and blame. Framing medical conditions as involuntary is important because it honours the way diseases really do impair patients' function. It also helps

[4] Talcott Parsons, *The Social System* (Free Press, 1951).

[5] On the other hand, sick people may falsely play well, whether to avoid burdening others, and sidestep the risk of being shamed by the medical boundary patrol.

[6] The term 'illness behaviour' entered scholarly discourse with David Mechanic's 'The Concept of Illness Behavior', *Journal of Chronic Diseases* 15, no. 2 (1962): 189–94.

prevent unproductively holding patients responsible for their disease. But telling patients they have an involuntary problem can make them feel passive and weaken their efforts to get better.

Drawing a bright line between involuntary and voluntary ignores the fact that every conscious choice is also the product of biological processes. Because I specialize in mood and movement disorders that affect the brain's voluntary action system, my patients and I constantly grapple with the ambiguous standards by which we call a behaviour a choice. The same problem exists, though more covertly, in every branch of medicine. Dentists traditionally stereotyped redheaded patients as wimps, not knowing that the melanocortin receptor mutation that causes bright red hair also causes lidocaine insensitivity. Cigarette-induced lung cancer gets dismissed as a bad choice.

How we distinguish being sick from acting sick has far-reaching practical implications. Caregivers' judgements of whether a person in bed is truly ill or just needs to try harder shape their decision to feel pity or cast blame, and such decisions can drastically affect the sick person's employment and family life. Judgements about volition guide treatment and can also lead it astray. People usually treat behavioural problems with attempts at changing motivations through argument or psychotherapy; conversely, they treat traditional medical problems with pills or surgery. Yet obsessive-compulsive behaviour can improve with pills as well as behaviour therapy. Heart disease can improve with exercise and healthy food choices as well as pills.

We can empower patients and their family to play an active role in their illness by addressing the cultural forces that discourage their participation. A good place to begin is with the English language itself, which subtly undermines patient agency. Terms like 'doctor', 'nurse' and 'aide' are all active verbs as well as nouns, denoting people who do, while 'patient' (from the Latin *patior*, to suffer or endure) is inherently passive and has no verb form. An active verb for being sick is a first step in empowering patients to act. Reviving the old verb 'to ail' gives sick people linguistic agency, and makes possible the parallel construction of 'carers' and 'ailers'. Just as some people with cancer prefer to be described as cancer survivors rather than cancer victims, some sick people will prefer 'ailer' to 'patient'. The goal is not to replace the word 'patient' – to do so would be to ignore the painfully involuntary aspects of illness – but to complement it.

It is not just the sick role that includes both willed and unwilled behaviours. Carers' behaviour is both a choice and the mechanical product of biochemical interactions; for instance, twin studies show emotional empathy is about twice as heritable as cognitive empathy.[7] I propose that we should broaden the

[7] Lior Abramson et al., 'The Genetic and Environmental Origins of Emotional and Cognitive Empathy: Review and Meta-Analyses of Twin Studies', *Neuroscience & Biobehavioral Reviews* 114 (2020): 113–33.

scope of the term 'illness behaviour' to include not only ailers' 'first-person' illness behaviour, but also carers' 'second-person' illness behaviour – their dispassionate or sympathetic reactions to an ailer's symptoms. Second- and first-person illness behaviour are usually enmeshed, as when a caregiver's disinterest makes a patient complain more loudly, which makes the caregiver withdraw further from a patient they see as histrionic. The way we react to our own symptoms can affect the way we react to another's symptoms. For example, when a carer makes an effort to stoically repress her own pain so that she can do her job, she may have less sympathy for an ailer who does not do the same.

For simplicity's sake, this chapter focuses on the interactions between ailers and carers. In real-world medical environments, those first- and second-person illness behaviours are also influenced by third-person illness behaviour: that of observers who include bosses, schoolmates and insurance claims adjustors. This audience of medical dramas can respond with scathing criticism and stigmatize what it sees as inauthentic performances, and it also has financial control through withholding sick leave and healthcare benefits.

Should ailers act naturally?

When sick people seek advice about how to interact with doctors, they may be told to 'just act naturally'. (For instance, doctors may explicitly advise patients not to dramatize or read about their illness.) In Chapter 1 of this book, McGinnis and Kleinman demonstrate why this advice fails doctors. But the advice misleads patients as well. To understand why, it is helpful to unpack what 'acting naturally' actually means.

All animals have evolved characteristic illness behaviours that serve two purposes: preventing further injury and recruiting aid from troupe members. In humans, cross-cultural studies confirm universal and primal pain reflexes that include wincing, grimacing and shrieking. Even children who are deaf from birth, and thus have never heard a scream, scream in pain. But we can and must learn to modify those reflexes. Despite the hard-wired nature of primal illness behaviour, it is nevertheless essential for human survival to consciously learn how to modify those reflexes. 'Naturally' acting sick is what babies do, and babies often do things that alienate caregivers or put themselves at risk. Babies scream after a minor injury, even if they are in a concert hall or their family is hiding from pursuers. As children grow older, they soon learn the negative consequences of acting naturally.

Why, then, might a caregiver tell a person in pain not to consciously modulate her performance? One reason is that many doctors assume that that the primary goal of skillful pain behaviour is more likely to be deception, not cooperation, that impedes efforts to understand the ailer's problem. More sympathetic carers may also want to spare the ailer, already burdened with illness, from having to consciously plan their illness behaviours. Despite these risks and difficulties, sick people should try to act thoughtfully, not naturally. For instance, to recruit aid in ways that are socially appropriate, adults often need to both signal their pain and simultaneously convey that they are not the sort of person who signals pain too often. One British study found the most effective way to convince an observer of one's pain was not through primal winces, grimaces and shrieks, but through gestural signs of pain suppression such as keeping the eyes wide open to prevent a wince, or pressing the lips tightly together to suppress a grimace.[8] Any medical performance must take account of the culture in which the illness is staged. Because cultural conventions about how to appropriately communicate pain can vary greatly, ailers who are not members of the dominant culture are at a disadvantage.

In any culture, caregivers often have inaccurate ideas of what chronic pain behaviour looks like. When judging pain severity, observers typically look for signs of acute pain, reflexes like pallor or sweating. In cases of chronic pain, however, these reflexes habituate and disappear. Chronically ill people thus have the extra burden of compensating for their lack of what observers believe is objective proof of real pain. In every human interaction, our character isn't just what we bring into a room, it is what we and the other person in the room make together. What happens when a patient with chronic pain tells his doctor at each appointment that his pain is worse, but the doctor sees no other change in behaviour? The doctor may dismiss the eternal crescendo as hyperbole, or, slightly more charitably, tell the patient that current pain is always more vivid than remembered pain. Ailers have strategies, too. Instead of saying their pain was eleven out of ten last month but is twelve out of ten now, they might quantify the effects of the pain. 'Last month I could take my daily walk around the block; now I can barely make it to the front gate.' They may find it useful to describe times they are not in pain, as a comparison: 'I only come here when things are bad. Last week I had a really good day; we even drove to a park.' The sick person gains by enacting more of himself than just his current pain. As the actor and director Konstantin Stanislavski once wrote, monotonous actors lack perspective: they only think 'of the immediate ... action, feeling or thought

[8] Amanda C de C Williams, 'Facial Expression of Pain: An Evolutionary Account', *Behavioral and Brain Sciences* 25, no. 4 (2002): 439–55, https://doi.org/10.1017/S0140525X02000080. It's worth noting, of course, that societies vary greatly. This British study might be relevant for someone seeking help in a culture that values stiff upper lips, but it might lead to undertreatment in more expressive societies. Any medical performance must take account of the culture in which the illness is staged.

without relation to the whole'.[9] Of course, that is harder advice to follow when you're exhausted and in pain.

Doctors, to sidestep the hard job of diagnosing patients by what they say and do, usually turn to objective data such as laboratory tests. However, objective tests add crucial information only about 20 percent of the time, while patients' verbal and non-verbal behaviour provide the diagnosis in over 80 percent of diagnosed cases.[10] Patient's efforts to convey their symptoms – the loudness of their words, whether they pace the room or double over in pain – are crucial contributions to assessing the cause and severity of a medical problem. It is therefore crucial that ailers gain competence in enacting their pain. Before they can tailor interactions to suit different caregivers, they need basic scripts and scenes to begin with. Understanding how and where they learn those initial routines – whether through family, media, or healthcare experience – can clarify which scripts might need to be unlearned and replaced with more helpful ones.

Learning the sick role

We first learn to perform illness as children, when our families and schoolmates give us feedback as we try to recruit aid from others while not being seen as a crybaby. This early education is as good as the teachers are. Anxious parents who try too hard to take children's minor complaints seriously may only entrench the child's belief in their bodies' fragility. A child with neglectful parents may find he only gets attention if he screams as if he is dying. As an adult, he comes to new treaters with over-dramatic narratives, and his yelp during band-aid removal may cause treaters to visibly pull back and become less responsive to his complaints. That may drive him to complain even more loudly, setting up a vicious cycle. We shouldn't blame the patient for starting with a learned script – he has to start somewhere. But both parties have failed to notice the counterproductive effect of their behaviour and to adapt their scripts to the situation.

Along with personal experience, people learn how to ail from the media. Because art imitates life and life imitates art, books, TV and film can not only mirror but change real-world illness behaviour. Television medical dramas, in which high-risk procedures like cardiac resuscitations are much more successful than in real life, influence viewers to make unrealistically optimistic decisions about their own end of life care. Cosmetic surgery reality shows such as *Miami*

[9] Konstantin Stanislavski, *An Actor's Work*, trans. Jean Benedetti (Routledge, 2017), 479.

[10] J. R. Hampton et al., 'Relative Contributions of History-Taking, Physical Examination, and Laboratory Investigation to Diagnosis and Management of Medical Outpatients', *British Medical Journal* 2 (1975): 486; Fumitoshi Fukuzawa et al., 'Importance of Patient History in Artificial Intelligence-Assisted Medical Diagnosis: Comparison Study', *JMIR Medical Education* 10 (2024): e52674.

Slice helped fuel the boom of aesthetic procedures over the past fifteen years. Stories are powerful, and dangerous, teachers.[11]

'High' art likewise has a powerful effect on illness behaviour, though for most ailers its effects are indirect. Notable exceptions include creative artists and the academics who study the arts. Because my clinic has an outsized number of such patients – they come to see me because I wrote a book about the neurology of writer's block – I've learned they often have distinctive troubles when acting sick. Creative writers don't act the way most patients do. They often speak with unnatural eloquence. This can backfire. On average, patients do better when they avoid overly literary phrases and when, if they are giving a history they have recited to many different doctors, they add pauses that sound as if they are giving their words some thought. Unused to treating writers, doctors and home caregivers alike sometimes judge their polished and highly coloured complaints as artificial. Other times, they make the opposite mistake, taking writers' heightened imagery at face value. One writer described his pain by saying, 'I'm suffering like Jesus on the cross' with such pathos that the doctor, unaware of the patient's literary training and penchant for poetic speech, thought he was delusional.

Unlike artists, academics are more likely to underact than overact. Their years of practice seeming rational can make their case presentations seem bloodless. A literature professor I knew once, for example, told me that her internist repeatedly ignored her descriptions of severe back pain. When I asked how she brought the pain to his attention, she replied that she knew better than to act like a hysterical woman. She waited until he was through with all his questions, and then – I imagine him with one hand on the doorknob as he ushered her out – she told him, in a carefully controlled tone, 'I still have that back pain.' I suggested she present her problem early in the visit and show its importance by letting some of emotion creep into her voice. Medical performances do not have to be particularly complicated, but they should take into account their audience's expectation that people in pain sound pained. Of course, neither over-stoic nor histrionic pain behaviour is restricted to artists and academics. All of us should, to the best of our ability, be aware of our tendency to overact or underact – keeping in mind that our current audience, not our own preference, is the final judge of what counts as too much or too little.

People don't learn their illness behaviour entirely from experience and stories about others' experience. Nonfiction books and websites teach ailers what to do when they are sick, although the emphasis is on diagnosis and treatment, not how to get a professional to diagnose and treat you. The explosion of accessible medical knowledge has made it possible for some people with

[11] Peter Brooks, *Seduced by Story: The Use and Abuse of Narrative* (New York Review of Books, 2022).

rare syndromes to know more about their condition than their doctors do. But meetings with doctors make many patients without advanced degrees careful about how they convey their knowledge. Doctors may respond defensively to a patient who acts like an expert, or they may offer patronizing advice such as 'Don't read about your illness, it will only make you anxious.' Ailers may avoid riling such doctors if they credit their medical knowledge to another physician: 'My friend who is a doctor said that apixaban would be a safer blood thinner for me than warfarin.' Invoking a doctor friend has a motivating effect on your doctors. Once they think another doctor has an eye on your medical care, they will try harder to do a good job. You aren't really lying when you attribute your knowledge to a doctor because, as the meme goes, 'Dr Google is your best friend.' Although the internet lures a few patients into echo chambers or nutraceutical infomercials, research shows that, on average, people who consult the internet for information about their condition get more out of their doctors' visits and have better health.[12]

Social media video posts are a new source of explicit teaching on how to act sick, as in the video post 'Hanging Upside Down While Calling Out Sick Apparently Helps Sound More Believable'.[13] While that is disturbing, some posts' content addresses real difficulties patients face when trying to interact with doctors. For instance, a Black medical student and TikTok influencer advised patients facing discrimination that when their doctor told them their headache or abdominal pain was normal, they should ask, 'What's your differential diagnosis?'[14] In the absence of any more specific information about the scenario, this is a useful line when speaking with doctors. The appropriate use of doctors' terminology for a symptom's possible causes shows the patient has some medical sophistication, forces the doctor to voice dangerous possibilities that need ruling out, and reminds the doctor that she risks malpractice if she misses one of those dangerous causes.

To my mind, the number of social media posts on getting doctors to listen is much less disturbing than the lack of serious effort that health educators

---

[12] 'Dr AI', even with its tendency to hallucinate, already answers patients' questions more accurately than Google, and more helpfully than a control group of human doctors (John W. Ayers et al., 'Comparing Physician and Artificial Intelligence Chatbot Responses to Patient Questions Posted to a Public Social Media Forum', *JAMA Internal Medicine* 183, no. 6 (2023): 589–96, https://doi.org/10.1001/jamainternmed.2023.1838).

[13] Try it; somehow it works. Cat Country 107.3, 7 February 2018, https://youtube.com/watch?v=iWY0KbYXfJY. Infuriated doctors and employers may take such posts as arguments against teaching ailers how to act. But all knowledge is double-edged, as doctors know first-hand. Learning how to save lives is also efficient instruction in how to kill people.

[14] TikTok, @dor_the_grayt, 3 November 2021, www.tiktok.com/@dor_the_grayt/video/7026473683074043182.

have made to give patients communication tools.[15] Some sick people, through painful and extensive experience, do learn impressive caregiver management skills. When I think with pride that I have been a good doctor for a patient, it is usually because they have been skillful ailers, able to redirect me from my stereotypical responses so I can learn to do what they really need.

II. THE PERFORMANCE OF CARE

Emotional labour

Let's now turn from ailers' first-person illness behaviour to carers' second-person illness behaviour, their reactions to another's symptoms. Since other chapters of this book discuss healthcare professionals, here I will focus on family members and close friends. Most of us care for a sick person at some point in our lives. Carers perform physical tasks but they also need to engage in what the sociologist Arlie Hochschild has called emotional labour, the process of regulating their feelings to facilitate their caregiving.[16]

Hochschild divides emotional labour into two components: surface acting and deep acting. In surface acting, emotional labourers display emotions they do not feel, as when a waitress chats enthusiastically with a customer she dislikes. In deep acting, the waitress tries to change her inner feeling, with techniques such as focusing on the customer's one likeable feature or reminding herself that all humans deserve love, so that the reworked feeling generates the expression she wants to display. However, both deep acting and surface acting are inadequate for the more complex and prolonged role of being a family caregiver. A richer alternative is the Meisner technique, a school of acting in which actors do not look inwards on what their own character's emotions should be, but focus outwards, paying attention to and reacting to other actors. Meisner's perspective may reassure those who fear acting is deceptive and it shows how a caregiver's bedside manner can blend practised skill with authenticity.

Caregivers often find deep acting very difficult, especially with antagonistic ailers. Even when they can generate empathy by attending to and reacting to their ailers, it may not easily lead to appropriate action. Feeling another's pain may make sensitive people flee the sickroom. The limits of empathy in driving

[15] One notable exception, written for patients with low health literacy, is the valuable and underused *How to Talk to Your Doctor HANDbook*, available in both English and Spanish (UAMS Center for Health Literacy, 2023, https://healthliteracy.uams.edu/kb/how-to-talk-to-your-doctor-handbook/).

[16] Arlie Russell Hochschild, *The Managed Heart: Commercialization of Human Feeling* (University of California Press, 1983).

the performance of altruistic action have been well articulated by scholars,[17] but this message has not percolated to the general public. As a young doctor, I sometimes asked mentors for rules of thumb to help me know when my putting a hand on a patient's arm would be comforting, and when it would seem threatening. Their advice to put myself 'in the patient's shoes' didn't help me, and it doesn't help family carers – especially when the sick person is delirious or psychotic. As carers, we need better stage directions to guide us.

One place to start is to for caregivers to try to discern their own objectives and those of their patient. When a daughter asks her elderly father to get dressed, is it because it depresses her to see him in that ratty bathrobe all day? Is it so he won't be late for his doctor's appointment? Does he want to go to that appointment? She could borrow the theatre technique called 'actioning', in which she considers which non-verbal actions could accompany her question to achieve her objective and help align her father's with hers. When objectives don't align, care work can be antagonistic and frustrating. Often, though, the main reason a sick person doesn't want to do a thing is merely that that the carer, by instructing him to do it, has decreased the ailer's sense of agency. An alternative approach is for the carer to step back and affirm to the ailer that it is his body and his choice. The carer may then help the ailer to express his own objectives and to think through how to achieve them.

Just as in a theatre ensemble, to act well together, carer and ailer have to demonstrate that they are on the same side. A family member who sees her job as acting can step away from a hierarchical carer–patient framework and reframe the interaction as two actors who collaborate to shape the scene. In improvisational theatre, actors make what are called 'offers', proposals, in the form of action or dialogue, about how a scene will advance. If one actor says he is in a laundromat, other actors may respond with actions involving detergent or a broken change machine. In medicine, an offer may indirectly present a version of how someone will be after a certain course of treatment. When a caregiver says 'Let's get you in the shower', the implied future self may be different only in being cleaner. When the caregiver says 'I'm going to take over keeping your pills straight', the implied future self is someone with less self-efficacy who may be involuntarily medicated. Even when the plan is not phrased as an offer, the ailer usually has the ability cooperate or reject it. The carer's job is to help the ailer understand the ramifications of various offers and how they relate to both of their goals.

---

[17] See, for example, Alex Mermikides, *Performance, Medicine and the Human* (Bloomsbury, 2020); and Doris Sommer, *Proceed with Caution, When Engaged by Minority Writing in the Americas* (Harvard University Press, 1999). A rare example written for a general audience is Paul Bloom, *Against Empathy: The Case for Rational Compassion* (Ecco, 2016).

Learning the carer's role

Informal carers are often in the same plight as ailers, first shoved into a role without knowing the playscript, then learning how to act through trial and often painful error. Family caregivers cannot take the bedside manner classes offered to medical students, although they sometimes learn skills second-hand by watching professionals help their family members.

Home carers, unlike ailers, cannot easily get stage directions from watching TV doctor show, because home care is rarely shown.[18] Its quotidian routines are, by nature, undramatic – lacking the plot progression and climaxes that drive soap operas and medical thrillers. The performative nature of daily supportive care is more closely related to a far older genre that represents the antithesis of modern plot-based theatrics: namely, religious devotional ritual. Acts of care such as feeding, bathing and placing a hand on a feverish forehead can become deeply moving and even transformative when performed mindfully.[19] Caring acts form powerful emotional bonds between individuals and put both ailers and carers in touch with ancient, performative healing rituals that exceed the more narrow and modern preoccupation with effecting a cure.

For those who mistakenly equate performing a ritual with mechanical action – 'going through the motions' – it is worth keeping in mind that going through the motions often produces true emotional investment. We nurture what we love, but we also learn to love what we nurture. As I admitted earlier, I entered medical school with few caring emotions to drive my actions with patients. My aim, initially, was to do my job well. To that end, I worked hard to help sick people by relying on the very few physical actions med students are permitted to perform, such as putting the patient's call bell within reach and replacing my habitual deadpan with a look of concern and saying earnestly 'That must be hard for you.' The sincere gratitude patients showed in response to my mechanical actions moved me. Gradually, acting as if I were compassionate gave me compassionate thoughts. Performing is the first step towards becoming. I learned what scientists and acting theorists have long known, that our facial expressions can change our emotions as well as vice versa.[20] Where

---

[18]Although the dementia epidemic is driving awareness of family caregivers, they are still so under-represented in the media that their presence is highlighted only by niche lists on caregiver websites such as this one: https://caringacross.org/blog/2022-care-moments-on-tv.

[19]Arthur Kleinman, *The Soul of Care: The Moral Education of a Husband and a Doctor* (Viking, 2019).

[20]The reciprocal link between surface acting and inner emotion is explained by the Perception-Action Model of empathy (Stephanie D. Preston and Frans B. M. Waal, 'Empathy: Its Ultimate and Proximate Bases', *Behavioral and Brain Sciences* 25, no. 1 (2002): 1–20). Even the subtlest forms of emotional empathy stem from the mirror neuron system that both generates and perceives external behaviors. This system ties our sensory inputs about others' motivated actions to our physical tendency to imitate those actions (as when two people walking together tend to walk in step) and

the body goes, the mind follows. When I was not feeling connected to a patient, consciously mirroring their expressions helped me to feel the emotion we were both displaying. As the filmmaker and photographer Corinne Botz writes in Chapter 13, 'acting can give birth to feeling, and artifice can expose the real'.[21]

When I was a patient myself, I loved the way the quiet of the sickroom, so different from the clatter of life outside, pushed nagging work problems far away. My pleasure made me feel guilty because, in the medical battle narrative, cure is the victory and it is traitorous to take any pleasure in being sick. When I found that being a home caregiver let me experience a similar consolation in the asylum of the sickroom, I felt less guilty. Plot-based medical stories offer only the illusion of cures: the person we care for will always, in the end, die. Well-rehearsed physical rituals of care, as when an ailer lifts an arm so a carer can pull on a sleeve, coordinate two human bodies and help both be mindful of the fact that the here and now is all we have.

To acknowledge the consolations of the caregiving role is not to deny its punishments, which can be financially and emotionally devastating in cases of chronic or catastrophic illness. Caring for a pain we can't help only makes us hurt too. And family members may not be grateful for the kind of help we want to give them. In that respect, though, home carers have more opportunity to learn what individual ailers want than do professional caregivers, who, faced with rapidly changing and diverse patients, often develop a one size fits all bedside manner. The approach medical school taught me was unitary: patients find clinicians' pity degrading, what they want is calm empathic listeners who can be present with them in their pain. I belatedly began to suspect things weren't so simple when, in a hospital bed after being hit by a truck, I found I had no interest in making my caregivers feel my pain; I wouldn't have wished that on a dog. And I loved when they expressed pity because it seemed evidence that they would make an effort to fix my problem, to do something more active than bear witness to my suffering.

Caregivers must learn where, on a given day, to place themselves on that listener–fixer spectrum. When I'm trying to help a family member, a touchstone is the hilarious and sobering ninety-second video, 'It's Not About the Nail', in which one member of a couple can't stop offering quick fixes to a partner who only wants a supportive listener.[22] Many ailers don't expect family members will be able to fix their medical problem, but they do expect supportive care from a good listener. Unless the ailer is upper middle class, they have learned to expect a doctor who will minimize listening and briskly perform a procedure

expressions (yawn and the world yawns with you). Even when we suppress visible imitation of others' behaviour, we experience that urge as an empathic reflection of the other's inner motivations.

[21] Corrine May Botz, 'Bedside Manner', in this volume, 279.

[22] Jason Headley, 22 May 2013, www.youtube.com/watch?v=-4EDhdAHrOg.

the doctor thinks will fix their problem. For instance, doctors known for successful cures don't need to attract patients with a good bedside manner, and very successful doctors can get away with acting as rudely as television's Dr House. The resulting association of high status and abruptness in turn influences patient expectation of the famous doctor role, to the extent that patients may interpret a caregiver's kindness as evidence of low status. Young doctors then learn from patients' behaviour towards them that if they act too sympathetic they may be taken for a nurse. Thus, although caregivers' behaviour shapes patients' expectations, patients' expectations and reactions reciprocally shape caregivers' behaviour.

In every role, actions may speak louder than words, but communication is clearest when both modes harmonize. For instance, in response to patient complaints that open emergency room bays made them feel exposed, one hospital instructed staff to always pull the curtain closed when leaving a bay. That policy led to new patient complaints of feeling neglected and isolated. Only when the hospital instructed staff to also announce, as they pulled the curtain, 'I'm doing this to protect your privacy', did patients' complaints decrease. Of course, it would have been better still if carers had replaced recitation with interaction, and simply asked each patient whether they wanted the curtain open or shut. Home carers who are good listeners need to actively feed back what they have heard, both to demonstrate their understanding and to allow ailers to correct them when they misunderstand. Carers who fix a problem cannot, unless they also explain their behaviour, assume that an ailer will understand their good intentions.

Sharing and exchanging roles

Carers who act unilaterally, without inviting ailers' collaboration, may experience their dominance as a weight of social responsibility. They may resent that their role extends beyond supportive care to taking on the patient's normal role and chores. It can help caregivers to think of roles as fluid and collaborative, mutual activities that families can share or swap. A boy may outsource remembering his pills to his parents, but before he goes away to college, he needs to take that job back from them. They need to stop sending him anxious texts twice a day, so that taking a pill stops feeling like an obligation to him, and becomes his own choice. Collaborating to construct his sense of adult agency makes it more likely that in the future, when they get sick, he will choose to care of them.

Productive sharing and swapping roles can happen even within brief doctors' visits when sick people bring a family member. A spouse can take on the patient's role as complainer, telling the doctor how serious the problem is – 'Once it made him faint in the supermarket' – while the ailer demurs.

Collaborative outsourcing of complaints allows the spouse to seem (and be) caring and the ailer to seem (and be) brave, while still getting the care he needs. Even if the spouse says nothing in a visit, just outnumbering the doctor can offset the power differential.

Good caregivers go beyond empathically reading each other to active listening: the action is to communicate what they think they have heard. Instinctive kindness is not enough; carers must also know when to stop being so damned helpful. The challenges of the art of caring for others reflect those of the art of ailing, which is, after all, the art of caring for the self. And when those two arts intertwine, they create something much bigger and immensely more complex: the ensemble art of illness.

III. AILERS AND CARERS INTERACT

When ailers act in ways that change carers' behaviour, and carers act in ways that change ailers' behaviour, the feedback loops can amplify a faint behavioural echo into either harmony or cacophony. How can patients and caregivers learn to augment each other's abilities rather than spiral into destructive cycles?

Conscious reflections

A deceptively simple way of redirecting highly charged human interactions starts with mirroring another's expressions as a way to communicate understanding and create interpersonal connection. Mirroring is an instinctive social response: most of us do not need to be taught to scream and run when others do because it is a hard-wired reflex that helps members of a group all respond quickly to danger. However, just as it can be counterproductive for patients to behave instinctively when they are in pain, mirroring needs regulation too. Most of us try to suppress emotional mirroring to avoid fanning the flames of another's strong emotion, and medical school explicitly taught me to maintain a neutral expression when others express anger or fear.[23] But there is a middle path between emotional contagion and suppression. Conscious mirroring, choosing when and to what degree you mirror another's strong expression of emotion, is more powerful than either reflecting the other's emotion or remaining calm and opaque.

[23] Some physicians have argued that one benefit of face masks is to hinder such mirroring, so that, before a difficult operation, patients won't see their doctor shares their fear (see, for example, Kent Sepkowitz, 'Behind the Doctors' Mask, a Little Room to Maneuver', *New York Times*, 2 October 2007). During the COVID quarantine, millions of non-doctors took comfort in the same false belief. In fact, masks are not good at hiding fear, which is expressed most clearly in the eyes (Celine Ramdani et al., 'Communicating and Reading Emotion with Masked Faces in the COVID Era: A Short Review of the Literature', *Psychiatry Research* 316 (2022): 114755).

One of the most masterful family caregivers I've ever met is the poet and human rights advocate Rose Styron. I met her through her husband, the novelist William Styron, who was my patient during the last years of his life.[24] About a year after we met, he was admitted for depression and weight loss to my Boston hospital. Three weeks into the admission, his health was improving, but he was still very ill. Rose told me that his eightieth birthday party, a 500-person Manhattan gala thrown by the *Paris Review*, was coming up. Rose then told his inpatient psychiatrist that she thought going to the celebration would have a wonderfully anti-depressant effect, and suggested that Bill leave Boston for the party. The doctor, shocked, replied in an over-loud voice that her plan was dangerous. Rose didn't try, as I would have, to reply in a calming voice. Instead, she raised her voice a bit to partially mirror his agitation back at him, and said 'You are right! Bill is too sick to go home.' I feared her tone would make him raise his voice more. Instead, he visibly relaxed. She followed up less intensely, by saying, 'Naturally you're anxious about the risk. We'd *all* feel better about the party if he were safely in a Manhattan hospital, where he can just leave on a pass for a few hours.' Then she adroitly changed the subject. Over the next few days, as their discussions continued, I saw that every time the doctor's behaviour became agitated, she would mirror his agitation as she agreed with him, then gradually calm her tone and redirect him. In the end, Rose's diplomacy changed the doctor's emotions and beliefs, and he arranged for Bill's transfer to a Manhattan hospital.

Rose's motive for mirroring her interlocutor's anger confused me at first. To calm someone down, shouldn't I act calm even if the other person isn't? I asked a colleague with more social skills than me – a psychiatrist – for guidance. She told me that it is a mistake not to mirror another's negative emotion. Remaining calm can make you seem cold and uncaring. Even reflecting the other's words and not their non-verbal intensity can backfire – to calmly tell an angry client 'I know how upset you are' can sound patronizing. My colleague, seeing I looked doubtful, put on a concerned look too. 'Naturally you're sceptical!' she said. Then, smoothly softening her worried face into a smile, she recommended a research study with counterintuitive evidence that anxious patients who are told positive test results are more reassured when the doctor delivers the good news in an anxious tone than when the doctor uses a happy tone.[25] She explained that the anxious tone comes across as concern for the patient and shows the other person that you understand how important

[24] The Styrons, who both felt that secrecy around mental illnesses only intensified their stigma, encouraged me to speak publicly about our interactions.

[25] Judith A. Hall et al., 'Communication of Affect Between Patient and Physician', *Journal of Health and Social Behavior* 22, no. 1 (1981): 18–30, https://doi.org/10.2307/2136365.

their problem is. Smiling and saying 'Relax! Everything's fine!' is more likely to sound dismissive, and may even drive the patient to ask for more tests.

I protested that I had been taught to act calm in order to avoid escalating others' emotions. My colleague granted that knee-jerk imitation of another's behaviour – as when a patient facing an angry caregiver yells back 'I hate you too!' – can be disastrous. The goal is to be reflective, not reflexive: to verbally and nonverbally acknowledge the other person's emotion, by saying 'You hate me!' Often, once the other feels you recognize how deeply upset they are, they will no longer need to yell. Consciously reflecting another's emotion differs from instinctive emotional contagion because it doesn't oblige you to share the other's state, it communicates that you recognize that state and its intensity. Then, once they sense that you are vibrating on their wavelength, you can both start to change the wavelength. Conscious mirroring is not rote mimesis, it is a way of signalling recognition, a non-verbal form of active listening, and the first step towards a new state for both of you.

Just as a core technique of narrative medicine is for a doctor to listen to a patient's story and develop empathy, a core technique of performative medicine entails carers and ailers sharing embodied reflection of others' actions. Whereas empathy is an invisible inner state, behavioural mirroring is visible and often recursive. Like any powerful human interaction, mirroring can disrupt connection as well as strengthen it. If two mirrors magnify the image of the other, the result can be a performative ricochet, a dangerous feedback loop that can distort both actors. This vicious cycle is one reason many of us hesitate to share our problems with loved ones. When a mother feels and mirrors her child's pain more intensely than the child does, and the child who sees the mother's distress feels more pain himself, the emotional chain reaction can overwhelm both, triggering a meltdown. When ailers and carers consciously modulate their reflections of each other, they can calm each other with reverberating images that are progressively smaller and dimmer. Far from being merely play-acting, intentional gestural communication can connect people even as it protects them from each other.

My colleague recommended mirroring as an excellent way to calm angry schizophrenics in the emergency room. Cautiously, I tried it out first on my young daughter during a breakfast tantrum. My yelling 'You hate oatmeal!' made her burst out laughing. Had she seen through my clumsy ploy? Whatever; she was no longer angry. Later, I faced a doctor's appointment with a new primary care physician (PCP) and tried another toned-down form of mirroring. After reading a research paper which showed that highly empathic people imitate emotionally neutral gestures more than those with low empathy,[26] I decided to try what I thought of as the 'nose rub test' to assess this new

[26] Tanya L. Chartrand and John A. Bargh, 'The Chameleon Effect: The Perception–Behavior Link and Social Interaction', *Journal of Personality and Social Psychology* 76, no. 6 (1999): 893.

doctor's empathy. During the meeting, I intermittently rubbed my nose during conversation and noted how often my doctor mimicked the gesture. She did so pretty reliably, though I worried she might have thought I was signalling she had a smudge there. When I told my psychiatry colleague about my new nose rub test, she laughed, and asked if I couldn't directly sense whether another person wanted to help me. People with high social skills, like my colleague or Rose Styron, naturally see the nose rub test as silly. For those of us whose social intuition is imperfect, it can be a useful tool – as long as we remember that empathy and helpfulness don't always go hand in hand.

Simple strategies can help in situations where carers and ailers who are new to each other must assess their ability to form alliances, especially across cultural differences where intuition alone may fail. Social mirrors are two-way mirrors that influence the object they reflect. The nose rub technique does more than read out another's empathy, it can also change it. If your new doctor is not mimicking your gestures, you can subtly mirror hers. Even if her crossed arms or lack of eye contact seem distancing, by doing the same you will likely make her feel more connected to you. As you attend consciously to her body language, you may even find yourself feeling more empathetic toward her. This technique mirrors theatre warm-ups, such as Meisner's repetition game, where actors pass words and gestures back and forth to build rapport and attentiveness. Conscious mirroring isn't manipulative when aimed at strengthening genuine bonds – it is doing a basic human behaviour mindfully, rather than reflexively. Good treatment relationships emerge from giving good performances with a responsive co-actor.

Connection and commitment do more than foster emotional support; they influence physical outcomes. If you and your orthopaedist do not make any human connection, she may still methodically set your broken arm well, but may have less motivation to help when you call a week later about a complication. In psychotherapy, the specific treatment method has significantly less influence on the patient's health outcome than has the quality of the therapeutic alliance – the relationship between clinician and client.[27] Although ailers and carers' feelings of empathy are invisible to each other, their interactive mirroring sets the stage for collaborative acts of healing and caring to continue.

Mutual care

Two-way mirroring is just one of many practical acting techniques available to ailers and carers. Another simple method is using the improvisational theatre mantra of saying 'yes, and' instead of 'yes, but' to avoid shutting down a

[27] John C. Norcross and Michael J. Lambert, 'Psychotherapy Relationships that Work III', *Psychotherapy* 55, no. 4 (2018): 303.

conversation.[28] A more difficult one is to help medical interactions emulate the exploratory environment of theatre. That is limited by the ways in which the real medical world is dangerous: in hospitals, scalpels don't retract into their handles when plunged into someone. But there are also ways to reshape medical practice that encourage open reporting of errors and that provide safe spaces for the rehearsal of difficult scenes. There is much scholarly work to be done, by people with more knowledge of theatre than me, to explore other aspects of acting and stagecraft that can shape the interactions of ailers and carers.

Performing in a drama is public and effortful, unlike the private acts of reading and writing. But the public nature of acting, even when terrifying, is also what makes it possible for interacting to bridge the gaps between human beings, the empty spaces that open up when an illness destroys the shared activities that formerly kept a couple close. While journaling about the experience of loss may bring consolation, shared daily actions such as feeding, bathing and trying to work the new nebulizer can create a new and stronger intimacy. Illness can shrink the ailer's and carer's world to the size of a sickroom, but their responses to the illness can connect them both to a wider community of ailers and advocates. Encouraging patients and home caregivers to act together can become the first step in a transformation from one-way care and dependence to ensembles of care and an interdependence that may be much richer than their former freedom.

In families, illness does not cut off an ailer's responsibility to reciprocate and help their carer, even though it may limit how the ailer can return that care. Mutual care might seem one more burden to cast on patients, but many sick people crave a way to restore balance by supporting those who support them. An ailer's sincere gratitude and efforts to minimize the carer's burden may seem pitifully small to the ailer, but a strong bond between the two will make the ailer's gift precious to the carer. Like all humane interactions, the interchange of care must be negotiated. A convalescent who cannot walk safely to the bathroom needs to remember that doing so without calling for her husband will, if she falls, only give him one more burden. Her husband, rushing to her side when he hears the thud, should temper his anger with the belief that she was trying to diminish his burden.

In contrast to the ideal of family care as an interdependent gift economy, the doctor–patient relationship can feel cold and transactional. Yet, even within a hospital's structured world, acts of generosity still have an important place. In

[28] Ankit Mehta et al., 'Improv: Transforming Physicians and Medicine', *Medical Science Educator* 31 (2021): 263–66. Though see also Frederic Jameson, *Brecht and Method* (Verso, 1998), for a discussion of the importance of the 'not, but' in theatre – as a way of preserving alternatives and virtual decisions that were not taken but are still important to recall as part of a process of arriving at a performance. This is one of the avenues I suggest that theatre theorists might pursue.

The Gift, Lewis Hyde movingly describes Walt Whitman's volunteer work with dying Civil War soldiers, illustrating that the deepest art of caring is found in what we give freely – practices that transcend the fee-for-service model of modern medicine.[29] My medical training, though, emphasized the postulate that generosity should only flow from doctor to patient. Accepting physical gifts from patients was thought to weaken doctor–patient interpersonal boundaries. As a young doctor, then, I self-righteously refused ailers' small gifts. Later, when a doctor saved my life, I learned how painful it was to not be able to offer her a gift. The third-party insurance reimbursements she would get felt irrelevant; I yearned to reciprocate in an emotionally richer currency.

Belatedly, I saw that by rejecting my patients' presents, I had been shoring up my illusion of independence by making my patients feel dependent and powerless. Now I effusively thank ailers for their gifts, whether maple syrup from a Vermont farmer or a plastic cow marked with bovine acupuncture points from a Chinese veterinarian. Patients who aren't able to give material gifts should keep in mind that many caregivers find heartfelt praise the most valuable present of all. It is such a powerful tool that it can turn a lacklustre clinician into a diligent one. When patients I haven't done much for nonetheless expresses fervent thanks, my embarrassment at the undeserved praise makes me work harder to help them.

Patients often help caregivers back by educating them, either explicitly or by example. One elderly mechanic kept offering to let me use his basement machine shop to make things. When I finally gave into my temptation, I learned a good deal of metalwork from him, but even more about flexible roles of mutual care. It turned out that I was only one of many regular pilgrims to his fairy wonderland of tools. His basement strongly resembled a site in the Australian Men's Shed movement, an organization that sets up community workshops to improve the health and wellbeing of isolated older men. My remarkable patient dispensed free repairs to neighbourhood lawnmowers, free political opinions to adults, and candy to neighbourhood children. He also gave those he helped the gift of letting them help him back, even allowing a recently widowed in-law, desperate to regain a sense of purpose, to do him the anxiety-provoking favour of reorganizing every tool in his densely packed workshop. After he grew too frail to keep his shop open, his small house remained as busy as ever. A seemingly endless stream of family and neighbours brought him hot meals, drove him to medical appointments, and during his final days, kept vigil.

Is it unrealistic to hope that modern healthcare could ever return, even in part, to such a capacious net of mutual aid? There are times when carers and

---

[29] Lewis Hyde, 'A Draft of Whitman', in *The Gift: Imagination and the Erotic Life of Property* (Vintage Books, 1983), 237–314.

ailers do need to disentangle themselves and strengthen the boundaries between their roles. Doctors should not accept expensive gifts or sexual relations from patients because such exchanges don't decrease power imbalances but make them even more fraught. But the network of gratitude that held my machinist's life together is within the reach of many people. Too dense a network of interdependence can limit individual freedom, and that is something that every ensemble must constantly renegotiate. But one thing worse than too tight a safety net is no safety net at all.

Nurturing the art of illness

This chapter has argued that patients and home caregivers benefit from learning to play their complex roles effectively – which means playing them together. The way in which educators expose students to the concept of theatre may be important. Students with an arts background may have no hesitation in embracing Shakespeare's and Goffman's position that all the world's a stage. Learners who privilege the natural sciences and see the teachings of art as untestable may reject theatre analogies as rhetorical trickery. For those students, it may be better to ease them into discussing the crucially performative aspects of illness by way of sciency synonyms for 'acting' such as 'non-verbal communication'. After all, the art of interaction includes talking in a language that the other will listen to. Whatever the language used, the message is the same: to communicate our selfhood and intentions to others, we need to seem as well as be who we are.

REFERENCES

Abramson, Lior, Florina Uzafovsky, Virgilia Toccaceli and Ariel Knafo-Noam. 'The Genetic and Environmental Origins of Emotional and Cognitive Empathy: Review and Meta-Analyses of Twin Studies'. *Neuroscience & Biobehavioral Reviews* 114 (2020): 113–33.

Ayers John W., Adam Poliak, Mark Dredze, Eric C. Leas, Zechariah Zhu, Jessica B. Kelley, Dennis J. Faix, Aaron M. Goodman, Christopher A. Longhurst, Michael Hogarth and Davey M. Smith. 'Comparing Physician and Artificial Intelligence Chatbot Responses to Patient Questions Posted to a Public Social Media Forum'. *JAMA Internal Medicine* 183, no. 6 (2023): 589–96. https://doi.org/10.1001/jamainternmed.2023.1838.

Bennett, Alan. *The Madness of King George III*. Faber, 1995.

Bloom, Paul. *Against Empathy: The Case for Rational Compassion*. Ecco, 2016.

Brooks, Peter. *Seduced by Story: The Use and Abuse of Narrative*. New York Review of Books, 2022.

Butler, Judith. *Gender Trouble*. Routledge, 1999.

Chartrand, Tanya L., and John A. Bargh. 'The Chameleon Effect: The Perception–Behavior Link and Social Interaction'. *Journal of Personality and Social Psychology* 76, no. 6 (1999): 893.

Fukuzawa, Fumitoshi, Yasutaka Yanagita, Daiki Yokokawa, Shun Uchida, Shiho Yamashita, Yu Li, Kiyoshi Shikino, Tomoko Tsukamoto, Kazutaka Noda, Takanori Uehara and Masatomi Ikusaka. 'Importance of Patient History in Artificial Intelligence-Assisted Medical Diagnosis: Comparison Study'. *JMIR Medical Education* 10 (2024): e52674.
Goffman, Erving. *The Presentation of Self in Everyday Life*. Doubleday, 1956.
Hall, Judith A., D. Roter and Cynthia S. Rand. 'Communication of Affect Between Patient and Physician'. *Journal of Health and Social Behavior* 22, no. 1 (1981): 18–30. https://doi.org/10.2307/2136365.
Hampton, J. R., J. M. Harrison, J. R. Mitchell, J. S. Prichard and C. Seymour. 'Relative Contributions of History-Taking, Physical Examination, and Laboratory Investigation to Diagnosis and Management of Medical Outpatients'. *British Medical Journal* 2 (1975): 486. https://doi.org/10.1136/bmj.2.5969.486.
Hochschild, Arlie Russell. *The Managed Heart: Commercialization of Human Feeling*. University of California Press, 1983.
How to Talk to Your Doctor HANDbook. UAMS Center for Health Literacy, 2023. https://healthliteracy.uams.edu/kb/how-to-talk-to-your-doctor-handbook/.
Hyde, Lewis. *The Gift: Imagination and the Erotic Life of Property*. Vintage Books, 1983.
Jameson, Frederic. *Brecht and Method*. Verso, 1998.
Kleinman, Arthur. *The Soul of Care: The Moral Education of a Husband and a Doctor*. Viking, 2019.
Mechanic, David. 'The Concept of Illness Behavior'. *Journal of Chronic Diseases* 15, no. 2 (1962): 189–94.
Mehta, Ankit, Belinda Fu, Erica Chou, Suzanne Mitchell and David Fessell. 'Improv: Transforming Physicians and Medicine'. *Medical Science Educator* 31 (2021): 263–66.
Mermikides, Alex. *Performance, Medicine and the Human*. Bloomsbury, 2020.
Norcross, John C., and Michael J. Lambert. 'Psychotherapy Relationships that Work III'. *Psychotherapy* 55, no. 4 (2018): 303.
Parsons, Talcott. *The Social System*. Free Press, 1951.
Pickering, Andrew. *The Cybernetic Brain: Sketches of Another Future*. University of Chicago Press, 2010.
Preston, Stephanie D., and Frans B. M. Waal. 'Empathy: Its Ultimate and Proximate Bases'. *Behavioral and Brain Sciences* 25, no. 1 (2002): 1–20.
Ramdani, Celine, Michael Ogier and Antoine Coutrot. 'Communicating and Reading Emotion with Masked Faces in the Covid Era: A Short Review of the Literature'. *Psychiatry Research* 316 (2022): 114755.
Sepkowitz, Kent. 'Behind the Doctors' Mask, a Little Room to Maneuver'. *New York Times*, October 2, 2007.
Sommer, Doris. *Proceed with Caution, When Engaged by Minority Writing in the Americas*. Harvard University Press, 1999.
Stanislavski, Konstantin. *An Actor's Work*. Translated by Jean Benedetti. Routledge 2017.
Williams, Amanda C de C. 'Facial Expression of Pain: An Evolutionary Account'. *Behavioral and Brain Sciences* 25, no. 4 (2002): 439–55. https://doi.org/10.1017/S0140525X02000080.

5

The ensemble arts of healing and learning: Forum Theatre and Pre-Texts

DORIS SOMMER

The Brazilian theatre artist Augusto Boal knew that learning and healing require acting and proposed to that end that 'spect-actors' could be catalysts of change. He coined the term when he and his theatre troupe began to recruit passive spectators of their dramas as creative companions. In Forum Theatre, spect-actors moved by tragedies make moves to interrupt tragic patterns. First, non-professional actors perform a skit illustrating familiar and apparently intractable predicaments, then the 'joker', a facilitator, invites the audience – we who watch – to play unscripted roles in replays that alter the drama. These 'spect-actors' respond by changing a speech or a gesture of the single-track plots that, as tragedies do, go from bad to worse and end disastrously. In Boal's community-based improvisatory art, bad endings signal possible beginnings for improving the scripts. Tragedy, on his watch and ours, is a social pathology that demands collective creative therapy. The interventions don't stop with one good try, or with two; they multiply, to explore options and to experience art as a platform for generating many responses rather than reaching one right answer.

Boal was concerned with the notion of empathy and how the phenomenon is misused. He thought that a spectator who passively feels empathy for a protagonist should become a spect-actor who explores why a tragedy occurred and how it can change. Boal used theatre to help the oppressed – a category that can include not only poor people but students, and patients – gain perspective and a sense of agency. Forum Theatre stages 'a rehearsal for the revolution' against authoritarianism, so a spect-actor might intervene in the entire dynamic of the theatre, such as by turning rows of seats into circles.[1] In this context, rhetoric and denunciations are not endpoints but points of departure. Boal's spect-actors embody Victor Shklovsky's well-known concept of artistic defamiliarization, in which art presents common things in strange ways, to grant us new perspectives.[2] Becoming a spect-actor helps decrease reliance on the power and authority of outsider-experts who, however, well meaning, often exacerbate rather than alleviate suffering. Forum Theatre skits thus empower communities to tackle almost any subject, including health crises, gaining a sense of agency and finding their own solutions to what ails them.

This chapter presents a series of case studies to unfold the ways that Forum Theatre and my related educational project, Pre-Texts, can affect health and emotional well-being. I begin with Boal's work with psychotic patients in Paris, then turn to a recent application of Forum Theatre to address the tuberculosis epidemic in Lima. I then describe my own work, with the Pre-Texts programme combatting depression among school children in Nairobi, and worldwide, and with an application of Forum Theatre by community leaders in Santiago brought together by concern over suicide and ultimately (re)focused on a response to domestic violence. Finally, I describe how lessons learned from using Forum Theatre and Pre-Texts in developing nations were applied to teaching medical students in Boston how to change from being passive information consumers to becoming spect-actors.

I. EXCISING THE COP IN THE HEAD: PARIS

Boal developed his interactive artform in Peru while in exile from Brazil's dictatorship (1967–85), recognizing the psychotherapeutic potential of theatre in the 1970s in Paris, his provisional home after Peru. Far from Brazil's murderous regime, he was shocked to learn that in first-world Europe, more people were

[1] Augusto Boal, *Theatre of the Oppressed*, trans. Charles A. & Maria-Odilia Leal McBride (Theatre Communications Group, 1985), 98,, originally published in 1974 as *Teatro del oprimido*.

[2] See Viktor Shklovsky, 'Art as Technique', in *Russian Formalist Criticism: Four Essays*, trans. Lee T. Lemon and Marion J. Reis (University of Nebraska Press, [1917] 1965), 3–24. Shklovsky writes, 'The technique of art is to make objects "unfamiliar", to make forms difficult, to increase the difficulty and length of perception.'

dying of suicide than of crime. In Brazil, he quipped, the enemy was visibly out there, while in Paris he wondered, 'how these "cops" got into our heads, and [how] ... to dislodge them'.[3] The distressing revelation about self-inflicted violence led him to explore the possible benefits of interactive theatre for people battling the 'cops' in their heads, particularly the mentally ill. Boal began to use Forum Theatre in a Parisian psychiatric hospital, offering *Flic dans la tête* (Cop in the head) as a workshop for patients at the hospital and then applying it as a standard technique in *Theatre of the Oppressed* (1974).[4]

As psychiatric patients participated in his workshop, Boal witnessed something dramatic. On stage, mentally ill people knew that they were acting and saw that they could choose to act differently. This was a revelation for everyone involved. Even severely afflicted actors who had been stuck in single-voice narratives for themselves could, while performing for other patients and for doctors, budge beyond their static stories. Taking the stage meant taking artistic distance from oneself, becoming an actor. The improvised artists watched themselves act and saw others watching them as well, creating layers of observation which made room for new manoeuvers. Boal was an attentive student of the participatory educator and philosopher Paolo Freire, who had observed:

> Problem-posing education affirms men and women as beings in the process of becoming – as unfinished, uncompleted beings in and with a likewise unfinished reality. Indeed, in contrast to other animals who are unfinished, but not historical, people know themselves to be unfinished; they are aware of their incompletion. In this incompletion and this awareness lie the very roots of education as an exclusively human manifestation. The unfinished character of human beings and the transformational character of reality necessitate that education be an ongoing activity.[5]

Boal's version of Freire's reflection on incompletion lands embodied on the stage, a defamiliarizing space where actors and spectators interact through unfinished scripts. This fictional space separates narrator from narrative to

---

[3] Augusto Boal, *The Rainbow of Desire: The Boal Method of Theatre and Therapy*, trans. Adrian Jackson (Routledge, 1995). 'In Paris, at the beginning of the 1980s, I led a workshop which ran over a period of two years, *Flic dans la tête* (The Cop in the Head). I started from the following hypothesis: the cops are in our heads, but their headquarters and barracks must be on the outside. The task was to discover how these "cops" got into our heads, and to invent ways of dislodging them. It was an audacious proposition' (8). See also *Legislative Theatre*, which begins with a report on work in a psychiatric hospital in England (Augusto Boal, *Legislative Theatre: Using Performance to Make Politics*, trans. Adrian Jackson (Routledge, 1998)).

[4] Boal, *Theatre of the Oppressed*.

[5] Paulo Freire, *Pedagogy of the Oppressed*, 30th anniversary edition, trans. Myra Bergman Ramos (Continuum, 2005), 84.

generate something new. It estranges habitual stories to reinterpret them from unfamiliar points of view. Multiple perspectives made possible on stage strain the limits of the kind of locked-down life stories familiar to therapists, which they have heard and expect to hear again.[6] The strain on these limits is felt in glimmers of new details. They dislodge familiar narratives with fresh attention to previously undervalued information.[7] After acting, Boal reports, patients worked better with their therapists. The improvement owed, on his reflection, to the aesthetic space that separates the stage from the audience:

> Only the human being is tri-dimensional (the I who observes, the I-in-situ and the not-I) because it alone is capable of dichotomy (seeing itself seeing). And as it places itself inside and outside its situation, actually there, potentially here, it needs to symbolize that distance which separates space and divides time, the distance from 'I am' to 'I can be' and from present to future; it needs to symbolize this potential, to create symbols which occupy the space of what is, but does not exist concretely, of what is possible … So, it creates symbolic languages: painting, music, words.[8]

In contrast to standard interpretations of 'narrative medicine' that encourage practitioners to develop empathy and intimacy by reading creative literature – as if fiction delivered reliable messages – Boal's theatre features aesthetic distance as an enabler of therapy.[9] For him, care should not count on closeness

---

[6] See Jon Elster's discussion of the relationship among constraints, aesthetic value and creativity in Part III of *Ulysses Unbound: Studies in Rationality, Precommitment and Constraints* (Cambridge University Press, 2000).

[7] Boal describes it in this way in *The Rainbow of Desire*:

> This movement forward in space and time is, in itself, therapeutic, since all therapy, before proposing the exercise of a choice, must consist of an inventory of possible alternatives. A process is therapeutic when it allows – and encourages – the patient to choose from several alternatives to the situation in which he finds himself, the situation which causes him unwanted suffering or unhappiness. In enabling, and indeed requiring, the patient to observe himself in action – since his own desire to show obliges him both to see and to see himself – this theatrical process of recounting, in the present, and in front of witnesses 'in solidarity,' a story lived in the past, offers, in itself, an alternative. (25)

[8] Ibid., 14.

[9] See Rita Charon's work in 'Narrative Medicine: A Model for Empathy, Reflection, Profession, and Trust' (*JAMA* 286, no. 15 (2001): 1897–902, https://doi.org/10.1001/jama.286.15.1897) and *Narrative Medicine: Honoring the Stories of Illness* (Oxford University Press, 2006). Several responses explore the contested connection between empathy and clinical care: see a recent example from Eugenia Stefanello, 'Narrative Medicine and Empathy: A Phenomenological Perspective' (*Journal of the British Society for Phenomenology* 55, no. 2 (2024): 167–83, https://doi.org/10.1080/00071773.2024.2314119). See also art therapists who dispute a privileging of process over product, pointing out that real art plumbs beyond the surface: 'But this attitude of acceptance, which is essential in all therapy, must not dull the artist's capacity for discrimination.

with another person but on a liberating distance. If caregivers 'feel into' their patients empathically, they may lose the perspective needed for effective interventions. Boal argued that the feeling of empathy doesn't generate real-world action. Instead, it collapses two people into one and reduces the room for agency. In Boal's words,

> As we have seen in 'Aristotle's Coercive System of Tragedy', *empathy* is the emotional relationship which is established between the character and spectator and which provokes, fundamentally, a delegation of power on the part of the spectator, who becomes an object in relation to the character: whatever happens to the latter, happens vicariously to the spectator.[10]

The protocol for Forum Theatre outlines hard work in preparation: to share personal problems, identify points that overlap and others that do not, stage distress and then consider reasonable interventions. Compared to this laborious process, empathy seems like a shortcut, and Boal actually calls it coercive because empathy entices spectators to forfeit critical thinking. Applying Boal's approach to the clinic, we might say that good clinicians know the benefits of maintaining some degree of distance from characters on stage: distance allows both patient and provider to notice new pathways. From this theatrical distance, clinicians are compassionate 'spect-actors' who accompany afflicted characters on a path that should get beyond being stuck. A clinician's compassion can be 'good empathy', in Boal's lexicon, but the good meaning should stay clear of the 'emotional orgy' that forgets oneself in the heat of another's passion.[11] The therapeutic encounter counts on estrangement of one person from another; it is dialogic and dynamic. Patients interact with doctors and doctors respond to patients. Their performances adjust to one another's improvisations. This interaction amounts to ensemble drama.

II. THE TRAGEDY OF PREVENTABLE DISEASE: LIMA

Forum Theatre began in Peru, Boal's first stop in a series of improvised homes during exile. Peru is a country with deep knowledge of collective tragedies, including conquest, colonization, terrorism, state-sanctioned

The teacher must preserve her integrity as an artist in order to be able to distinguish between the fake and the genuine, between blocks and limitations, regressions and progress, superficial pretense, and genuine communication' (Edith Krämer, *Art as Therapy: Collected Papers*, ed. Lani Alaine Gerity (Jessica Kingsley, 2000), 18).

[10] Boal, *Theatre of the Oppressed*, 84.

[11] Ibid.

massacres and a persistent disease, tuberculosis. Despite improved treatment and expanded clinical training, Peru still faces chronic and new cases of tuberculosis, one of the leading causes of death from infectious disease worldwide. What accounts for the stubborn scourge? Many clinicians blame patients' fear of the disease's stigma, which made them underreport infection to save face or save jobs.

In January 2018, over eighty local participants staged Forum Theatre in Carabayllo to explore the barriers to tuberculosis treatment. The theatre was facilitated by local organizations, Mercedes Becerra, a Partners in Health epidemiologist and members of the Cultural Agents Initiative at Harvard University. Many of the participants were survivors of tuberculosis, some were family members of patients under treatment, a few were nurses. When each person identified their most urgent and intractable problem – the first step of Boal's Forum Theatre protocol – we discovered that stigma was indeed an obstacle. But it was not the only one, nor the most salient.

Other difficulties not considered until then included violence on the street that prohibited circulation from home to health centres and abuse against women who tried to leave home to reach the clinic. Add to these obstacles high levels of drug and alcohol addiction, and one may appreciate the community's complex hurdles for healthcare. After everyone identified problems and staged their skits for spect-actors to witness and to replay, sometimes with liberating laughter and acute observations, Dr Becerra commented that we had learned more about this community in one morning than social scientists would have discovered over lengthy residencies. The clinicians were frankly impressed by the lay volunteers who offered persuasive interpretations and ingenious recommendations, and, further, the volunteers rose in their own self-esteem. Everyday people displayed efficacy in public on stage: they could diagnose social complexity and recommend mediations for stubborn challenges. That day, Forum Theatre became a resource for public health in Carabayllo.

III. PEDAGOGY AS ANTI-DEPRESSANT: PRE-TEXTS FROM NAIROBI TO HOLYOKE

Education is an overlooked but central component of medical treatment, and schools sometimes need to take on medical roles. Mental health challenges, in particular, are real and urgent concerns in schools both nationally and globally. The question is not if we need to address the challenge, but rather how best to do so. A traditional medical approach treats students as chronic or potential patients for clinicians who provide mostly individual treatments. However, there are seldom enough providers for the growing number of distressed young people, and observers have begun to worry that the clinical approach in schools is not only impractical, given the numbers, but also actively harmful in its focus on pathology.[12] A second approach addresses students' growing need for attention by empowering non-professional facilitators to offer mental health 'first aid'. Teachers, counsellors, community leaders and parents can now access information about preventing crises and about identifying signs of distress that require intervention. The expanding online network makes mental health resources accessible to many more first-line caregivers than professional clinicians could represent.[13]

Inspired by Boal's application of the theatre arts to healthcare, I have developed a third approach, Pre-Texts, whose mischievous name nods to the irreverent process called art-making. Pre-Texts is a pedagogical protocol that actively promotes mental health in groups of students by using arts-based activities which integrate students' reading, creativity and connection to their community.[14] An activity typically takes place for a set amount of time over a given period – an hour a day for a week, or an hour a week for a month. Pre-Texts presents challenging texts – not just from literary sources, but drawn from science and politics as well – as raw material for art-making and group interaction that supports cognitive and emotional development. With this approach, Pre-Texts has turned classrooms into stages for therapeutic intervention in schools around the world. It can seduce even reluctant young people to master daunting texts and to experience the pleasure of self-efficacy.

This student-centred version of Boal's 'rehearsal for revolution' is an international 'class struggle' in that it constitutes a campaign to change classroom culture and climate. It begins by rearranging schoolrooms from hierarchical rows to democratic circles, dismissing the 'cops' in student heads by rotating leadership among teachers and students. With one acupunctural prompt, 'Make art from this text', the protocol activates a cluster of faculties. The text, sometimes a difficult or dry one, is read aloud by one or more of the students. The creative challenge posed by the prompt ignites critical thinking, emotions, interpretation and communication in the listening students. Students may be indifferent or even hostile to the text, but they are often eager to make art. Stigma recedes with Pre-Texts because it engages whole classrooms in a shared activity without singling out sick people. As documented in a 2023 *Lancet* article, when clinically depressed and anxious Kenyan youth in the Kibera slum of Nairobi were

---

[12] See, for example, the work of journalist Abigail Shrier in *Bad Therapy: Why the Kids Aren't Growing Up* (Swift Press, 2024); public awareness of this concern is evident in the title of a recent *Boston Globe* article, 'Is Focusing Too Much on Mental Health Making Our Kids More Neurotic? Mental Illness Shouldn't Be Stigmatized, but It Shouldn't Be Celebrated Either' (Chris Ferguson, 29 April 2024).

[13] See 'Empower' in Dr Vikram Patel's 'Mental Health for All Lab', https://mentalhealthforalllab.hms.harvard.edu/empower.

[14] See www.pre-texts.org, and Jose Luis Falconi and Doris Sommer, *Pre-Texts International* (Harvard University Press, 2024).

given a week's experience with Pre-Texts, their depression and anxiety scores dropped more than twice as much as a control group. Even a month later, they were still 30 per cent lower than their baseline scores.[15] Follow-up prompts confirm the student-centred approach by rotating the facilitator role among the students. When young people work on individual or collective art projects after interrogating a text – rather than being interrogated about it by a teacher – self-expression and self-efficacy can surface even among clinically depressed and anxious students.

An experience of relief and inclusion is typical for Pre-Texts interventions. When it was employed in Holyoke, the poorest city in Massachusetts, one public school teacher sent a report of Pre-Text's effects on a child in her fourth-grade class. The child had been experiencing unusual stress because her father had been diagnosed with cancer and had become increasingly quarrelsome with her mother. The COVID quarantine had recently ended, and the girl's classmates no longer wore masks, but she had to mask everywhere to avoid infecting him. The child refused to participate in class and hardly spoke. 'During the implementation of the Pre-Texts methodology', the teacher reported, 'she gradually became more receptive and by the third day she was actively participating and enjoying the activities with a smile on her face. Her mother, a counsellor at the school, was frankly surprised by the change and very happy'.[16]

During a week of Pre-Texts, participants typically learn to feel the personal pleasures of making something original, which displays their irreplaceable particularity, and a collective admiration for classmates. Competition among peers relaxes to allow for collaborations. A welcome consequence for teachers is to lighten the burden of classroom management, because students help to manage themselves and to regulate one another. In this adaptation of Forum Theatre, as in others, afflicted people thus become agents of their own therapy.

IV. DOMESTIC VIOLENCE: RE-ACTING IN SANTIAGO

In Chile, suicide is more familiar than murder. Boal would have been devastated to learn that Latin America has caught up to the first world on this count. Severe depression that can lead to self-extinction has become a priority for politics as well as health organizations or mental health professionals. It is the most urgent issue for the mayor of Maipú in Greater Santiago, for example, outstripping unemployment, drug abuse, domestic violence and street crime.

---

[15] Tom Osborn et al., 'An Arts-Literacy Intervention for Adolescent Depression and Anxiety Symptoms: Outcomes of a Randomized Controlled Trial of Pre-Texts with Kenyan Adolescents', *eClinicalMedicine* 66, 102288 (December 2023), www.thelancet.com/journals/eclinm/article/PIIS2589-5370(23)00465-0/fulltext.

[16] Olatz Etxebarria, email to Doris Sommer, 4 March 2024.

The predictable consequence of this concern has been public health efforts to expand clinical services, though most people understand the structural limits of this advance. More clinicians and longer hours cannot keep up with the growing need for psychological support.

In 2023 I joined a coalition of psychiatrists, economists, designers, engineers, media experts and educators to address mental illness in Santiago.[17] With Forum Theatre our coalition managed to let some light peek through the limitations of conventional therapy. The night before our first meeting with Maipú's community leaders, who included clinically depressed victims of domestic violence and lonely senior citizens – for whom suicide was a familiar option – we decided to stage 'rehearsals' for life with no previous preparations. As usual with Forum Theatre, no one predicts what the plays will portray or how the issues will be explored. The only prediction is that each participant has an urgent or nagging problem that may begin to untangle with interventions.

One survivor of domestic violence was reluctant to relate her experience, even to the small company of like-minded spect-actors who had come together around a shared concern about gender abuse. The flexible and organic nature of Forum Theatre came to the fore, as more time to talk than the allotted fifteen minutes was in order, and still more time to create a skit that would represent her traumatic experience of beatings and sexual abuse by her father. The victim chose not to act, but to direct the action in a carefully curated choreography. That decision put her agency on view even before the actors took the stage. The performance was unnerving for the public, and perhaps especially for the visiting Harvard engineering professor who played the abusive father, surprised by his own good performance. Then, spect-actors entered the fray. One embarrassed the shameless man, another removed the girl to a friend's house, and both inspired more interventions. An occasional chuckle at overacting gave welcome relief to the tension of outing a prohibited but haunting memory.

In another skit, a mother could not console her sleepless newborn after several nights of noise invasion from neighbours who dealt in drugs and regularly revelled with clients. Confronting them in the original skit ignited a retaliation of more noise and so much violence that the conflict played out on the defenceless infant body, collateral damage in a duel of adults. During one of the replays, a spect-actor offered a win-win scenario of home cooking in exchange for a midnight curfew. Another intervention began with a visit to the rowdy neighbours by the mother, babe in arms, accompanied by a policeman.

[17]For more information on the Chile–Harvard coalition in Maipú, see Bárbara Sarria De la Vega, 'Crean la primera Coalición de Alto Impacto Social con el fin de prevenir enfermedades de salud mental en Maipú', *El Mostrador*, 9 August 2022, www.elmostrador.cl/agenda-pais/2022/08/09/crean-la-primera-coalicion-de-alto-impacto-social-con-el-fin-de-prevenir-enfermedades-de-salud-mental-en-maipu/.

The next day, we met in a circle to hear each other reflect on challenges and survival strategies. A particularly distressed participant shared that her determination to join the meeting made her skip medication she normally took, because it relaxed her to the point of prostration with no desire to move nor mental clarity to think. In another very personal engagement, throughout the two-hour session (enough time for each of us to speak and to hear everyone else), the nine-year-old son of a participant sketched our circle of sufferers and supporters, as we hovered between intimacy and public performance.

V. TEACHING DOCTORS TO HEAL

The concepts taught by Freire, staged by Boal and activated by everyday spect-actors inspired a current course at Harvard Medical School, 'Rx: Arts for Global Mental Health'. Piloted in 2017 by myself in collaboration with Harvard's Global Health Education and Learning Incubator, over a typical semester we review deformations with Michel Foucault's *Discipline and Punish* (1975) and Zygmunt Bauman's *Liquid Modernity* (2000), literature on loneliness including *Project UnLonely* by Jeremy Nobel (2023), responses to oppression such as Boal's *Rainbow of Desire* (1995), and speculations on scalable remedies including my own work on art as therapy. True to the therapeutic promise of art-making that convenes us, the course begins with making art. We stage Forum Theatre, unannounced and unrehearsed. Starting on stage provides a shared creative space that animates reflections and suggestions for more readings and guest lectures. This first session serves as an agora among students who do not yet know each other but do know that each one chose to be an active citizen at the intersection between creativity and well-being.

The skits performed during the recent fall 2023 session featured, as usual in Forum Theatre, psychological deadlocks recognized by clusters of participants. On stage and playing parts, our locked-down inhibitions morphed into useable artistic elements and even prompts for acting out traumatic experiences. One skit performed the mental breakdown of a wife after learning, long distance, of her husband's sudden death. The inconsolable shrieks of pain we heard pierced the air and our hearts. Played by her daughter, the mother's crisis gripped us like a knot of compound disasters, because the actor had lost not only her father but also the sanity of a helpless mother who could not support her developing child. In another skit, adult sisters fumbled as they felt useless to address the surprisingly advanced dementia of a mother who had deteriorated since their last visit, evidently too long ago. How does one make up for lapses of love? How do you beg forgiveness from a parent who no longer remembers her children?

In these skits and in others, we learned about each person's passions and about our collective dedication to care for one another. Personal feelings became prompts for collective explorations. They neither stagnated through guilt nor stayed paralysed by limited emotional resources. Thanks to the artistic protocol of Forum Theatre and the emotional space it created, our private passions, liberated from the loneliness of personal pathologies, could become public concerns.

CONCLUSION

Augusto Boal knew the importance of co-creation and brought it to disciplines outside traditional art. He understood that mental health is a group activity that should start in early childhood and continue in lifelong learning. To prevent depression and to treat it, theatre arts can train us to step back from unhappy habits and try out alternative behaviours. Those unhappy habits include those created by authorities whose hidden curriculums can intensify depression and aggression – doctors who pressure their patients into passivity and teachers who force submission on students. Traditional communities block the top-down effects of power when they meet in circles and face one another. Circles survive through collaborations in artists' workshops and in 'innovative' pedagogies. When we diverge from a linear hierarchy to come face to face with fellow actors, we recognize each person and ourselves as members of an ensemble.[18]

The dramas enacted in Forum Theatre and the texts brought to life by Pre-Texts promote mental health and justice not just by the content of their interactions but in their collaborative forms of engagement. Boal recognized that art *is* therapy.[19] Making something new means making decisions, using judgement. Whether or not an artwork has intrinsic value, the therapeutic effect of making – which requires deciding about colour, form, rhythm and so on – is to recognize oneself as an active agent. When we see that we are acting, we learn that we can act differently. Forum Theatre can demonstrate functional connections between art-making and problem solving, between personal injuries and political disaster. The connection between authoritarianism and depression is a hint that repressive cops, dogmatic physicians and bigoted teachers continue to bully people inside the victims' own heads. Boal's dynamic art beckons us to step back and try out manoeuvers to dislodge them.

REFERENCES

Boal, Augusto. *Theatre of the Oppressed*. Translated by Charles A. and Maria-Odilia Leal McBride. Theatre Communications Group, 1985.

---

[18]The phrase 'face to face' is Emmanuel Levinas's shorthand for ethics. See 'From Existence to Ethics', in *The Levinas Reader*, ed. Sean Hand (Basil Blackwell, 1989), 82–4.
[19]Augusto Boal, *The Aesthetics of the Oppressed*, trans Adrian Jackson (Routledge, 2006).

Boal, Augusto. *The Rainbow of Desire: The Boal Method of Theatre and Therapy*. Translated by Adrian Jackson. Routledge, 1995.

Boal, Augusto. *Legislative Theatre: Using Performance to Make Politics*. Translated by Adrian Jackson. Routledge, 1998.

Boal, Augusto. *The Aesthetics of the Oppressed*. Translated by Adrian Jackson. Routledge, 2006.

Charon, Rita. 'Narrative Medicine: A Model for Empathy, Reflection, Profession, and Trust'. *JAMA* 286, no. 15 (2001): 1897–1902. https://doi.org/10.1001/jama.286.15.1897.

De la Vega, Bárbara Sarria. 'Crean la primera Coalición de Alto Impacto Social con el fin de prevenir enfermedades de salud mental en Maipú'. *El Mostrador*, 9 August 2022. www.elmostrador.cl/agenda-pais/2022/08/09/crean-la-primera-coalicion-de-alto-impacto-social-con-el-fin-de-prevenir-enfermedades-de-salud-mental-en-maipu/.

Elster, Jon. *Ulysses Unbound: Studies in Rationality, Precommitment and Constraints*. Cambridge University Press, 2000.

Falconi, Jose Luis, and Doris Sommer. *Pre-Texts International*. Harvard University Press, 2024.

Freire, Paulo. *Pedagogy of the Oppressed*. 30th anniversary edition. Translated by Myra Bergman Ramos. Continuum, 2005.

Krämer, Edith. *Art as Therapy: Collected Papers*. Edited by Lani Alaine Gerity. Jessica Kingsley, 2000.

Osborn, Tom, David M. Ndetei, Pier Luigi Sacco, Victoria Mutiso and Doris Sommer. 'An Arts-Literacy Intervention for Adolescent Depression and Anxiety Symptoms: Outcomes of a Randomized Controlled Trial of Pre-Texts with Kenyan Adolescents'. *eClinicalMedicine* 66, 102288 (December 2023). www.thelancet.com/journals/eclinm/article/PIIS2589-5370(23)00465-0/fulltext.

Shklovsky, Victor. 'Art as Technique'. In *Russian Formalist Criticism: Four Essays*, translated by Lee T. Lemon and Marion J. Reis. University of Nebraska Press, [1917] 1965.

Stefanello, Eugenia. 'Narrative Medicine and Empathy: A Phenomenological Perspective'. *Journal of the British Society for Phenomenology* 55, no. 2 (2024): 167–83. https://doi.org/10.1080/00071773.2024.2314119.

6

Rehearsing failure: What theatre can teach medicine about being present

BIANCA DAHL AND PHILIP DAVY MCKEE

You're on Earth. There's no cure for that.

(Samuel Beckett, *Endgame*)

This essay explores the relationships that theatre and medicine have to making meaning of suffering, highlighting limits to extant cultural narratives around healing, empathy and vulnerability while reflecting on the different ways theatre and performance could contribute to medical education. As others are doing in this volume and in medical humanities more broadly, we seek better insights to address how patients and doctors each make sense of, and live with, chronic illness. Many scholars have praised the integration of theatre techniques into medical training as a remedy for medicine's shortcomings in sensitivity and care. They accommodate what Arthur Kleinman, in Chapter 1, has identified as theatre's capacity for 'witnessing', that is: 'feeling something akin to awe before the unfolding of a singular human experience – a drama'. This formulation credits theatre and drama with the power to 'inspire medical students' empathy, their interpretative critical thinking, and reflective practice, ... thus enabling them to become both competent and compassionate practitioners'.[1]

[1] David Ian Jeffrey, *How Shakespeare Inspires Empathy in Clinical Care* (Palgrave Macmillan, 2024), 22.

After reflecting on our own professional and personal experiences, however, we have grown cautiously sceptical of theatre's potential to transfigure – whether its audiences, society as a whole, or medical practitioners in particular. In another context, theatre scholar Martin Harries has identified similar practices as the dream of 'destructive spectatorship': the belief that authentic witnessing to suffering must involve a radical and spectacular unmaking of the subject.[2] Despite widespread calls for medical students to cultivate empathy through crafting 'better' scripts, we worry that the typical use of theatre in medical training actually inhibits the most powerful connections between doctors and patients, or impedes meaningful contributions to narratives about patient suffering. The problem is not that medical practitioners simply need to be better versed in the art of theatre, we suggest, but instead that the capacity of live theatre – in the broadly realist mode that predominates in North America, much of Western Europe and other parts of the world that have been influenced by realist dramaturgy – to make meaning of suffering is itself limited. Any meaningful integration of the medical humanities must first grapple with the limitations of both medicine and theatre. Armed with this recognition, we argue that interventions in medical training and practice would instead be better served by a reorientation around the post-dramatic theatrical notion of 'presence'.

Playwrights and actors who illustrate living within limits, the inescapability of suffering, the capacity to endure the demands of the role, and the risk and experience of failure, instead offer more valuable insights for bridging theatre and the ensemble drama of illness. The concept of 'presence' captures a quality of self-conscious immediacy where performers are 'notably focused or "in the moment" ... convey[ing] strong engagement with themselves, their roles and/or their work, a particular quality of concentration, and a special "aura"'.[3] In contemporary theatre aesthetics, a preference for '*presence* over *representation*' is identified with post-dramatic theatre, which foregrounds shared embodiment, the co-presence of actors and spectators, over storytelling and role-playing.[4] Notably, most medical humanities approaches embrace realist theatre precepts rather than post-dramatic ones, and we argue this orientation may even worsen medicine's so-called empathy problem. By contrast,

---

[2] Martin Harries, *Forgetting Lot's Wife: On Destructive Spectatorship* (Fordham University Press, 2007).

[3] Paul Allain and Jen Harvie, *The Routledge Companion to Theatre and Performance* (Routledge, 2014). While the concept of presence has drawn merited critique from performance theorists and others, we nonetheless use it here to capture the qualities of '"immediacy", "spontaneity", "intimacy", "live-ness", [and] "energy"' that improvisational actors must cultivate. Cormac Power, *Presence in Play: A Critique of Theories of Presence in the Theatre* (Editions Rodopi, 2008), 15.

[4] Hans-Thies Lehmann, *Post-Dramatic Theatre*, translated and with an introduction by Karen Jurs-Munby (Routledge, 2006), 109.

'presence' is closely woven into the actor's confrontation with shame[5] and the possibility of failure, as well as their capacity for improvisation, vulnerability and connection – and here is where we see the greatest promise for medical practitioners.

We propose presence as a value and a framework that are opposed to many forms of narrative. Both traditional live theatre and medical practice perpetuate the myth of a tidy resolution to experiences of suffering, and so their merging in medical humanities education risks reinforcing this dynamic. The shared desire of doctors and patients for diagnosis and cure echoes a broader cultural longing for stories where hardship is heroically overcome. However, the promise of the actor's confrontation with shame and failure lies precisely in their ability to arrest the unhelpful and, at times, harmful teleology that implicitly subtends traditional theatrical and medical narratives. This offers a model for integrating suffering, uncertainty and endurance into medical practice.

Our methodology in this essay is primarily autoethnographic, as our approach to enhancing patient–doctor communication and empathetic connection stems from both professional expertise and personal experience. Professionally, Bianca is a socio-cultural medical anthropologist whose teaching included inaugurating a mixed-level seminar in medical humanities and ethics (for MD, MPH and BA/BS students); Philip is a theatre director, playwright and psychotherapist who has also provided drama therapy for patients with lived experiences of addiction and/or mental illness. Personally, we also draw on our experience navigating disability, chronic pain and medical errors as a patient (Bianca) and her partner (Philip). Our trajectory is illustrative of moments that challenge the mechanical reliance on medical 'scripts' and narrative conventions (such as the protocols governing how to break bad news to a patient), which lead us instead to prioritize responsiveness and presence in patient–doctor interactions. We see more potential here in the renunciation of medical scripts – in an embrace even of anti-narrative – than in their rote repetition and mastery. Notably, the most meaningful breakthroughs in our experiences with the Canadian and UK healthcare systems came from instances where doctors abandoned their scripts, allowing themselves to experience and recognize their fallibility. We maintain that these moments were less about doctors experiencing empathy[6] – widely

[5] Here we take inspiration from Marlene Goldman's revisiting of shame, in which she contends that 'conscious re-enactments of shame which facilitate an empathic response have the capacity to mitigate against shame's destructive and, at times, lethal effects'. Marlene Goldman, *The Social, Aesthetic, and Medical Implications of Performing Shame: Interdisciplinary Approaches* (Routledge, 2023), 4.

[6] We note that the term empathy is often used imprecisely. Where it is defined, it is regularly delineated into different subtypes, for example: emotive, moral, cognitive and behavioural (Zak Kelm et al., 'Interventions to Cultivate Physician Empathy: A Systematic Review', *BMC Medical*

claimed by medical humanities enthusiasts to be the most important skill the subdiscipline can teach doctors – and more about practitioners who challenged their sense of themselves as infallible experts. In these instances, by cultivating a genuine sense of presence, doctors departed from the standard playbook, opened up space for resistance to traditional narratives and enabled both affective and material support for their patient to emerge.

By sharing this autoethnography, we also engage in an exercise in vulnerability and self-reflection. When narrating our story to various listeners, we have been disconcerted to discover that our account appears to constitute a coherent whole, leading to expectations of narrative resolution on the part of our friends and community. These are the very conventions that we find so problematic, and which fail to capture the experience of living with chronic pain and create impossible expectations for resolution for doctors and patients alike. This again puts us in conversation with Kleinman, who argues for an 'authentic relationship grounded in the presence of the practitioner eliciting the presence of the family and the patient' rather than steering them towards some wished-for or institutionally mandated closure. In fact, rather than experiencing resolution, we find ourselves still in limbo. Writing these reflections proved more challenging than either of us anticipated. They represent our effort to step outside our own spaces of professional comfort: an exercise in the very practice for which we are advocating.

THE LIMITATIONS OF THEATRICAL TECHNIQUES AND SCRIPTS IN MEDICAL CARE

Suffering remains a foundational obstacle for doctors and patients. In our experience we recognized the outlines of previous humanistic attempts that have been made to equip doctors, and patients to deal with suffering, so we begin there. Contrary to the dominant presumptions of medical humanities, however, we suggest that the obstacle of suffering benefits less from attempts at cultivating empathy in doctors or teaching them effective scripts and more from galvanizing their ability to remain present.

Broadly speaking, North American cultural attitudes toward medical suffering convey the impression that it can – and should – be overcome. Persistent suffering is therefore an interpretive problem, one that challenges doctors,

Education 14 (2014): 1–11). In this essay, we are discussing the dominant vision of empathy that emerges in much of the medical training literature, as the capacity to recognize and understand the feelings of others. Our intention in this broad definition is to encompass the general usage of the term across medical training.

patients and their broader networks. Chronic or unresolved suffering usually appears devoid of value or meaning. When medicine fails to deliver a diagnosis or treatment, patients often experience this as a violation of cultural scripts, influenced by medical dramas that glorify the heroic doctor who resolves illness. In other words, both patients and doctors can experience suffering – particularly ongoing or chronic suffering – as a failure or narrative rupture, a problem of signification.[7] When suffering is acknowledged, it is regularly framed in terms of familiar tropes: the martyr or hero who overcomes pain through sheer willpower, or the admirable sufferer who meets pain with stoic endurance. These narratives reflect a cultural discomfort with witnessing suffering in its raw, unmitigated form, pressing us instead to transform it into stories of triumph or redemption.

Alongside the cultural work being done by the transformative narrative refiguration of suffering, empathy is continually championed as a crucial skill for clinicians, albeit one that worryingly decreases during the course of medical school and residency.[8] The medical humanities are increasingly promoted as a necessary corrective to this trend. The logic seems to be that since doctors are always already actors in a drama, we might as well teach them to be *good* actors.

These are commendable goals, but the version of theatre typically promoted in medical humanities programmes often ends up having the opposite effect.[9] Training in scripts and role-play, in fact, risks producing a further entrenched *lack* of empathy on the part of doctors, by reinforcing the distance between doctors' expertise and patients' desires for meaning-making. Anthropologist Janelle Taylor's ethnographic research highlights how role-playing medical encounters actually teach doctors-in-training how to *repress* their emotional response – their potentially unruly empathy or presence – when faced with patient suffering in real-life clinical settings.[10]

---

[7] Paula Treichler, *How to Have Theory in an Epidemic: Cultural Chronicles of AIDS* (Duke University Press, 1999).

[8] Melanie Neumann et al., 'Empathy Decline and Its Reasons: A Systematic Review of Studies with Medical Students and Residents', *Academic Medicine* 86, no. 8 (2011): 996–1009.

[9] See Janelle S. Taylor, 'The Moral Aesthetics of Simulated Suffering in Standardized Patient Performances', 'Ethnographies of Clinical Training', *Culture, Medicine and Psychiatry* 35, no. 2 (2011): 134–62; Goldman, *Performing Shame.*

[10] Taylor, 'The Moral Aesthetics of Simulated Suffering'. The emphasis on verisimilitude in SP performances ironically introduces what Taylor calls a 'moral aesthetic of inoculation', where the emotional impact of an SP performance is designed to prepare – or 'inoculate' – students against the weight of 'future encounters with suffering' (134). The ultimate intention of these interactions is thus not necessarily to cultivate empathy but rather to temper it, teaching medical students to regulate or restrain their emotional responses.

SUFFERING AND NARRATIVE EMPLOTMENT IN MEDICINE

In recent ethnographic research that Bianca has undertaken with chronic pain sufferers participating in social media-based patient support groups, she found that participants devote a lot of time to discussing strategies for convincing doctors to take their experiences of pain seriously. The goal seems to be both to win understanding from their doctors and to gain a diagnosis that will provide an authentic claim on compassion and narrative legitimacy for their suffering.

One participant – whom we'll call Lisa – divulged her strategy in seeking diagnosis of a condition she believed to be a rare and difficult-to-diagnose genetic disorder. On the online patient support group, Lisa posted a four-page document detailing every medical symptom she had experienced in the previous three days. She explained that she had prepared the document for her upcoming first consultation with a new specialist. Her goal, Lisa said, was to impress upon the doctor the severity of her suffering by the sheer volume of her complaints. To strengthen her case, she wrote in the diagnostic language she had found online, intentionally aligning her symptoms with the criteria for the genetic condition she suspected.

This type of narrative differs significantly from the genre of illness storytelling typically discussed in the medical humanities, where 'patient stories allow making sense of their suffering and how it feels from the inside' as a mode of coping.[11] Instead, Lisa's approach hews more closely to a phenomenon that anthropologist Cheryl Mattingly described as 'therapeutic emplotment'.[12] This concept recognizes that 'physicians are creators as well as "readers" or interpreters of clinical stories. They establish a therapeutic plot for patients, as a course of treatment is set in action, and they "read" the unfolding "medical plot" determined by disease process and patient response'.[13] Doctors' narrative emplotments involve not only their words but also their diagnostic actions, treatment suggestions and interpersonal interactions with patients.[14] This is not a straightforward conversion of patient symptoms into diagnoses and treatments, either. Physicians often ask leading questions designed to reinforce the explanation they have already developed for a patient's suffering.

[11] Vera Kalitzkus and Peter F. Matthiessen 'Narrative-Based Medicine: Potential, Pitfalls, and Practice', *Permanente Journal* 13, no. 1 (2009): 81; see also Arthur Kleinman, *The Illness Narratives: Suffering, Healing, and the Human Condition* (Basic Books, 1988; repr. 2020).

[12] Cheryl Mattingly, 'The Concept of Therapeutic "Emplotment"', *Social Science & Medicine* 38, no. 6 (1994): 811–22.

[13] Mary-Jo Delvecchio Good, 'Cultural Studies of Biomedicine: An Agenda for Research', *Social Science & Medicine* 41, no. 4 (1995): 463.

[14] Mattingly, 'The Concept of Therapeutic "Emplotment"'.

On the other side, anthropologist Joe Dumit highlights a 'counter-politics' oppositional to the diagnostic power wielded by medical practitioners, where patients like Lisa strategically 'emplot' their doctors, 'telling them exactly what needs to be said to get what they want'.[15] Particularly when patients perceive a lack of recognition from doctors, they employ a range of strategies to elicit compassion. Lisa, for instance, didn't just craft her four-page symptom list; she also crowd-sourced feedback on it with fellow patients. Her goal was to strike a delicate balance between impressing the specialist with the severity of her suffering, while not threatening the doctor's hierarchical status by overtly appearing to have decided on a self-diagnosis already (which she admitted to the group she had in fact done).

What she sought was an experience of presence, recognition and legitimation from the gatekeepers of medical authority. It strikes us, however, that strategies like Lisa's often ironically inhibit moments of connection and presence between doctors and patients: her desire for legitimation led her to further quantify her suffering in ways that risked labelling her as a hypochondriac, as one poster on the forum cautioned.

What stands out in Lisa's case is that the genetic condition for which she sought diagnosis did not have any treatment beyond the symptom management she was already receiving. Her sole motivation for pursuing a formal diagnosis was to bolster her illness narrative, to seek recognition. Diagnosis holds signifying power: it legitimizes experiences of suffering and provides a sense of standing within the medical system. Admittedly, had Lisa met with more presence and recognition from previous clinicians, perhaps she would not have been so fixated on the absence of a diagnosis. But compassion alone was not her primary goal; she wanted the narrative legitimacy granted by an established disease category.

There is a striking gap in the academic literature on integrating theatre into medical education that materializes here, where the shared storytelling of the clinical encounter comes up short: this literature rarely addresses how both doctors and patients cope with patient healing trajectories that fail to achieve resolution, diagnosis, or cure. Even in work that acknowledges the limitations of script-based medical humanities training, such as a call for 'a broader understanding of performance theories and practices' by performance studies scholar Gretchen Case and internal medicine specialist Daniel J. Brauner, the focus often falls on the improved execution of medical scripts.[16] Case and Brauner

---

[15] Joe Dumit, 'Pharmaceutical Witnessing: Drugs for Life in an Era of Direct-to-Consumer Advertising', in *Technologized Images, Technologized Bodies*, ed. Jeanette Edwards, Penelope Harvey and Peter Wade (Berghahn Books, 2010), 56.

[16] Gretchen A. Case and Daniel J. Brauner, 'Perspective: The Doctor as Performer: A Proposal for Change Based on a Performance Studies Paradigm', *Academic Medicine* 85, no. 1 (2010): 159.

maintain, for example, that 'a complex understanding of performance is essential to the development of an empathetic imagination, a cognitive faculty that allows physicians to generate unique responses to given situations rather than employing reactions learned by rote in "communications training" '.[17] Implicit in their argument is an underlying assumption that applications of a largely realist understanding of theatre – if only better implemented – can serve as a transformative tool, perhaps even a panacea, for the shortcomings of medical practice.

This is where we differ from Case and Brauner. Lisa's fixation on finding a practitioner who could offer an explanation for her suffering reflects a desire to rewrite her own story, seeking narrative coherence where medical answers had failed her. However, in cases such as hers the standard medical script may always prove inadequate, even with the help of a new specialist or an attentive clinician. In a back-and-forth in the comments on Lisa's social media post, she acknowledged having 'caring' doctors who were managing her symptoms well. Again, what she sought was not empathy, per se, but an experience of agency and recognition in how the narrative emerges: a participation and coproduction in the legitimating forms of diagnosis. Lisa's unfulfilled quest underscores the importance of an alternative approach: telling stories that harness the power of signification, of meaning-making, even if they fail to match reassuring narrative markers. And that happens when doctors *and* patients both perform together in the interest of lucidity and complexity rather than premature closure.

We turn now to our critique of the standard, script-based medical-theatrical solution to the obstacle of suffering. To illustrate this argument, we explore several of our experiences in which a doctor was able to recognize their own limitations, feel an unexpected experience of presence with their patient (Bianca), and thereby make space for a shared project of meaning-making and coping – outside received scripts of diagnosis, treatment and recovery.

MEDICAL ERRORS AND PHYSICIANS' PRESENCE AND FALLIBILITY

In her late twenties, Bianca began to experience significant pain in her right hip. A sports medicine specialist diagnosed her with a torn labrum – the tissue that cushions and connects the ball and socket of the hip joint – and referred her to a surgical specialist. While waiting for the referral, Bianca's pain worsened to the point of being debilitating. She returned to the original specialist, who handed her a pair of crutches and instructed her to stop bearing weight on the affected hip. But when the referral finally came through, the new surgeon

[17] Case and Brauner, 'The Doctor as Performer', 159.

balked at scheduling her for a procedure, suggesting that Bianca's level of pain indicated a more serious pathology beyond the labral tear. He then referred her onward to another surgeon, locally recognized as 'the best' at the procedure in question: the person who had originally trained him, Dr Walker. (All names of health providers in our story have been anonymized.)

Dr Walker similarly refused to schedule Bianca for surgery, citing the complexity of her presentation. In one memorable interaction, Dr Walker, visibly frustrated, addressed Philip (ignoring Bianca entirely), proclaiming, 'I'm a hammer-and-nail kind of guy. I have one hammer, and I can hit one kind of nail. I'm good at that. I have really high success rates when we're just fixing a torn labrum. There's something else going on here. I don't want to operate.' He added that he had an endless list of patients with simpler cases and higher likelihoods of success.

Yet just a few months after this encounter, Dr Walker performed the surgical repair on Bianca's hip under an expedited timeline. What changed his mind? While we'd like to suggest it was our persistence, his empathy for Bianca's suffering, or her successful performance of a 'model' pain patient (one who remained physically active despite mobility limitation, who refused to take opioid painkillers and who daily practised physical therapy), our moments of breakthrough with Dr Walker unexpectedly occurred when he experienced shame and guilt himself. While we certainly aren't advocating for shame as a professional motivator, this form of vulnerability did cause him to connect with Bianca's experience and seek to alter it. In other words, he allowed himself to become present in a different and meaningful way.

The first of these moments occurred subsequent to a distressing diagnostic procedure conducted by a radiology resident, at Dr Walker's referral. The resident was tasked with injecting Bianca's hip with steroids and a numbing agent under fluoroscopy. The injection should have taken a matter of moments, but from start to finish the needle was in Bianca's body for over thirty minutes as the resident struggled to penetrate her joint. Bianca reported back to Dr Walker that the resident never actually penetrated into her hip capsule, a narrative that he immediately dismissed as improbable. Dr Walker instead referred Bianca to a rehabilitation medicine specialist, Dr Singh.

Upon hearing Bianca's account of the ordeal, Dr Singh responded with more credence, immediately volunteering to repeat the injection himself with ultrasound guidance. During the procedure, Dr Singh encountered the same rigid resistance to the needle the resident had faced, but he understood its significance. Within minutes, he had completed the protocol and was able to manipulate her leg under local anaesthetic. This revealed a radically limited range of motion caused not by pain, but by tissue damage. Dr Singh diagnosed adhesive capsulitis, a condition rare in hips, which more commonly appears as 'frozen' shoulder.

This new diagnosis, coupled with what both Bianca and Philip interpreted as a moment of guilt or responsibility on Dr Walker's part – whether for referring her to an unskilled resident, dismissing her account, or overlooking key aspects of her condition – marked a notable shift in Dr Walker's demeanour. Typically brusque and confrontational, Dr Walker displayed a rare moment of humanity and vulnerability. This wasn't empathy with Bianca's pain in any meaningful way, but it had an arguably more powerful effect: it led Dr Walker to offer to put Bianca on his surgical waiting list, a surprising reversal. The normal wait time was fifteen months, but he offered her an almost immediate cancellation slot. In a way, Dr Walker needed Bianca to have a(nother) diagnosis in order to categorize her suffering, though his techniques alone had been insufficient to uncover it. Notably, Dr Walker never physically examined Bianca himself, relying instead on X-rays, CT scans and MRIs to mediate his understanding of her condition. The technological mediation of his diagnosis reflected and reinforced his lack of presence with her. Yet, as it turned out, his initial reservations about the surgery proved warranted. While Bianca's pain improved post-surgery, it did not resolve entirely.

Six months later, her hip completely dislocated when she stood up from a table, leading to a night in the ER, a major relapse of pain and eventually to a diagnosis of Ehlers–Danlos Syndrome by another specialist. Ehlers-Danlos is a connective tissue disorder characterized by overly lax joints, chronic pain and other manifestations of collagen mutation. The diagnosis fully explained all her symptoms (and also many prior medical issues), creating a narrative container that rescripted her experience away from Dr Walker's lingering suspicion of hyperalgesia or central pain syndrome and toward a clearly identifiable biological pathology.

That was when Bianca and Philip decided to travel to the UK to consult a specialist in hip instability in young people, who worked extensively with Ehlers–Danlos Syndrome patients and had authored many publications on the topic. We hoped he might advise a hip replacement that could restore Bianca's quality of life. Mr Bates (surgeons in the UK are referred to as 'Mr/Ms' rather than 'Dr') had a different revelation and prognosis, however: Bianca's right hip was dysplastic, too shallow (another missed diagnosis), and this, combined with her hypermobile joints from Ehlers–Danlos Syndrome, was making her joint extremely unstable. He advised surgery, not for a hip replacement but for a far more aggressive procedure called a peri-acetabular osteotomy. The operation involves cutting apart the pelvic bone into pieces and rearranging them with large titanium rods, ultimately creating a deeper socket for the femoral head to rest within. With Bianca having already had only partial relief from the labral repair, Bates said something no other doctor had told her: 'I believe I know what's causing your pain, and I think I can fix a lot of it.' The recognition of suffering, and the offer of a solution, were major legitimating experiences for both of us, so much so that we decided to book the surgery under likely self-pay (while petitioning the Ontario Ministry of Health to cover its expenses, ultimately unsuccessfully).

But when Bianca returned to consult with her specialists in Toronto about the new treatment plan, she encountered distressing resistance. Dr Singh, who had previously seemed empathetic, memorably dismissed the surgery that Mr Bates advised as 'inhumane' and 'borderline barbaric'. Notably, he justified his critiques on the basis of supposed 'empathic' concern for Bianca's experience undergoing so major a surgery. He went on to say that he might consider supporting such a procedure only after Bianca had 'completely dislocated the hip at least seven times'. However, when Philip asked Dr Singh what other solutions or pathways he might advise in the interim, he had nothing to suggest. Despite his earlier display of seeming compassion, Dr Singh's failure to acknowledge the daily burden of Bianca's mobility limitations – or to help her find any pathway toward alleviating her pain – placed him in opposition to her quest for relief.

After this demoralizing meeting, Bianca braced herself for her next consultation with Dr Walker, anticipating even greater resistance from him. Bianca spoke with one of Dr Walker's residents before the specialist entered the consulting room, who whistled and said, 'Listen, he's not going to like this recommendation. Don't hold out hope for him to come on board.' Indeed, Dr Walker's initial reaction was similar in content to Dr Singh's, but angrier in tone. He loudly addressed his two residents, not Bianca, stating that no surgeon in Canada would perform this particular osteotomy due to its highly invasive nature and the brutal recovery. But once his high-volume rant subsided, it became apparent that his anger was less about Bianca's decision to undertake a procedure he wouldn't have recommended and more about the diagnosis of Ehlers–Danlos Syndrome that had been confirmed since her last appointment with him, after the hip dislocation. Dr Walker seemed incensed by the implication that he had missed a significant diagnosis – one that, given its relevance to his specialty, he might reasonably have been expected to identify. Bianca had never insinuated such a failure, but he responded as though she (or someone else) had.

Turning to Bianca, still near shouting, Dr Walker insisted that he had suspected Ehlers–Danlos Syndrome months earlier. Frustrated by what felt like a return to the adversarial tone of their earlier encounters, Bianca pushed back, insisting that he had never communicated this suspicion to her. In response, Dr Walker abruptly and wordlessly turned to the computer in the consulting room, then began scanning Bianca's medical file. This apparent retreat from the clinical interaction lasted several minutes, during which the two residents tried to add some information about the osteotomy, appearing uncomfortable with the specialist's silence. Bianca didn't know what Dr

Walker was doing, until suddenly he exclaimed triumphantly and directed everyone's attention to the screen. There was an image of what appeared to be handwritten clinical notes scanned in from some earlier consultation. In small letters at the bottom of the page, Dr Walker had written 'EDS?': shorthand for the connective tissue disorder (Ehlers–Danlos Syndrome) she had finally been diagnosed with.

For Bianca and Philip, this note held no significance. Dr Walker had not taken action to investigate the possibility of Ehlers–Danlos Syndrome, nor had he ever mentioned the suspicion to her, so a scribbled acronym that produced no follow-up was not meaningful in any way for her experience. But it *was* significant for Dr Walker, because he clearly felt 'proving' he had suspected the connective tissue disorder restored his authority, mitigated his sense of vulnerability and allowed him to respond differently. Ironically, he became present not so much through an engagement with his fallibility but a reinstantiation of his infallibility – which he felt had been called into question by the narrative of a missed diagnosis. He was only open to listening carefully to Bianca once he had established that she was working within a diagnostic script he had already proposed.

To the surprise of both us and his residents, Dr Walker again suddenly reversed course. Restoring his clinical authority had enabled him to recover from the narcissistic injury and freed him up to listen to Bianca – to really engage with her attentively – for what felt like the first time. Again ironically, it enabled him to be more present with Bianca's circumstances.

At the end of the consultation, Dr Walker not only endorsed her decision to do the procedure but – to Bianca's astonishment – volunteered to write a letter of support to the Ontario Ministry of Health in support of her petition to cover her out-of-country surgical costs. Although the petition was ultimately unsuccessful, this gesture marked a major shift in Dr Walker's approach. Doing so also allowed him to exit the stage and to leave the burden of narrative resolution to another doctor.

SUFFERING AND THE RISK OF FAILURE: INSIGHTS FROM THEATRE

Although we have signalled our concern over the transformative power sometimes ascribed to theatre, we believe that it has value nonetheless, not least because it can give suffering meaning, or provide an orientation toward it. This is the need with which so many patients like Lisa are obsessed – the value of a diagnosis for a chronic condition is often sought because it provides a container that legitimizes their pain. Bianca's story reveals that this is true not only for patients, but for specialists like Dr Walker as well. The diagnosis of capsulitis made him suddenly willing to operate on her, after he had previously refused;

the diagnosis of Ehlers–Danlos Syndrome similarly made him support her undergoing the major osteotomy. These diagnoses were significant because they opened up spaces of mutual presence and collaboration. But from what we can discern from the literature and our own research, this is not the focus in most adaptations of performance and theatre techniques into medical training.[18]

The dramaturgy that has shaped much of the medical humanities draws heavily on Aristotelian principles – the same backbone of 'well-made' realist plays that have dominated mainstream commercial Western theatre for over a century – structured around a script that delivers a coherent story with a clear beginning, middle and end. However, reality often defies such coherence, particularly in the realm of suffering and endurance. In conventional theatre, the story ends, just as each medical encounter has a finite duration. In life, the story continues, frequently failing to achieve the resolution that both doctors and patients desire and work toward. Seeking closure, suffering patients try to emplot the outcome that is archetypically provided by the narrative format. Patients find themselves repeating or revising the scripts they use with doctors, re-enacting their suffering and attempting different strategies to recruit the medical practitioner into their desire for a closure of the script/narrative. This can take the form of the quest for a diagnosis, as was Lisa's preoccupation, but even after diagnosis, pervasive uncertainty about the future trajectory of illness can keep resolution elusive. At this stage, sufferers are frequently seen by others around them as violating the 'sick role' by the longevity of their pain and its lack of resolution.[19] This frustrates everybody involved. For many patients with chronic conditions, the anticipated narrative resolution (in the shape of a diagnosis, cure, or treatment) never comes. The stakes of the 'performance' in the exam room, whether by doctor or patient, are thus very high. When the encounter fails – to provide a diagnosis, to proffer a cure, or, perhaps most crucially of all, to help a patient live with the weight of their ongoing suffering – the impact reverberates beyond the clinical setting.

There is potential here for a counter-thread in performance theory, one that could furnish a different contribution to medical practice. To do so, we will need to foreground a critical perspective reflecting on these meta-narratives – and on their power to recruit patients and doctors into often unfulfillable hopes for healing. Turning to post-dramatic or existentialist theatre can illuminate a version of performance that fosters presence, rather than distance, between doctors and patients. This approach provides a more supple and accommodating model for patients to cope with the unresolvable realities of chronic

[18] See, e.g., Case and Brauner, 'The Doctor as Performer'; Taylor, 'The Moral Aesthetic of Simulated Suffering'.

[19] See the introduction for a discussion of the 'sick role' as formulated by Talcott Parsons.

conditions, offering not an artificial creation of closure but a reorientation towards suffering itself.

In live theatre, an actor is not in mortal danger, even if their character is. However, there is always a risk – felt by both the actor and the audience – that they might mess it up or perform badly. This liveness, this excruciating openness to vulnerability, this willingness to be exposed in front of others, is why we celebrate theatre actors (and why many of us continue to attend live theatre performances in the era of Netflix). In Philip's experience as a theatre director, most stage actors strive to eliminate feelings of self-doubt and vulnerability before stepping in front of an audience. But from the perspective of a play's director, the opposite is true. To excel, a skilled theatre actor must embrace vulnerability and confront the possibility of failure – not only within their character's narrative but also in their own craft. They must collaborate with others who are similarly navigating the tensions of uncertainty and the very real risk of failure.[20]

In other words, it's the reality of live performance encounters, not (just) the script, that generates connection, transformation and breakthrough in live theatre. This approach, rooted in post-dramatic acting theory (though central to many other approaches to acting as well) underscores that the lived, unpredictable actuality of the performance is what creates the magic of the stage: an understanding that conflicts with common metaphors or persistent stereotypes about acting in much of mainstream theatre and the medical humanities. These encounters can also enable the basic goals of much theatre-inspired medical education, of improving communication ability and creating empathy. However, without being rooted in a politics of presence and a recognition of doctors' fallibility – a vulnerability they share with their patients – the application of role-playing and other theatre-adjacent encounters in medical education will continue to reproduce the hierarchical structures and erasures it has always reinforced.

Being open to the possibility of failure forces an actor to stay fully present, giving their performance a resilience in unscripted moments which builds connection. An actor, according to this method, should not anticipate rehearsed outcomes, but must observe and respond to the real events happening in the room – whether expected, unexpected, ideal, or otherwise. Accepting these failures and their unanticipated complications allows the actor to transform them into an unforeseen form of success. When an actor responds authentically to an unplanned event, the reality of their character's experience continues

---

[20] See, for example, Herbert Blau, *Blooded Thought: Occasions of Theatre*; Nic Ridout, *Stage Fright, Animals, and Other Theatrical Problems*; Brett Gamboa, *Shakespeare's Double Plays*, among other commentaries, for discussions of how failure, uncertainty and vulnerability are constitutive of theatre.

uninterrupted. The substance of the world experienced by the actors and audience will swerve, but connections are maintained, and a story continues (albeit in some way different than planned, or desired). In contrast, if a rehearsed outcome fails to materialize, and the actor refuses to see it, acknowledge it and respond to it, their connections to themselves, the other actors, the audience and the story are abruptly severed. Such a rupture may only last a few moments, but can compound across a performance when the actor retreats inside themselves to adhere to their vision of what they wish was happening. Ironically, by shutting themselves off in an effort to ensure success, the actor instead guarantees further ruptures, unravelling their performance. While others in the room – actors, audience, or directors – might attempt to ignore these disruptions, doing so comes at the cost of authentic engagement with the performance's unfolding reality.

To achieve this presence, an actor must be willing to be vulnerable when they step on stage. They are exposed to the possibility of things not going as planned, to making mistakes, to the mistakes of others, and any number of external variables beyond their control. They must relinquish certainty and embrace not yet knowing how things will unfold. This does not mean ceding professional authority or competence. But it does prepare them to deal with unexpected events. This requires tolerating a state of tension in which uncertainty defines their work. The conditions of their performance are not comfortable: they are unstable and unpredictable. Being present, acknowledging uncertainty, means the actor will experience stress and suffering.

Their work is hard. How does an actor train for this hard work? A script is, essentially, a plan. But here's the rub: actors exclusively trained in script-based rehearsal are much more likely to believe things will, and should, go as planned. In contrast, actors trained in improvisation, existentialist, or post-dramatic approaches understand that their most valuable skill is staying present. This presence requires a deep connection with both oneself and others. It demands being able to observe and respond to what is in the room. When such actors do perform a script, they can both execute a plan and respond to the unexpected. Rehearsal helps them master the plan while anticipating that things will deviate from the plan. By heroically embracing this contradiction, they can pursue a set of goals, a narrative, an outcome, while also allowing space for variation in every encounter. Each performance, like each patient, and each clinical presentation, is different, but maintains authenticity and hence is laden with signifying power: the potential for making meaning.

The prevalent emphasis in the medical humanities on learning and performing scripts not only fails to prepare the doctor to improvise, it can create deeper fissures and misrecognitions between patients and practitioners. This, as Janelle Taylor observed, produces conditions wherein script-based training leads doctors to 'inoculate' or inure themselves *against* their own empathy – the opposite of the medical humanities' goals.[21]

The key insight we want to apply here arises from the recognition that it is not just patients or 'actual' people who suffer: both doctors and actors risk forms of failure that make them vulnerable, but also create opportunities for genuine presence, connection and, ultimately, narrative meaning-making.[22] Effective doctors, like effective actors, learn to harness this vulnerability to create meaning that resonates for actual people who suffer 'in the real world'. Ultimately, we argue that doctors' willingness to acknowledge their limitations can serve the patients in their quest to alleviate suffering. While there is undeniable value in using pre-existing 'well-made' dramatic narratives to shape and give meaning to medical experiences and to shifts in embodiment, we argue that adapting theatre to medicine must also incorporate additional, alternative techniques and practices.

BREAKING THROUGH THE SCRIPTS: CREATING PRESENCE AMIDST ANOTHER MEDICAL ERROR

A few months after Bianca's last consultation with Dr Walker, she underwent the peri-acetabular osteotomy at an elite, private London hospital.[23] Surgery went as expected, and Bianca woke up in recovery, groggy but painless with both intravenous medication and a catheterized pain pump at the incision site, which numbed her pelvis and leg. Philip was also in her private room when Mr Bates came to do his post-operative assessment. This involved having Bianca wiggle her toes, move her legs and then gently lift each knee off the bed. But try though she might, she couldn't make the right knee move at all.

Another doctor arrived, along with two nurses. A huddled consultation followed another assessment, and then Mr Bates told us his concern that the femoral motor nerve didn't seem to be firing. There could be a series of reasons for this, but the first course of action was to remove Bianca's local anaesthetic

[21] Taylor, 'The Moral Aesthetics of Simulated Suffering', 134.

[22] Heather Nichol et al., 'Navigating the Paradox: Exploring Resident Experiences of Vulnerability', *Postgraduate Medical Education* 58 (2024): 1469–77.

[23] It is worth noting that patients in the National Health Service (NHS) in the UK, which is funded through general taxation, would almost certainly encounter a different level of care than in the private hospital system we accessed, and we don't wish to present our experience as normative. While we aim to draw a broader lesson from our experience in an exclusive system, the principles are inclusive for all carers: the presence, vulnerability, modesty and tolerance for irresolution demonstrated by Mr Bates is a disposition and an ethic that everyone involved in healthcare can cultivate. Finally, Mr Bates also performs this surgery in the NHS system (at a different hospital), maintaining both public and private practices simultaneously. Many patients Bianca interviewed undertook their initial referral to Bates through the private system for the faster timeline, then switched back to his services in the public one for the operation itself.

pump. 'It's possible that the catheter is right on the femoral nerve and is numbing it such that signals can't travel to your leg', he explained.

Mr Bates came by later that evening to check if the leg had returned to normal function. He was there again first thing in the morning and continued to check on her multiple times throughout each subsequent day. On the third day after the surgery, Mr Bates came into the room, asked Philip to sit down and told us that it was now apparent there had been significant damage to Bianca's femoral nerve during the procedure. While the damage would likely reverse itself fully or partially, this would take time – likely many months – and would radically complicate her recovery from the osteotomy. She would be unable to use any of her quads muscles, to extend her knee or flex her thigh at the hip joint, or to bear weight during the recovery – a fact that could (and indeed did) affect her bone growth in repairing the cuts in her pelvic bones created by the surgery. One of those breaks has never fully closed, leaving her with a permanent non-union fracture.

Although Mr Bates had of course dealt with patients who experienced complications from surgery before, this particular issue was novel terrain for him. Motor nerve damage is always possible with an osteotomy, but despite doing between forty and seventy of these procedures each year during a long career, he had never had a patient emerge with this issue and he couldn't figure out what on earth had gone wrong in this case.

As a specialist surgical consultant, Mr Bates was well trained with a repertoire of medical scripts to manage the communication of bad news. Most such scripts emphasize speaking with compassion, being gentle, ensuring the patient has family there to help absorb the news, focusing on positive next steps and emphasizing whatever hope might be possible. Mr Bates more or less adhered to those best practices, proving in many ways the opposite of Dr Walker's blunt and even combative communication style. But when Mr Bates tried to inform us of the diagnosis and prognosis, neither of us reacted. Nobody had read *us* the script for this sort of event. In a bizarre moment of inversion, Mr Bates found himself having to convince us that this was a major complication, to elicit an affective response that demonstrated we recognized the import of what he was saying. After his initial long explanation was met by our blank stares, he urged in a pleading tone, 'I need you both to understand that this is really, really bad.' This was not part of his original script, and in fact was the opposite in tone and content from the positive, compassionate recitation he had just narrated. The moment of delivery of bad news was marked by his clear display of distress, concern and his effort not to downplay the seriousness. It was also marked by his ability to throw out the script and improvise.

The medical script also did not dictate what he did next, though his affective response continued to shape ours. The following evening, a Saturday, Mr Bates came into the hospital even though he had previously said he wouldn't be working. He felt compelled to check on Bianca. That morning he had been driving with his wife to a wedding, he said, and had to pull over off the highway, on the verge of tears, to take deep breaths. He told us he felt so wracked with responsibility that he couldn't focus on the road. For Bianca in particular, that expression of shared suffering was an immense source of support, one that continued to comfort her during the months and years that followed. She read him as expressing solidarity and partnership in the arduous recovery ahead of us.

But as we reflect on those early days after the surgery, we realize that Mr Bates wasn't exactly expressing empathy with us. Instead, he was admitting his sense of vulnerability at his own error. Still, that created presence and connection. Even though his communication style was radically different from Dr Walker's, both proved able to grapple with the narcissistic injury from a medical error and to acknowledge their fallibility. What Mr Bates did extraordinarily well was to be present with his affective reactions and not to try to defend, downplay, or dismiss his responsibility. In responding to his ego damage by acknowledging that he, too, shared vulnerability and suffered alongside us, Mr Bates effectively parlayed our capacity to cope with a paralysed leg. The creation of connection was highly effective – Bianca felt compelled by what seemed to be an experience of shared suffering and shared vulnerability. He hurt Bianca; Bianca was hurt by him; and this hurt him too; both were implicated in the tragedy of the situation. Mr Bates never attempted to distance himself from responsibility for the mistake. In fact, he even expressed doubt when other specialists opined that it was Bianca's Ehlers–Danlos Syndrome that had ultimately caused the problem, not anything he had personally done or failed to do.[24]

Bates's reaction wasn't only emotional, it is crucial to note; he took important and concrete actions. Cheryl Mattingly's argument that action also crafts narrative is relevant here.[25] He gave us his personal cell phone number, set up appointments with a prominent neurologist consultant and a pain specialist, wrote prescriptions for the vomiting and nausea that were caused by

[24]The explanation suggested by an anesthetist was – in layman's terms – that Bianca's Ehlers–Danlos Syndrome rendered her collagen too elastic to provide resistance to overstretching during the procedure. The motor nerve ripped because it is composed of fibers that could not stretch like the rest of her connective tissue. Mr Bates did not challenge that medical explanation on its merits, but when Bianca discussed this theory with him, he did not embrace the absolution of responsibility that she thought it offered him. Then, a year after she returned to Toronto, her Canadian neurologists discovered both that she had damage to a second motor nerve (the obturator) and that her body was rejecting the titanium screws, which they believed were now causing the pressure palsy on the obturator. While Bates immediately offered to operate to fix the issue, he said he thought the obturator damage had likely been from his original procedure, and claimed responsibility even though colleagues in Canada thought it was not 'his fault'.

[25]Mattingly, 'The Concept of Therapeutic "Emplotment"'.

Bianca's parasympathetic nervous system's response to the nerve damage, saw her at least monthly during the following six months in which we remained in London, weighed in on imaging and nerve conduction test results after we returned to Canada, and eventually performed a second surgery on Bianca a couple of years later (and at a slightly reduced cost) when that proved necessary. He also significantly changed his intake consent forms, as Bianca later discovered, to include detailed and protracted discussion of the risks of nerve damage. The assumption of shared vulnerability created a narrative bond that supported Bianca long after the medical event had passed.

FROM NARRATIVE BOND TO ANTI-NARRATIVE

Both Mr Bates and Dr Walker, in their very different affective responses, allowed themselves to struggle with and be open to their vulnerability to medical error. If the account we have told is compelling, it is precisely because it has elements of dramatic narratives, with twists, turns, complications and satisfying moments of denouement. We know the appeal of these kinds of medical tales. In fact, the costs we faced from two self-paid surgeries in London were offset by a crowd-funding effort that several of our friends set up – without Bianca's foreknowledge – which raised about $30,000 in the space of two weeks.[26] This is a testament to the profound kindness of our community; it is also, inescapably, a testament to the power of these kinds of narratives.

But our story has not ended with the tidy resolution we want from our medical dramas. The promise Mr Bates had made of being able to ameliorate Bianca's pain proved mostly true: she is in far less pain today, has a more active life and was able to carry a baby to term (things that often seemed totally out of reach during the years seeking diagnosis and treatment). Since her surgeries, she has twice completed an open water swim from Alcatraz Island to mainland San Francisco. But she still walks with a forearm crutch and a limp, and the nerve-damaged leg still sometimes collapses under her, recently causing long-term tissue damage to one of her fingers during the subsequent fall. On a regular basis, both of us encounter friends and acquaintances who ask why Bianca 'still' needs a gait aid, or express confusion about 'when' she will be 'normal' again. This is the effect of the narrative promise we have bought into, that medicine solves suffering and makes people better. Of course, we all know many medical problems do not resolve. While elements of Bianca's experience – misdiagnosis, medical error and surgical complications – form a compelling story, only small parts of our lives over the last ten years qualify as contributing toward

[26]We were and are deeply moved by such generosity from friends, family and total strangers. For us, that care was the most profoundly meaningful part of this ordeal.

a coherent plot. The lack of narrative resolution is disappointing not only to us, but also to our broader social networks. A relatively young and otherwise fit person relying on a mobility aid represents 'matter out of place', to borrow anthropologist Mary Douglas's phrase.[27]

The challenges of unresolved stories differ for doctors, patients and their social networks, but we are all enmeshed in a collective mythology and propaganda around medicine's ability to heal. The disavowal of suffering is understandable; it is difficult to experience, anticipate experiencing and to witness. Doctors may seek greater distance through appearing to be unhelpful or unsympathetic, or by discharging a patient altogether. Patients, in turn, may keep trying with another doctor, or grow ever more desperate to perform their suffering such that its authenticity is recognized. Ultimately, doctors' and patients' mutual goal of seeking health is not well served by rote, depersonalized scripts, which break down in the face of the uncertainty and terror of illness. Instead, what Kleinman might call the 'awe of illness' demands our presence as individuals, as people who are open to a deep sense of each other's humanity. By acknowledging the reality of inconclusive suffering we might in fact find ways to go on, bearing the non-resolution with humour and a determined commitment to holding human connection.

Although viewing medicine through the lens of theatre helps doctors to recognize illness narratives as valuable in treating patients, we crave space to resist the ingrained cultural belief that performance is only 'successful' when it culminates in narrative resolution. As our own unresolved story underscores, a focus on scripts returns us to the conundrum of inherited expectations about theatrical performance. As a medical anthropologist and a theatre director and psychotherapist, we are attuned to the performances that caregivers give and how patients respond to them – and, of course, we are unusual patients in that regard. We also know well theatre's capacity to innovate out of static conventions, tapping insight or creativity found in the becoming-together of presence. The performance theory derived from Philip's craft as a director, which emphasizes presence and connection among the ensemble to prepare for the unexpected, has tremendous potential for doctors seeking a method to stay in the story when it 'fails' to reach the conventional resolution of healing or recovery. Alongside the tools of narrative medicine, then, a more impactful or comprehensive training for doctors might equip them to develop and maintain presence with their patients.

This could have a profound outcome for patients. Although our story did not unfold as anyone had hoped, the sense of collaboration and respect for Bianca's agency when she experienced a doctor truly being present with her

[27] Mary Douglas, *Purity and Danger* (Routledge & Kegan Paul; repr. 2002).

became crucial in helping her cope with pain and disability. Presence runs both ways in the medical encounter, opening space for subjectivity and agency on the part of a suffering patient: acceptance and endurance, though difficult, can foster profound connections and a deeper humanity in both patients and doctors. The medical humanities could do well to coach medical practitioners to have a different confrontation with their own – and their patients' – vulnerability.

REFERENCES

Allain, Paul, and Jen Harvie. *The Routledge Companion to Theatre and Performance*. Routledge, 2014.

Beckett, Samuel. *Endgame*. Faber & Faber, 2012.

Case, Gretchen A., and Daniel J. Brauner. 'Perspective: The Doctor as Performer: A Proposal for Change Based on a Performance Studies Paradigm'. *Academic Medicine* 85, no. 1 (2010): 159–63.

Colas, Kelly. 'Unexpected Intimacies: An Exploration of the Physician–Patient Relationship during the COVID-19 Pandemic'. *Anthropology in Action* 27, no. 2 (2020): 20–7.

Douglas, Mary. *Purity and Danger*. Routledge & Kegan Paul, 1966. Repr. 2002.

Dumit, Joe. 'Pharmaceutical Witnessing: Drugs for Life in an Era of Direct-to-Consumer Advertising'. In *Technologized Images, Technologized Bodies*, edited by Jeanette Edwards, Penelope Harvey and Peter Wade. Berghahn Books, 2010.

Fainzang, Sylvie. *An Anthropology of Lying: Information in the Doctor–Patient Relationship*. Routledge, 2015.

Goldman, Marlene. *The Social, Aesthetic, and Medical Implications of Performing Shame: Interdisciplinary Approaches*. Routledge, 2023.

Good, Mary-Jo Delvecchio. 'Cultural Studies of Biomedicine: An Agenda for Research'. *Social Science & Medicine* 41, no. 4 (1995): 461–73.

Harries, Martin. *Forgetting Lot's Wife: On Destructive Spectatorship*. Fordham, 2007.

Jeffrey, David Ian. *How Shakespeare Inspires Empathy in Clinical Care*. Palgrave Macmillan, 2024.

Kalitzkus, Vera, and Peter F. Matthiessen. 'Narrative-Based Medicine: Potential, Pitfalls, and Practice'. *Permanente Journal* 13, no. 1 (2009): 80–6.

Kelm, Zak, James Womer, Jennifer K. Walter and Chris Feudtner. 'Interventions to Cultivate Physician Empathy: A Systematic Review'. *BMC Medical Education* 14 (2014): 1–11.

Kleinman, Arthur. *The Illness Narratives: Suffering, Healing, and the Human Condition*. Basic Books, 1988. Repr. 2020.

Lehmann, Hans-Thies. Post-Dramatic Theatre. Translated by Karen Jurs-Munby. Routledge, 2006.

Mattingly, Cheryl. 'The Concept of Therapeutic "Emplotment"'. *Social Science & Medicine* 38, no. 6 (1994): 811–22.

Neumann, Melanie, Friedrich Edelhäuser, Diethard Tauschel, Martin R. Fischer, Markus Wirtz, Christiane Woopen, Aviad Haramati and Christian Scheffer. 'Empathy Decline and Its Reasons: A Systematic Review of Studies with Medical Students and Residents'. *Academic Medicine* 86, no. 8 (2011): 996–1009.

Nichol, Heather, Jennifer Turnnidge, Nancy Dalgarno and Jessica Trier. 'Navigating the Paradox: Exploring Resident Experiences of Vulnerability'. *Postgraduate Medical Education* 58 (2024): 1469–77. https://doi.org/10.1111/medu.15426.

Nie, Jing-Bao, Yu Cheng, Xiang Zou, Ni Gong, Joseph D. Tucker, Bonnie Wong and Arthur Kleinman. 'The Vicious Circle of Patient–Physician Mistrust in China: Health Professionals' Perspectives, Institutional Conflict of Interest, and Building Trust Through Medical Professionalism'. *Developing World Bioethics* 18, no. 1 (2018): 26–36.

Pasquini, Mirko. 'Mistrustful Dependency: Mistrust as Risk Management in an Italian Emergency Department'. *Medical Anthropology* 42, no. 6 (2023): 579–92. https://doi.org/10.1080/01459740.2023.2240942.

Power, Cormac. *Presence in Play: A Critique of Theories of Presence in the Theatre*. Editions Rodopi, 2008.

Schmidt-Sane, Megan, Elizabeth Storer, Santiago Ripoll and Tabitha Hrynick. 'Exploring Medical Mistrust: From Clinic to Community'. *Journal of the British Academy* 11, no. 6 (2023): 1–12.

Stefanello, Eugenia. 'Your Pain Is Not Mine: A Critique of Clinical Empathy'. *Bioethics* 36 (2022): 486–93. https://doi.org/10.1111/bioe.12980.

Taylor, Janelle S. 'The Moral Aesthetics of Simulated Suffering in Standardized Patient Performances'. *Culture, Medicine and Psychiatry* 35, no. 2 (2011): 134–62.

Treichler, Paula. *How to Have Theory in an Epidemic: Cultural Chronicles of AIDS*. Duke University Press, 1999.

PART THREE

Caregivers

Caregivers are essential members of the ensemble who are often overlooked in descriptions of care that focus on the doctor and the patient to the exclusion of the vast network that enfolds them. In this section, several experienced caregivers occupy centre-stage. The three caregivers featured here draw on theatre and performance as metaphors, as practices, as supplementary training and as rhetorical tools. They also deliver much-needed direction to their fellow caregivers, doctors and patients. To frame the stakes of our project and these caregivers' original and important perspectives, we draw on the insights of literary theorist Lauren Berlant (1957–2021), who recently died of cancer during the COVID epidemic. Her writings provide an invaluable foundation for reimagining contemporary forms of care and caregiving – for self and the other – during health crises. Berlant, who so often has her eyes on questions of what makes life worth living (or not worth living), enables us to recognize how structures designed to save us may also be complicit in destroying us – spiritually, and often bodily.

Berlant's recognition that something we desire and, in some cases, require can be antithetical to our flourishing or even survival highlights the stakes of our performative intervention. In her view, people become attached to ideals or fantasies of 'the good life', even when these ideals are unattainable or harmful. The American Dream, for example, constitutes a form of cruel optimism instigated by the entropic and withering forces of neoliberal capitalism. According to Berlant, we cling to impossible dreams as a survival strategy in a world that has increasingly limited people's real-world agency. In the context of healthcare, in Berlant's view, the most serious threat conveyed by illness and disease is 'the revelation that … one has only been loaned a name and biography and personality and meaningfulness, and that that loan could be recalled not just by death, but by the cruel forces of life'.[1] Although these forces may be random, they are also frequently 'predictable, systematic, and world-saturating'.[2]

As the three interviews that follow attest, properly understood, care can partly counter the structural 'cruel forces of life'. While it includes attention and instrumental and mechanical tinkering with the body, care also prompts performative gestures, rituals and intimate conversation that preserve and even enhance personhood in the face of annihilating and depersonalizing structures that mobilize around people coping with illness and disease. Care opens a space in which we paradoxically become 'both stranger and intimate' to ourselves.[3] In the liminal space of illness and caregiving prior identities and attachments mutate, and that also affords the potential to connect with ourselves and people who care for us, with a newfound mutual awareness of vulnerability.

As the caregivers who explore their histories and their approach to caregiving confirm, illness can prompt what Berlant calls a 'desperately improvised pedagogical process' that includes a space for unlearning unkindness.[4] During this process, previously healthy people learn how to assume the illness role and how to suffer. Their friends and family must also learn how to collaborate with someone who is suffering without effacing themselves or the other person. For the caregivers interviewed in this section, this vertiginous, defamiliarizing intra- and interpersonal process of character deformation and reformation is part of their (extra)ordinary experience.

These experiences also resonate affectively, and caregivers must regularly cope with overlapping affects of care including resentment, joy, compassion, uncertainty, numbness and exhaustion, often all at the same time. Consciously and unconsciously, caregivers turn to theatre for guidance because theatre does not merely accommodate contradictory affects, it normalizes complex responses. The caregivers featured here likewise draw on theatre's affective capaciousness and its tolerance for ambiguity and ambivalence.

In the service of healing, the contributors featured in this section deploy an array of improvised, embodied, performative tactics. Reflecting on the performative elements of her role, Adele Vogelsang, a nurse, explains that like a seasoned improv actor, she had an uncanny gift for walking into a room, recognizing the dynamic qualities of the situation and joining the action. Recalling Berlant's emphasis on the life-sustaining qualities of conversation, Vogelsang

[1] Lauren Berlant, *Cruel Optimism* (Duke University Press, 2011), 91.
[2] Ibid
[3] Ibid., 61.
[4] Ibid., 58.

repeatedly accepted the task given to her by doctors, who were unwilling or unable to initiate an intimate conversation, of inviting her patients to reflect on their performance of the illness role and how they might want to modify it to enhance its curative and healing effects. Thanks to her willingness to intervene, what would otherwise have amounted to a stern monologue from the doctor was transformed into a compassionate dialogue that restored both personhood and agency to frightened and angry patients, who were often not merely coping with illness, but also with stigma and shame.

In addition to underscoring the inherently embodied, theatrical dimensions of caregiving, Vogelsang's insights balance the first section's approach to presence. She reveals, for instance, the way that a caregiver – particularly a female nurse – needs to oscillate between affording presence and setting boundaries to avoid becoming the target of overly intimate or inappropriate comments and gestures. Put differently, the systemic violence that threatens to diminish the patient's personhood also takes its toll on caregivers.

The theme of violence links all three interviews. George Anderson, an experienced home aide, explains how he brings to his practice of caregiving a lifelong, first-hand knowledge of the ongoing shattering of the sovereign self. This ongoing crisis was something he experienced early on as a child sentenced to adult prison, and, later, as a caregiver to wealthy, entitled, cantankerous, terminally ill men – many of whom were former Harvard professors. Anderson's clients were teachers thrust into the role of student, forced to relinquish control and learn how to suffer and die.

Our final contributor in this section, Marcus Coates, is a performance artist who has worked with and on behalf of communities to imagine solutions to seemingly intractable social problems. His practice is situated between social and personal care and the arts. It inspires us because, in keeping with Berlant's emphasis on healing as opposed to cure, it complements traditional western medicine by offering patients opportunities to restage and, in the process, reinterpret their experience of illness and the psychological and physical violence associated with stigma, and shame. As our interview with Coates demonstrates, the patients in palliative care and recovering psychotics who work with him unlearn unkindness and regain a sense of agency. His collaborators are frequently patients who are usually unavailable to conversation as conventionally understood. This partly explains why he offers up his own body as a medium and a projective surface for their experiences.

The collective value of these caregivers' performances lies in their ability to 'operate' differently than the doctor–patient clinical encounter. To some extent, they serve as a goad and a guide to doctors – a supplement to clinical care and, at times, a force that influences it. In contrast to doctors who are leashed to evidence-based medicine, engaging with things that can be measured and tested, caregivers have more opportunity to rely on conversation, ritual and embodied gestures to engage the intellect and the imagination in the service of healing.

REFERENCE

Berlant, Lauren. *Cruel Optimism*. Duke University Press, 2011.

7

Nursing tactics: Voice, touch, scent

AN INTERVIEW WITH ADELE VOGELSANG

In accounts of the clinical performance, scholars focus almost exclusively on the doctor–patient dyad, eliding the crucial role played by nurses and their insights into bedside manner. To remedy this oversight concerning the ensemble drama of illness, we turned to Adele Vogelsang, an inpatient nurse in Boston, Massachusetts. (She requested that we refer to her pseudonymously.) This print interview is based on many hours of conversation with her, two recorded interviews and her published writing. Vogelsang presents her unique, embodied and largely improvisational approach to the drama of inpatient life. She explores the ways she has been both an actor and director, sometimes explicitly coaching doctors and patients on better ways to present themselves and interact with each other.

Vogelsang's nursing experience began early, as she began caring for sick family members at the age of six. She got her first job as a nurse's aide in a nursing home when she was only fourteen, having reported her age as sixteen. After nursing school, Vogelsang worked on neuroscience and oncology wards for over forty-five years. Although she describes the skills she relied on in nursing as instincts honed in childhood, she is also articulate about the way she has used her voice, gestures and even nursing uniform to help patients. In addition to her nursing degree, Vogelsang trained as an opera singer (Boston Conservatory of Music) and was well known for singing to patients as a way of calming or inspiring them. Outside the hospital, Vogelsang works as a fragrance journalist and award-winning writer on the science of scent. She continues to professionally evaluate and collaborate with perfumers. Her expertise in this area likewise contributed to her skillset as a nurse. On the wards, she could discern the smells of specific microorganisms, stages of disease and experiences of fear and pain. She describes her use of perfume with her patients as restrained – 'insidious and innocuous' – but effective in calming pain and anxiety.

Whereas the prevailing view in medical education holds that doctors must hone their empathic skills to establish greater intimacy and trust, Vogelsang's childhood experiences alerted her to the opposing need to establish boundaries with patients and clinicians that she can expand and contract as necessary. Vogelsang's improvisational strategy constitutes a tactical play between closeness and distance, tactics that recall performance scholar Joseph Roach's insight into what we look for in actors, namely, presence and 'unbiddability' associated with the actor's charismatic relationship with the audience – an enigmatic oscillation between presence and absence.[1]

I. PREPARATION AND PERFORMANCE

Can you tell us what performances, personae and tactics a nurse needs to bring to the job?

Adele Vogelsang (AV): As a child, tact was absolutely essential for my wellbeing. Having honed this skill caring for family members, I knew nursing was going to be a piece of cake for me.

Can you give an example of a clinical situation that called for tact?

AV: Once I met with a very young patient on behalf of the attending doctor who was too busy and likely too uncomfortable to approach the patient himself. The young man was still in high school, but he had developed neurosyphilis because he didn't practise safe sex. His mother was with him, and he was very anxious. Having been the mother of two gay sons, I sat down, and I said, 'You are aware what you're here for, right?' We talked about it, and I said, 'I don't want you to be embarrassed. I'm a mother. I've got sons like you. And we have lots of the same things we had to discuss. One thing, however, that is really critical is, going forward, it would be really helpful if you insert anything anywhere to cover it up first.' This very shy boy broke out in laughter. His

[1] Joseph Roach, *It* (University of Michigan Press, 2007), 178.

mother was immensely relieved. And I said, 'Really, this is all that anyone is asking you to consider before you have any kind of sexual relations.'

Did you need to prepare yourself physically or mentally before you approached the young man, or did you have to think about how you needed to perform or your role before going to enter the room?

AV: All of my experience and my life experience prepared me for it. I've always had a gift for walking in cold into a really conflagratory or potentially conflagratory situation and being able to defuse it. I didn't really need any preparation. I didn't really know the young man, I just happened to pick him up on my morning assignment. And this was early in the day, like 8 o'clock, when doctors round. I made the decision that the doctor was already burdened, and this was something I could handle for him. Nothing will stand you in good stead better than previous experience and understanding of the disease entity. So that's where I come from.

For the most part, my job was to walk into a room and read the situation – emotionally – to sense what was going on. The only times I felt that I needed to perform or assume a persona is when I was handed patients that no one else wanted to touch, including physicians. And people who didn't know anything about boundaries. There were occasions when I actually had to use a name tag that said *Mrs V.* instead of my first name. As Mrs V., I was no less sympathetic, I was no less kind, but I was very aware that if I was going to deal effectively for myself and for the patient – for their wellbeing – I had to set that little boundary. Because if you can't call somebody by their first name, that sets the playing field there.

I didn't like having to set those boundaries. But sometimes that was the only way to manage very difficult, untenable situations. That for me was performance. Also with physicians with whom I did not see eye to eye or get along with.

You've explained how you've used performance to impose boundaries, and that you've brought props like name tags into those performances. Are there other aspects of self-presentation that you bring to your work as a nurse?

AV: The only part of performance that I totally endorsed was how I presented myself to the patients. Now, I have never come in like an unmade bed. I always felt that I owed it to my patients and to my fellow staff to come in hygienic, pleasant, in a decent humour, so that the patient had a sense that here's a person who has some self-respect and respect for me because they're not coming in looking like they just had been out all night. That part of performance is important. I think it gives the patients confidence, and it gives the physicians confidence.

At work I made it an absolute point that I wore a buttoned-up uniform I had received in nursing school. For a celebration of the school's centennial, they gave us all a variation of Florence Nightingale's uniform. It had black and white gingham, a pinny that was starched, black lace-up clinic shoes and black stockings, without the seams at the back. It had seven-button cuffs (see Figure 7.1).

All the other hospital nurses had fancy little nursey shoes and short skirts. I walked around in black clinic shoes, and everything I wore was below the knee and buttoned up to the chin. I had really long hair almost down to my knees, and could get a migraine from braiding it into a tight bun above my high collar. I made sure that I looked like someone to be treated with a certain degree of respect.

II. LEARNING HOW TO ACT

In previous conversations, you mentioned a powerful role model at your first job at the nursing home when you were fourteen. Can you tell us more about her and her influence on your personae as a nurse?

AV: Yes, she'd been an army nurse – a career army nurse. She was efficient and compassionate and wonderful. She was a little Irish lady in her sixties, hard as nails, who wore white clinic shoes. The administrators called her 'Peanut the Cop' because she was just the tiniest thing of a woman. She knew what she wanted and what she expected of her assisted personnel. This woman was the soul of compassion with patients, no matter how challenging they were. Her speech with us might have been clipped and terse, but her approach with the patients was something to see. I thought, 'That's the kind of person I want to be.'

So you've modelled your performances on nurses you admire. Have you also served as a model to others?

AV: There were several physicians over the years who knew their shortcomings. There were times when I would privately say, 'Would you object if I helped communicate what you wanted to say to the patient?' And they would say, 'Oh please, I'm so uncomfortable.' So then there would be the attending doctor and myself with the patient in a conference, and I would be translating what the doctor said, and also presenting it in a more compassionate way.

Did you ever have to counsel a patient on how to perform to ensure she received appropriate care?

AV: Oh yes! I recall having a very histrionic, very Goth, and very opinionated female patient who was gravely ill, and her doctor asked me to teach her how

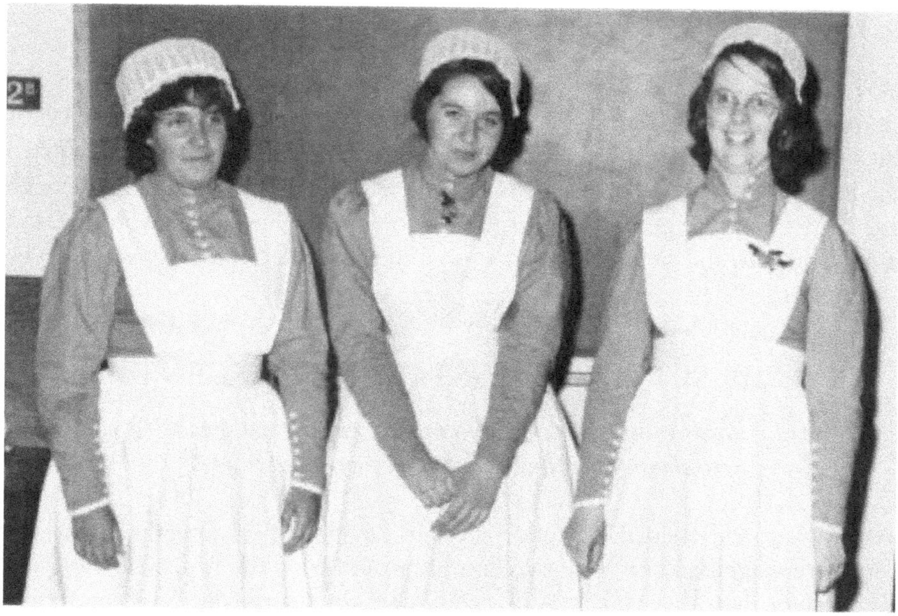

FIGURE 7.1 Classmates of Adele Vogelsang, buttoned into in the Massachusetts General Hospital of Nursing School's 1973 centennial uniform. Courtesy of the Massachusetts General Hospital Archives & Special Collections.

to interact with her medical team. He was a well-meaning but exasperated male doctor. He took me aside and said, 'Can you have a word with this young lady? Because I recognize that her illness is absolutely bona fide, but the rest of the team are not willing to take her seriously.' I had to sit down and very gently explain to her about how the system works. That it is unfair, and that women still, to this day, suffer and are questioned more than men about the veracity of their suffering.

With her, I developed a rapport very early because I'm not very judgemental. Yes, she had a Goth appearance and told people she was a witch. She had scary opinions, and it was off-putting. I sat down with her and said, 'I was just talking to the attending, the lead doctor on your team, and he believes that something is seriously wrong with you. His concern and mine is that women who present themselves as in any way challenging to male doctors – and sometimes female doctors – tend to be overlooked, and he wants you to get the care that you need.'

'Perhaps you could be a little less confrontational and think about it before you speak. If you can do that, I think that they will hear you. Right now we have a bunch of people who aren't listening to you and they're not hearing you. That's unfair, and it shouldn't be, but we want you to get the care that you need.' And that was how I approached it.

Was it just female patients, or did female nurses also need coaching?

AV: Yes, I saw a lot of lovely young women go through getting harassed and dumped by doctors, and it was painful to watch. I started work in the 1970s and the early 1980s, and it was a different environment – the whole sexual environment was very different. I did try to help support these girls through the stuff they were going through. I tried to advise them that maybe it wasn't a good idea to shit where you eat. I put it kindly because nobody wants to be dictated to.

III. SETTING THE STAGE WITH SCENT

Can you say more about how your early experience sensitized you to the needs of both female patients and nurses?

AV: As a young child, I had poor eyesight. Smell helped compensate for my terrible eyesight very early on. My mother would open the fridge and hold out a container that was just shy of its expiry date or past the date, and say, 'How long is the milk good for?' And I just would know. I'd say, 'Well, we've got three days for this and two days for that, and it's already off', but nobody else could really smell it.

My household was a very volatile environment. All three adults in that environment could go off at any time. I had to learn very early, probably younger than two, to take the emotional temperature of the household. I learned what their intention was by the cadence of their walks. I learned what kind of odours they emanated and what each augured. I noticed that when adults had certain intentions, they smelled differently. My father smelled a certain way when he was going to be inappropriate with me. My mother smelled a certain way when she was going to beat me.

You've won an award for publishing an article that traces how lavender, gardenias and jasmine mimic the effects of tranquilizing drugs such as Valium on the human brain. Can you tell us how you relied on smell in to change the atmosphere or set the stage in your work with patients?

AV: The main goal is to soothe and appease the savage beast. My approach was to be insidious and innocuous, and I found that with jasmine my colleagues and the patients were more relaxed. I never blew it. I never went too far. You have to be subtle. You have to be judicious in how you approach things. Otherwise, you'll call attention to smells, something that everybody insists they don't want in this current 'perfume and scent free' era.

You've talked about the importance of using scent and the voice with patients and doctors. How did you use touch with patients, many of whom, as you've explained, were fearful of being touched?

AV: I would just very gently, very unobtrusively put my hand on their arm or their shoulder, and I could see their tension melt away. This is part of how I tried to ameliorate the tension in the room, the indecision. It was a lot easier to get information from them or from the family, then, which we needed to complete their history and care for them properly. I never thought of it as being someone else. It was just part of who I am. Being someone else, for me, isn't a 'performance' in the sense of a calculated sequence of actions that's intended to elicit an effect. I'm describing something instinctive – how, from childhood, I was conditioned to act. My instinctive responses are inseparable from the performances I engaged in to survive.

IV. THE VOICE

Besides nursing school, you also did conservatory training as an opera singer. You often sing to your patients. Can you describe how you use your voice – a familiar and beloved tool of all actors?

AV: The voice is everything! If you can channel the right voice for the specific circumstances – soothing, authoritative, friendly – whatever is called for, you can affect all kinds of subtle and not so subtle changes. I would adapt my voice to a soothing tone for people who were extremely agitated. I used my voice as a tool.

I first used it when I was nineteen as a student nurse to help orthopaedic patients in horrible pain – people who were literally held together with pins. My voice could make a patient's pain threshold a little higher than it had been before I walked into the room. Patients were able to tolerate more because they naturally felt soothed, and they felt safe.

Keeping an even, measured tone is helpful. People prefer the lower tones, not necessarily very low, but you don't want to be a squeaker. I use a more mellifluous kind of speech. I actively listen and respond on that level, so the person feels heard, but not in a contrived way, as if I'm trying to mimic or position myself in any way. It's sincere, and it reads as non-threatening and soothing to the often brain-injured individual in the room. You have to reach them on a very primal level.

Can you tell us about the songs you've used to soothe or motivate patients?

AV: I sang a lot of lullabies – not the usual ones, some really fabulous ones – to brain-injured people who were very distressed and perceived my cadence more than my words. But I sang other things, too. I had a patient who was a professor, who had a horrible head injury. He was on a ventilator for months. Most of the nurses had written him off, so he played dead when they came into the room. Then I noticed that his eyes were tracking me. I knew from his family that he lived for baseball and Mozart's *Magic Flute* in German. So I sang *The Magic Flute* to him for months. I sang the whole opera from beginning to end, so many times. Then, one day, he looked like he wanted to talk. I put my finger over his ventilator tube, so he could talk, and he said to me, 'Bei Männern welche Liebe fühlen' ('With men who feel love'). In German, which was not his primary language, he had identified the opera's duet between Pamina and Sarastro.

I used my voice often in hospice care, because it was known that if somebody was brought from the ICU to die on our floor, which happened a lot, I was the best person. They wouldn't give the palliative care patients to the young nurses who were terrified of giving the really strong painkillers to relieve pain or symptoms, so they would under-medicate them. So I'd come in and patients and family were really miserable. I could tell.

Even though I'm an opera singer, I'm not a musical snob. I was open to all kinds of things. I would sing lyrics about the meds I gave patients. When patients needed anxiety medicine, I'd sing to the tune of 'Oh Christmas Tree', 'Lorazepam, lorazepam, do I look like I'd give a damn? I'm going to give you tiny pills, to cure neurotic little ills. Lorazepam, oxazepam, and for the worst … clonazepam.'

I used to make up songs on the spot about diseases. I would sing to get patients motivated to do their physical therapy. We'd do King Julian from the movie *Madagascar*, singing, 'You got to move it, move it! I like to move it, move it.' Then the patient would try and lift the extremity – the song just broke the ice and eased the mood. It made the patient feel, 'Okay, I can do this.'

We also had a lot of seizure patients (we had a special unit for that), and some of them were very frightened of having grand mal, tonic-clonic seizures. Some of them were brain-injured, severely brain-injured. They were so tense. I created a song to Little Eva's *Loco-Motion*. It was called Do the Tonic-Clonic. And so I would march around the patient's room, knowing a seizure was coming, singing, 'Everybody's doing a brand-new dance now. Come on, baby, do the tonic-clonic.' And we would laugh, and it would help them relax.

How did you reach out to people from other cultures?

AV: I grew up in a very diverse neighbourhood. So I was familiar with lots of cultures before there was required cultural competence training; I thought that training was the biggest joke in the world, because my life gave me that training.

I had a Belgian guy from Brussels, who spoke Flemish. He had a difficult family, and they were very upset. I sang a Flemish song very quietly into his ear while I was getting him ready to pass. If he was the least bit sentient, there was the possibility that he would know somebody was taking care of him in a very particular way that would be comforting to him, given his culture.

I could sing in different languages. So even if I couldn't speak to a patient, there was a really good chance that I could sing to them in their natural language, which put them more at ease in an unfamiliar environment that they perceived as hostile culturally. For example, I don't speak Portuguese, but I would try to string together my Italian, my French, whatever Spanish and Ladino on top of that to create an environment where someone just felt, 'Oh, I can breathe. I can be at ease with this person.'

REFERENCE

Roach, Joseph. *It*. University of Michigan Press, 2007.

8

What part of the stage are you standing on?

A CONVERSATION WITH GEORGE ANDERSON

Over 90 per cent of patient care comes not from doctors but home caregivers and nurses, but to date the medical humanities have shamefully neglected their perspectives. Narrative medicine, as Arthur Frank pointed out in *The Wounded Storyteller*, favours plot-based tales of recovery or tragedy. These don't fit the cyclic, repetitive work of care for chronic illness. A better model is the far older theatre of religious ritual, in which daily acts such as cleaning and soothing the patient gain deep meaning because of their recurrence.

This conversational interview was conducted by Alice Flaherty with a home-care provider, George Anderson, whose interactions with patients have been much broader and deeper than that of most physicians. Many doctors, who see a new patient every fifteen to thirty minutes, rely on generic bedside manners that they tailor only slightly for each new patient. They can turn off that manner at the end of each clinic session or when speaking with subordinates. Home aides may spend all day for years with the same client.

Although most home care is provided by women, Anderson tells of his life in a world of mostly male care. His early experiences, in an elite school, reform schools, prisons, farms and as a state mental hospital orderly, were in institutions that stressed custody over care. For the past twenty years he has played an impressively fluid role as a personal companion to a series of elderly and strongly opinionated male academics. Those relationships have been true ensembles of illness, in which care and knowledge radiate both ways.

Anderson has learned to inhabit a remarkable range of personae which he uses to help patients. Rather than view these personae as artful constructs, he describes them as aspects of his true self. In the interview that follows, he offers anecdotes that highlight his ability to integrate his caring persona with an assertive and courageous persona that calls out authority figures who abuse their power. Along with the rituals of daily care, Anderson also creates a meaningful and formal ritual, of which his clients are aware, of writing their eulogy during the last years of their life. After their deaths, he gives his carefully worded but honest eulogy publicly at their memorial service.

The text of this interview draws on many hours of informal conversation with Anderson, two recorded interviews and his written eulogies. We also include an excerpt from written notes he took on interactions with one client, to update the client's wife. George's awareness of the drama of care appears not only in the content of his patient notes, but also in their form. He structured them as a play script that includes dialogue, description, and stage directions.

I. HEALING PERSONAE

Alice Flaherty (AF): George, you've been a caregiver in so many different settings: as a mental health aide, looking after children, taking care of people who are elderly and disabled. Do you have a general term for what you do?

George Anderson (GA): Companion … death doula … I think I'd say my favourite is a companion. I haven't had to do any physical health aid for years. Maybe I would drive my companions somewhere or prepare a meal. I would sit with them. Mostly I have been a companion for elderly men who are faced with end of life issues, basically dying. Some of them, I took care of them for years, and the whole time they were confronting death.

AF: And you got to observe that drama?

GA: I was their companion in it. I learned about their approaching death along with them, what it's like to face it. And I learned about their lives. Life for me is an ongoing learning process.

AF: I guess I was trying to ask a leading question, because I wonder what you think about the connection between theatre and medicine.

GA: You mean, am I playing a role for people? Yes. I share some of my life stories, like what I learned in prison or my study of the Quran. They don't know the whole me because we have so many different personae that we present. I try and find something my companions can interact with and relate to. That changes all the time. I don't think a different persona changes the core me. It's just that if I want to assist somebody, I have to do it in a way that they can feel comfortable with. So to me, that's part of theatre. And I don't have any problems with it.

AF: Could you give some examples of personae you've used?

GA: What immediately comes to mind is the idea of being non-threatening. My background is not my companion's background. I grew up and lived in a world with 99 per cent male companionship. I learned that being non-threatening to people is a survival technique.

AF: Can you say more about the need to be non-threatening?

GA: My first encounter with authority, I was probably around seven years old. Teachers thought I had potential, they sent me away to a fancy school on an island in Boston Harbor.

It was at a very young age. I either thought I wanted to be, or I felt I was, a healer – which is different from a doctor. Part of my problems were with that. I ran onto the radar of a group of people who felt, yeah, this kid might have something special to him. 'He could be a healer, but ... .' I'd only be allowed to be a healer if I did it under their auspices. I'd have to perform how they liked.

The way I see it, when I was young, adults diagnosed me with a life-threatening disease they called potential. Good or bad potential, once having that diagnosis there was no way I could get out from underneath. They always thought, well, you know, he hasn't done anything lately, but he did this and that before. He has the potential to do something more, so you have to keep an eye on him. Eyes on me meant I had to look non-threatening to do what I think I can do without getting in trouble for it.

In the remedial school I was supposed to act one way. I didn't, I rebelled. So they sent me to different places. Custodial care came by stages of them taking me away from my family, then making me a ward of the state. That journey took me into a detention centre when I was about eleven. And then when I was fifteen, I was in adult prison, in a world of powerful men. They said they tried me as an adult to 'teach me a lesson'.

AF: Is that the lesson you learned? Or a different one?

GA: Somehow I learned how not to get hurt. At first I thought maybe no one hurt me because I was young, so much younger than everyone. Prison became my new school of life and humanity. I learned to adapt. Then there was another very young prisoner. Men beat him; they used him as a sex toy. He often asked me what he should do. And I didn't know.

There was compassion there. I listened to him. But I couldn't help him. Anything I told him to do, he would have been killed. One day he told me he was going to hang himself. I thought about whether I should try to stop him. But how could I stop him? I couldn't save him. Then he hung himself.

The prison psychiatrist was on me about that. Whether I was upset, whether I felt guilty for not stopping him. I said 'You people make the prisons this way, you make him live like that, and then you ask me if I feel guilty that I didn't save him? I couldn't save him. Only you could.' You can bet the psychiatrist got mad, he put a lot of things in my chart. That was one of my learning experiences about doctors.

AF: Did you need a new persona when you went from school to prison?

GA: It wasn't so different. I was a child, I didn't know anything. All the older prisoners had lives. So my persona was just to sit and listen to their stories. I couldn't contribute because I had no story. But at the same time, trying to find and learn my identity, well, I was in a learning process in that sense. I was still in school. Prisons were different then, in the 1960s. Prisons had libraries, we had different classes to learn new roles. I worked on a farm, I learned computers and then I taught computers in classes to women in a different prison, I worked in a state mental hospital. Besides prison classes, there were also the inmates and guards, they were teachers.

II. PAIN AND THE PERFORMANCE OF HEALING

AF: Was the hospital work your first experience as a caregiver?

GA: I would say the farms were. The first farm, across the street from a prison, was the horse farm of the Lancers. They had been a cavalry militia troop in the past, but by then they were just ceremonial. I took care of the horses; I rode again; I put on a uniform and rode in parades and drill exhibitions as a trooper (see Figure 8.1).

One day I had gone over to work in the stables and I couldn't find one stallion, Woody. I didn't see him in the yard. I thought maybe he had escaped, so I went looking for him. I found him lying down in a field near the road, tangled up in barbed wire fencing. He was cut up and bleeding from the wire, and the more he struggled, the more he got ripped up. I had no tools to cut the wire, I didn't have anything. But I felt the need to calm him, so I just sort of stayed with him, to keep him from hurting himself more.

Imagine the side of the road, a country road across from the prison. There were a lot of glass beer bottles and whatnot thrown off the highway, broken, shattered. I was trying to keep the stallion from moving around. I sat and moved his head on my lap so I could be between him and the glass. We were both lying in this. The horse was bleeding more than I was, but I was just embedded and my legs were glassed. This was before cell phones, and we lay there for a couple of hours before a trooper found me and called the vet. They got us untangled, cleaned us up and sutured and everything like that. They pulled out as much glass as they could find. Well, we got written up in the newspaper for that. Drama in real life and all that.

AF: It seems like you helped the horse the way you are a companion to your clients. We doctors aren't companions, we dart into a patient's room with the hope that we can perform a dramatic cure. When you know all you can do is care, does that make the act of being with a patient, staying with them, more painful?

GA: I recognize they are in pain. Their pain is not my pain to bear; that's different. A couple of weeks after trying to help the horse, I was loading hay one day with another man. I went to wipe my forehead from the sweat, and my hand comes out bloody.

And he says, 'Yeah, you're bleeding, George. What's up?'

I said, 'I don't know. What is it?' He saw it was a piece of glass that had made its way out through my forehead. This is two weeks after the horse drama.

The man called the vet and told him about it. The vet came by and he pulled it out for me and said, 'Somehow we missed this piece of glass and it got buried in your skin and it floated its way up and came up to your head.'

I said, 'That's been travelling my system? But it didn't do any damage?'

He said, 'No, you're lucky.'

So there are two things I learned from that drama. One, I could not have just walked away to get help; I was the help at that moment in time. Two, a reminder of the Law of Unintended Consequences. There was the glass working through my system, the hurt is part of the healing. Then, there was the prison transfer. Because of the newspaper article, because they knew I could take care of a horse, they sent me to a different prison that had a herd of dairy cows. One of the young prisoners up there had thrown bleach in one of the cows' eyes. They told me it was good if I went there and worked with the cows. They thought I could role model for the others. Now, I didn't ask for this. It wasn't something I sought out. It was something that somebody decided I could do. And I said, 'Yes, I can do that, I think.' So I helped cows for a while. A learning experience, you know, helping cows, learning from new people. Part of healing others, and being healed, is learning I could do 'good things' in spite of having been taught how to do 'bad things'. Those were freeing and empowering lessons.

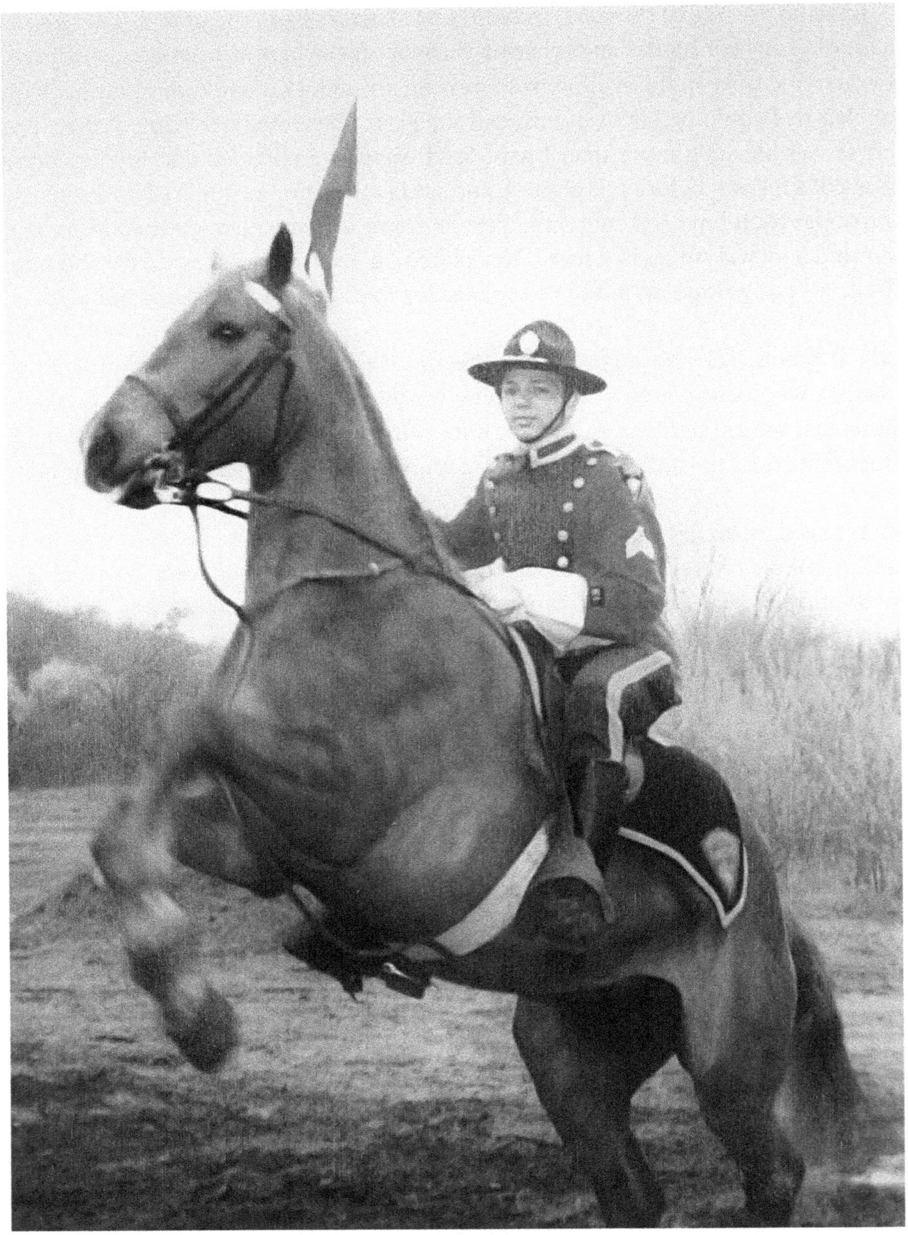

FIGURE 8.1 George Anderson before a Lancers parade, *c.*1972. Hospitals, prisons and the military are three of the few remaining organizations that use formal costumes to assert rank. Credit: Pauline Mariam Anderson.

III. CUSTODIAL CARE

AF: When was it you worked in the hospital?

GA: After the farms they sent me to work in a hospital, a state mental hospital, and I learned about a new kind of prison. It was like the experiments that they did on college students being prisoners and being gods.

AF: Gods? Oh! I see, you mean 'guards'. It's your Boston accent; you pronounce it 'gahds', so for a minute I thought you meant 'gods'.

GA: Yes; that's what some of them think they are.

AF: You were referring to the Stanford prison experiment? The one where the students were told to act like prisoners and guards, and they performed so violently that the experimenters had to stop the trial in only a few days?

GA: Playing 'gahd'.

AF: Yes. In prisons and state hospitals you're a captive population, a captive audience, so to speak. You can be experimented on so many different ways without you even knowing it. Do you know about the Fernald School oatmeal study?

GA: Can you tell me?

AF: It was a Massachusetts state facility where they put children who were disabled or just abandoned. Quaker Oats did nutrition studies on a group of boys there, they fed them radioactive oatmeal.

GA: The idea of theatre is the comedy and the tragedy and how they interact. Once you know you're just a subject in someone else's performance, once you get the joke, it might not be laughable, but you still know that it's a joke. Working at the state hospital was part of that joke. Even though I was still a prisoner, they gave me hospital work where I was basically a guard. Well, I wasn't one to want to be a god. I realized that every patient in that institution was just like me. You know, they had no power, they had no control, they had no autonomy. They were prisoners. Only their chains were chemical, and mine were physical.

AF: How did the state hospital compare with the state prisons?

GA: The hospital wards were calmer than the prison cell blocks. One reason was that in those days, before antipsychotics started in the 1960s, mental hospitals did a lot of lobotomies. Some of the patients were helpless old people who had been there for more than forty years. I also heard a rumour from an older patient that the police would pick up homeless boys from around the city and bring them to the hospital to be lobotomized.

That interested me. Part of the work I did there was clerical, so I went to the records room and looked up the boys' (now men) surgical reports. It was true.

When I learned those patients' stories, I thought, I wanted to help those men, but what can I do? How can I do anything? Just do the best I can. I told the social workers at my prison. I thought they were good people. They were appalled. They asked the hospital staff if that was true. Of course I got punished for illegally accessing files. It was not my place to help people.

The trouble had consequences. It was okay. I learned from it and I grew from it. But I can never go backwards.

One patient, he had been a ward of the state since he was maybe sixteen. I learned he had been scooped off the streets for his habit of going to a restaurant, getting breakfast, and leaving without paying. So they put him in the hospital and did a lobotomy.

He was in his early forties when I met him. I accompanied him when he was allowed to go off the hospital campus a short time. He'd go to the restaurant – it was still there – and he would still do the same thing. He'd go in, have a meal, and walk out without paying. So, the question was, how effective was performing the lobotomy? Talking with him and understanding that he had lost his whole life, the life that he could have had, because of medical care which doctors could do to him, to them ('them' being people who were in his condition). Do they teach that kind of history to doctors?

AF: We doctors were only taught that there was a dark past we emerged from. How do you see the difference between doctor and healer?

GA: A doctor can do a Fernald School, a Tuskegee, an Oregon experiment; a healer cannot. Doctors sometimes act like they're better than everybody else because they know what is wrong. They think they can make you better by experimenting with you. It's part of the theatre of doing what doctors do. I believe the whole world is a stage and we're all actors, so my question for people is, 'What part of that stage are you standing on? What part of that act are you in control of? Are you a director? Are you a character who writes your own script?'

AF: How much do caregivers affect the script?

GA: All that direction disappears when someone gets dementia. How do we treat and interact with somebody who's in that situation? They're no longer actors in control. Not just in the clinical sense of a doctor's visit, but the people who'll be there when someone wakes up in the morning? Understanding that they might be different than who they were last night.

AF: After all that you've seen and experienced, do you think doctors have a vocation to help people?

GA: Doctors can do some things, yet, in one sense, we're all doctors. So, how do we all learn just as human beings not to lose that humanity? To be more human? I didn't want to have a special 'vocation', so I didn't want to go to school. But I also had a talent or a knack that I could offer help, on an individual basis with people that I interact with. I think all of us are capable of all of those things.

To people like you who are trained to have a career at it, I can't say I envy you. I know you're necessary, but there's a price tag that happens to you. You can't trust a school to train you to be the best that you can be; that weight is on you. The two things when I think about doctors are, 'Do no harm', and 'Physician, heal thyself.' I'm not sure which has a priority. Both of those things – I don't know who teaches you. I do know we learn. We learn. But it's a mistake to expect a for-profit society to teach you how to do it successfully.

IV. COMPANIONS' LIVES

AF: After you went out on parole, you started a landscape company. And then for some of your clients you became a companion, right?

GA: They thought it was something I could do; I didn't seek that out. But I learned from them. The people I helped were mostly academics. One was in math and philosophy; one worked in a defence lab; there was a lawyer. They liked to tell me things. I would drive them to their seminars and sit in; I got to know their friends and have discussions with them. One of my companions described our relationship as being a part of my ongoing liberal arts education. I find no fault with that description. I was still able to ask them questions for which they had no ready answer.

I knew an affection for them that I would not call love and there were times and events where I very much disliked them. The differences between us in our social background, life experience and philosophy were always fertile soil for planting and weeding. Patients as amateurs at being disagreeable.

One of my companion's doctors said, 'You take such great care of mean old men. Can you teach me to be as tolerant of patients like them as you are?' I told her they really are nothing compared to the men that I grew up with. My companions were trying to act as professionals at being disagreeable when really, for me they were amateurs.

AF: How did being a prisoner and learning from fellow prisoners shape your work as a companion to mean old academics?

GA: Some of the prisoners who I learned from, except for the crime and the environment, could have been university deans, professors, or doctors. They were capable of having those skills, they could have had that success. They just did something that they got caught for. There are a lot of people that do bad things and don't get caught.

So there's really no difference between them. I look at a companion as a fellow human being and understand that they're just like me. They just haven't gotten caught.

AF: What was your role as they got sicker?

GA: I lived my life in environments where I was never in control in the sense my companions thought they had control. They never questioned their control because they'd never been in prison. When illness showed them that they were not in control, I could share and help them go through that by pointing out that in their own lives their education, their spiritual or religious backgrounds, gave them a different way of looking at things. Watching them come to understand their lack of control, I understood more too.

Being a companion is something that I've been learning to do all my life. Doing that, being a companion, is non-threatening because I'm not curing anything. To say 'I will cure you', that can be a threat. I'm not a doctor. I'm just helping people who are going through something of a process that I have an inkling of understanding for.

V. THE COST OF CARING

AF: How do you protect yourself from the pain of caring for someone sick?

GA: For every act you choose, there's a price tag. Getting involved with the patient, getting involved with somebody who's losing their ability to function in what we consider a normal, acceptable way – there's a price tag. Sometimes the cost of helping is becoming aware that I am also helpless, unable to cure myself or even change what happens next. I have to be willing to pay that price. I think that the price is worth it because it teaches us our humanity, and because we want somebody to do that for us.

AF: Could you say more about the price? Itemize it?

GA: There is empathy and emotional loss, physical and mental labour. Then there's payback to people who have helped or hurt you. The first time I heard Arthur Kleinman talk was at a seminar I took my companion to. Arthur talked about the book he wrote about taking care of his wife when she got dementia. Arthur said he had been the dominant spouse, while his wife took care of him and their children. She fed him, she picked out his clothes. When she got dementia, he saw it was time for him to repay his debt. He saw how important feeding and cleaning her was, doing that work every day; he said most doctors don't know about that kind of care.

AF: What is the link between 'paying a price' and 'paying back'?

GA: Well, there are different kinds of payback. If the dominant partner throughout a prolonged relationship has been abusive to the other partner, and then that dominant partner starts losing control of his abilities, the other partner then gets a chance to come into a payback position. Some people see sickness as a chance to get the other family member back. When I see that happening, I know that it's wrong. But how do I work to alleviate that in my companion and their partner?

One of my first landscaping clients was a woman I had known for years, a friend. Her husband, a defence researcher – he was one of the people you would call a mean old man. He had been dominant all those years, and, when he got sick, she didn't want to take that out on him as his caregiver. She felt she was just not capable of being a caregiver for him as a spouse should be. She asked me if I could step in, if I could deal with him. From my past experience working in the state hospital, I had decided that was not a job I wanted. The empathy and the involvement had been so unregulated for me.

AF: But then you did help. Why?

GA: Because she was my friend, and she needed help. I wanted to. Then after I got to know her husband better, I wanted to help him too. He couldn't move well, he was a prisoner to his illness. But he could still talk, so he told me a lot of stories. So, I listened.

VI. PROGRESS NOTES

AF: George, you have shown me the meticulous notes you kept for your client's wife. They are so much richer than a doctor's notes; more like a playscript.

GA: Here is an excerpt, a dialogue I had with my client from a day in 2006 soon after his wife had to move him into an assisted living facility.

Client: I asked [my wife] to come over to the October birthdays event, and she said no. She couldn't wait to get out the door and leave me here with people I don't want to be around either.
George: Yes, it sucks, but did you even bother to say to her thank you for coming over to see me, take care of yourself, I'll see you later, I love you?
Client: No.
George: Well again shame on you for not ... You sometimes want to act like everyone else's life has to stop, because you have gone to prison [the assisted living]. I say sometimes, because I think you are still aware enough to understand that thought position is just wrong ... You can talk with me about almost anything ... you can talk with a lot of people, but you never seem to be able to talk with your wife. So you tell me whether you think there is something wrong with the picture I have of you.
Client: Just because I listen doesn't mean I agree or accept what you say is true.
George: I have always understood that and have no problem with it.
Client: You don't always know what goes on between us.
George: That is true and that is how it should be.
(Staff came to call him for dinner here, about 5:05.)
Client: Well again you leave me with a lot to think on.
George: Just another day for us both.
(I left him at the dining hall.)

GA: And here are notes to my client's wife from several years later. It was right after my client had to move to a new room in the assisted living facility, on a floor where he would get more supervision.

I arrived at his new floor on Monday 09-08-08 at 7:45 p.m. He was in good spirits, tired from the day's activity. He was warmly welcoming to me and thanked me for my help in the room move. He was sitting in the lounge and watching TV. He tried to explain to me the plot of the programme he was watching, but could not smoothly verbalize. He was aware of the time as he said it was late for me to be visiting. I said I would be staying overnight with him. He said he thinks you told him about that plan, but ... he was feeling confused ... .

At about 8:30, he suggested tea for me and hot cocoa for himself. He got up from his chair (unassisted), and walked over to his room, looked in, turned around and tried the exit door. He walked back ... and walked up the corridor to a door that was approximately where his friend's room is located on the fourth floor. I said to him that he is now on the third floor and she is one floor above. He turned to me and said 'Oh, right', and came back and sat down. During this walking, his balance was good, almost no foot shuffling. Other than the grasping of the exit door knob and touching of the TV cabinet in passing, he used no aid and needed no assistance.

He and I watched TV until 10:00 when he told me that he was tired and ready for bed.

The next morning, on getting out of bed, he was able to give me morning greetings and ask of how my night was. He recognized that he had slept the whole night through. He went into the bathroom and used the toilet, washed his hands. He proceeded to make himself a cup of coffee, but could not start the microwave. He walked over to the bed side stand, picked up his glasses and went back to and did turn on the microwave. He came back to the bed area and standing in the middle of the room proceeded to do four stretch bends, bending from the waist and touching his toes … .

In summary, as we had discussed prior … I used a minimal physical assistance approach with him. He was pretty much able to 'do for self' throughout my twelve-hour time with him. He slept a good eight hours. He was alert, and though slow, his physical movements were balanced. That he was able to initiate and follow conversations, to grasp some idea of the stress involved over his situation for you, with … the room and status change, and my being there, shows his cognitive abilities to be functioning, much better than when I visited him at the rehabilitation hospital.

VII. FINAL ACTS

AF: You have given a eulogy at all your companion's funerals, right? You put a lot of thought into the writing and performance of them.

GA: I start writing my companions' eulogies during their lives. We can't control our lives, but we can learn things. I want to share what I learned. It's the final act of the drama.

AF: Do they know you're writing their eulogy? That you have the last word?

GA: They ask me to. One man who heard my eulogy for his wife, when later I became his companion too, he asked me to deliver a talk about him equal to what I had done for her. I told him that he was not her and I could make no such promise. He then promised not to haunt me if I did my best. Over the years, whenever he had a life event which reminded him of his mortality, he would ask me what I would write about him. I could only reply, 'I don't know.'

I knew him thirteen years. A few years before his death, I told him that I had started writing his eulogy, I asked if he wanted to make any closing remark to anyone who would hear his story and find cause to reflect on their own caring relationships. He sat in a long silence, sipping tea. He then told me that for better or worse, all he could say was 'Thank you'.

9

'I like to act vicariously on behalf of people'

AN INTERVIEW WITH MARCUS COATES

Marcus Coates is a London-based performance and visual artist who explores the lived experiences and realities of humans, non-human animals, and natural phenomena by entering into and re-enacting other states of being. His work is presented live, in video and film installations and often in service of asking questions or solving problems on behalf of specific communities. Coates bases his art in 'mental journeying' and contemporary Western shamanic practices, which performance and philosophy scholar Laura Cull has described as 'not concerned to reproduce some sort of "authentic" shamanic ritual (whatever we might understand that to be)' while being serious 'with respect to the *reality* of metamorphosis and becoming' and 'conducted with … diligence and care'.[1] He therefore draws on pre-modern medical practices in which theatre and healing rituals were cognate and entangled. As Coates also explains, his art is grounded in personal experiences of illness that helped to develop his unconscious imagination. By surviving long-term illness he believes, 'you've gone beyond the reach of the medicine available to your society – you've been deemed to have journeyed somewhere that other people haven't, and you've survived and come back'.[2]

[1] Laura Cull, 'Affect in Deleuze, Hijikata, and Coates: The Politics of Becoming-Animal in Performance', *Journal of Dramatic Theory and Criticism* 26, no. 2 (2012): 190.
[2] 'Marcus Coates', *Modern Painters* (March 2012): 15.

Coates rose to prominence in the UK art world of the early 2000s through performances in which he witnessed, communicated with, or partly transformed into non-human animals. In the interview that follows, Coates discusses two more recent projects: *The Trip* (2011), a long-term project that resulted in a film collaboration with one of the patients at St John's Hospice in London, and *The Directors* (2022), five short films that collaboratively present the experience of psychosis.[3] Created over the course of five years with Mark Banham, Lucy Dempster, Anthony Donohoe, Marcus Gordon and Stephen Groves (the 'Directors'), all of whom are in recovery from psychosis, *The Directors* was developed in consultation with psychiatrist and neuroscientist Dr Isabel Valli. During the filming of the discrete experiences of psychosis, Coates was given instructions over an earpiece from each 'director', which are also included in the soundtrack, and in each Coates inhabits the auditory, visual and tactile hallucinations described by a director without imitating or enacting them in any conventional sense. Mostly filmed at and originally shown in locations around a large housing estate, Churchill Gardens, in Pimlico, London, *The Directors* asks audiences to physically and emotionally empathize with the everyday world of each subject – and, in the case of Lucy, to sit on her bed in her apartment while watching her film.[4] By doing so, Coates proposes, the stigma and unfamiliarity of psychosis might be reduced.

In this interview, Coates addresses a variety of topics, including the opportunities for artists to bring their skills to medical environments, the undervalued role of the imagination in treatment, the centrality of the 'contract' in both performance and medicine, the ways that medical institutions invite and constrain interpersonal performances, and opportunities for mutual play and empathy in the relationship between doctor and patient.

I. AN ARTIST WALKS INTO AN INSTITUTION

To get us started, can you tell us how, as a performer, you've thought about the relationship between theatre and medicine?

Marcus Coates (MC): I can see that alignment quite clearly. I think quite early on – from doing or making performances – I understood that there is a social contract between myself and the audience.

---

[3] *The Directors* can be viewed at www.whatsgoingon.org.uk/, a dedicated site for access to the films, background info and support for individuals, communities and clinicians.

[4] Colin Martin, 'Art and Empathy: Five Lived Experiences of Psychosis', *The Lancet*, 9 October 2022.

My performances aim to be pragmatic, purposeful and enabling. Often I'd ask the audience to ask me a question and the performance would have to answer that question. I deliberately put a pragmatic, rational framework in there to test out what that relationship is between myself and the people I'm working for. Working towards an answer put a framework of usefulness around the activity, and an investment in the outcome. And I think what I find – and it is always quite surprising to me – is that as a performer I don't actually inhabit any power at all.

This goes against the myth of what a performer is. I realized I was becoming what the audience needed me to be in order for them to get what they wanted. So I enabled the audience to participate enough so that they could project onto me what they wanted in return, and for me to be alive to what they wanted, and for me to adapt it accordingly. I definitely wasn't the one in power, but at times this contract required me to embody the illusion of that. At other times, it required vulnerability, but what had to be rooted in these personas or states was an intentionality that was shared with the audience, a sense of collective purpose or enquiry.

After sitting in this for a while and working with this, I saw that dynamic in every aspect of culture: when I went to the doctor's, when I talked to a lawyer, and you see it with politicians on TV and you see it in all of show business. But I think art is interesting because you are not necessarily dependent on the audience or clients in the same way: as well as working for them you can also test that relationship, to reveal it and alter it.

Probably the same is true for medicine in a way that you're not dependent on the patient, but the roles are dependent or defined to a certain extent by the culture of the institution. That's where the institution, I think, is quite important. As an artist, I've tried to really play with that culture or framework, what that institution sets up as a context or a contract for that relationship. In my last projects, both of which have involved medical institutions, the institution was the thing I had to deal with most – to pick apart and find my way into, and maybe subvert or feed off it.

Which institutions do you mean?

MC: Well, I'm talking about a couple. For the project I made called *The Trip*, I worked in a palliative care institution, a hospice. I worked there for about two years. I'd go there one day every week and I'd meet the patients. I really didn't know what my role as an artist was. It was an artist residency that I'd set up with the Serpentine Gallery, called Skills Exchange, part of a wider programme of putting artists in different areas of society. And I was thinking, 'Skills Exchange', what do I actually have to offer here? So I'd sit down and have lunch with the day patients quite a lot and then go meet people in their rooms.

> And they'd say to me, 'So yeah, what are you doing here?'
> I'd say, 'Well, I'm an artist.'
> And they'd say, 'Okay, so you're going to draw some pictures with us. And do some painting?'
> I said, 'No, not really.'
> 'So what are you going to do?'
> I said, 'Well, I'm not sure.'
> And they said, 'Well, what can you do?'

It really forced me to think about my usefulness and purpose as an artist and my position within that institutional contract. The hospice is a very special place. I was expecting it to be a depressing and sad place, but I found it incredibly uplifting, because I think it was so truthful and honest.

Everyone there was in the same position. Everyone was going to die. Maybe within a month, maybe a year, but they all knew they were terminally ill. And that brought out this incredible sense of … I think pleasure in the moment, a need for the normal and a lightness actually, about what life is.

Once I started entering into that, I could say to them, 'Okay, yeah, these are the things I can do. I have an imagination. I want to use that for other people. I'm interested in your stories and I want to somehow be of service to you as an artist. And beyond that, I can't really explain or tell you until I see it or am in it with you. So if you allow me to, I'd just like to sit and talk every week with you.' Eventually, lots of stories started to come out about things people really had wanted to do in their lives, or still wanted to do. I thought maybe I could be of service in that way. Not necessarily in a practical way, organizing a trip somewhere, but actually looking at the value of the imagination in that context, and how powerful narrative could be.

This was true particularly with people in the hospice who had a vivid imagination and saw that as a significant reality for themselves – they dreamed about other places, they thought of these places a lot, and they inhabited these places day to day. They used these places when they were in pain, they really went to these places. So, these are the places that I got quite interested in.

There were five or six people who I talked to who came up with scenarios they'd asked me to inhabit on their behalf, vicariously, to go on a journey or a trip for them and come back and tell them about it. It was about me embodying their imagination, living it and them living it through me as a cipher for them. It was an eye-opener for me in terms of the power of narrative, mental imagery, and my vicarious action on someone's behalf. I went on a trip to the Amazon rainforest on behalf of Alex. He said it gave him another bend in the river and another conversation to have with the forest community on a trip that he had made many times in his imagination. It extended his inner world when everything surrounding him was getting smaller.

II. THE SCHOOL OF THE IMAGINATION

You mentioned you'd recently worked with other medical institutions as well.

MC: Well, I continued working with the imagination. I did another project called The School of the Imagination, where I worked with five people who answered a call-out, five members of the public who wanted to immerse themselves in their imagination and work from that place. It was basically a training week to help people use their imagination more productively in their lives. With this group of people, we spent a week looking at how to immerse oneself in the imagination and give it as much significance as consensus reality or external reality. We used that space to answer or give insight into problems people have, or social questions.

Quite a few of these people we were working with had experience of being homeless, or were otherwise vulnerable. We had a psychiatrist there just to make sure everyone was okay, because going deep into this immersive space could be triggering or problematic if there were mental health issues. The variety and scope of how people use their imagination is enormous. When some people close their eyes, it's just darkness, nothing, and with some people – it's very vivid and detailed, with some it's very absorbing and it's a big shift to return from it.

So that really interested me. The psychiatrist in that programme, Dr Isabel Valli, said, 'I'd really love for you to come meet my patients.' She works in the early intervention clinic at the South London and Maudsley NHS Foundation Trust, with people with early signs of psychosis. I started going there once a week, just sitting in with her in her consultations (she'd ask the patients if they'd mind me sitting in before they met me). We'd go in, and I'd sit there, and I'd hear her talk to her patients with genuine curiosity, which I became very interested in.

Her inquisitiveness and curiosity was infectious. She showed genuine interest and passion for her patients. I was really impressed with that. But I was quite taken aback by how much she entered into their narratives, and particularly their delusions.

And I said to her, 'Shouldn't you ... Isn't your job to be pointing out, they're not in reality, and this is a different world from the world they're imagining is real?'

'No, that's as real to them as this is to us', she said. 'And it's not my job to confound that or to stop that. I'm just finding out what's there for them and what are the threats and what are the issues and difficulties for them.'

And I found that quite intriguing because in all other walks of medicine that I've ever experienced, particularly as the patient, the idea of establishing the facts and establishing an objective truth is paramount for the clinician.

Whenever I'd spoken to a doctor, my narratives about my body had always been steered toward a singular standard pathology. I could see this was useful for a doctor and their assessment, but it wasn't useful for the narratives I had needed to create to deal with my own illness.

Usually you give a psychotic medication because you can't just talk someone out of their psychosis. Why do you believe she used this approach?

MC: She definitely wasn't trying to talk them out of psychosis. Her approach was an effective assessment and diagnostic tool for her to make decisions about which medication, what dosage, and what extra care was needed. After I had been going to the clinic for a while, I realized that there was a big issue that I had in terms of empathy. I found there were huge barriers for me personally to understand and engage in their experiences. I felt I didn't have the cultural tools to be able to do that. Also, I think there was a sense from the patients that I wouldn't understand anyway, even if they explained it to me. And of course there was a fear of judgement.

Did they also feel that Dr Valli wouldn't understand?

MC: I think they really felt like she got it. They really valued her because she was saying things like, 'Did you experience this?' She was almost predicting their experience. They were saying, 'Yes, yes, you understand.' I think she understood their pain and fear – but this wasn't necessarily understanding their experience, it was just that she had a vast experience of so many peoples' experiences of psychosis that she could use this to recognize traits and commonalities across patients.

What did you feel you didn't understand about psychosis?

MC: I felt like before I went there, to the hospital, I was quite scared. I didn't know what I was going to face. That's the stigma. But what was really happening was that I thought I had to be a certain way in that institution. I had to be almost a model of rationality and sanity. I had to show myself as rational, and I had to be sure about where this boundary was. I had to have very clear boundaries.

Where were these expectations coming from? Did anyone tell you or did you have cultural presets?

MC: I think this came from lots of different areas. My mum was a drama therapist, and she talked about her experiences in psychiatric units. Some of them were quite alarming. I think my expectations also came from films, TV, media, all of that; probably from my experience of being ill, being in hospitals, I thought that having these very formal boundaries was how it's done, maybe even a necessary protection?

In the clinic, I thought that as soon as I spoke I would unveil that I didn't know anything, that I'm going to expose a vulnerability somehow. But soon as I started talking to patients about what they wanted to talk about, what they were interested in as people, I realized: they're not illnesses, they're people. This is an institution where I could talk to people, have amazing conversations. That was a massive shift, which probably happened within the first few weeks.

How did that realization lead you to the idea that you could represent illness collaboratively?

MC: When I realized I didn't need to be defined by the stigma, when I started to share myself. We were simply people talking about music, about our interests, about our childhoods, just shared experiences. I thought, 'Okay, this is a basis for something. This is not what the doctor does. I'm not assessing them.' I think the patients understood and reacted to that immediately.

I thought, how can we use this in a way that's more useful for them? 'It's nice and everything, chatting, but how can this be a proactive thing that gives them agency within their illness?'

Within that context, it became clear that I couldn't develop the idea with the patients, there were too many obstacles – or if it was possible, it would have meant changing or introducing a new practice into the hospital, which would have been too time consuming. It wasn't until I started working outside of that institution, when I got in touch with the mental health charity, MIND, and the arts organization Artangel, that the possibility of working collaboratively emerged. We did a call-out to people with lived experience of psychosis that MIND knew and had worked with to help change public stigma of the illness. A few people contacted us, wanting to talk about their psychosis and wanting to tell their unique stories to challenge the public's stigma and attitudes towards themselves.

I talked to these individuals about how as an artist, I like to act vicariously on behalf of people, and use the imaginative space to do that. I told them that initially I just wanted to talk to them about their experiences and that a way of working together might emerge, but from us both. We spent a long time with each other, listening and discussing their stories, me trying to understand and them trying to help me understand. I think their prime motivation was to tell their stories in the way that they wanted to tell them and how they wanted them to be understood – and they didn't think that version of their stories had ever been listened to or heard before.

III. ALLOWING PEOPLE TO BE THEMSELVES

How did you decide which patients to involve in the project?

MC: Primarily this decision came from working with MIND and a group of professional individuals in the mental health and care sector, who were either clinicians or had lived experience of psychosis, assembled to support me and the project. All the people that contacted us were at different stages of recovery of psychosis. It was clear that some people weren't able to reflect in detail on their experiences, and they were able to make the decision for themselves that their participation was not possible for them. But there was a certain group who felt they were able to reflect without risk to themselves, and who wanted to establish a narrative that was authentic and useful for themselves and others. So, we started to have regular conversations that lasted from one to two hours at a time, where we began this process of trying to explain and understand.

I think what I felt in the hospital was that there wasn't really the language there to talk about this stuff. I found I could begin to relate to their experiences on an emotional level and this became a significant tool for us to connect to each other.

You've said that what they got out of this was a conversation. That seems different from making a film where you're projecting their experiences and you're serving as a conduit. How did that transition happen? How did you get yourself and the directors from the one to the other?

MC: I think if the work had remained as unrecorded conversations that would still have been significant, but part of their motivation was to get their stories out to a wider public. I was aware of that responsibility. As I was talking to them and imagining me inhabiting their experiences, I imagined myself up on stage or on a film set. I'm not sure why, but it kept cropping up for me, that I was the actor and they were the director coaching me in ways to inhabit the experiences.

The context of the film set would put us in positions where we'd have to deliver our experiences in a certain way for each other. The skills of a film director are very specific. It's not about telling people what to do, it's about allowing people to be themselves. Once we were in the situation of the cameras, and we were in the context that the directors wanted to be in – I was sitting on the sofa or walking in the park, or wherever it was – I'd start by saying, 'Okay, so what's happening? What's going on?' And they'd respond, 'Well, this is happening, that is happening.' The process was all about how we could explore the language we needed to both fail and succeed in relating across these extraordinary and difficult experiences.

How did you decide where to set the films? The locations are very specific and very different from each other: Lucy's room, the stage, Greenwich Park and so forth.

MC: That was decided on Zoom and was planned together. All Lucy's material was about the instability of reality, so we had the idea of a sort of doll's house. 'It feels like a set, my world feels like a set', Lucy said – in that Truman Show way. So, we thought, let's go towards that, see what we can do, and let's see how we can allow the audience into that instability too.

The directors had choice around the locations and they determined that the setting was metaphorical. It was *about* their reality rather than actually being their reality. One of the directors, Marcus Gordon, decided on the theatre. His experiences were centred on his sense of being interrogated, so the idea of the stage in theatre became very obvious in that sense.

In that situation, I was thinking, 'My God, my worst fear is standing on stage, people looking at me and I don't know what I'm going to say or do, there's no plan.'

And Marcus said, 'Yeah, there won't be any plan. This is great. There's no plan.'

Marcus told me he was going to really confuse me, in terms of my senses. For example, he told me how he feels hot and he feels cold. So, I talked to the theatre producers: what can we do to make me hot and cold? We brought in heaters and we got ice, and lots of it; I sat on a chair on the stage, watched by an audience as I was simultaneously heated up and rubbed with ice. But Marcus is the one deciding when and how it happens, and nothing we discuss is planned beforehand.

I knew some of what was going to happen, but there were other aspects I didn't know about – experiencing the smell of rotten meat, for example. I had told Marcus, 'Look, I need to keep some of it as a sort of shock for me. I don't want to know everything. I don't want to know how long it's going to go on for. I don't know what you're going to tell me or how I'm going to experience this, really. You've got to help me through that.' He really took on that role of being the guide to his hell. It's not that he relished it, but I think he really valued the idea: someone is going to go into that with him.

IV. VISUAL REPRESENTATION AND STIGMA

You've touched on what may be some of the impulses that led to a desire to restage and help other people witness. But in the films we don't actually see the people with psychosis. We hear both of you, but we only see you.

MC: I think that sight is where so much of the stigma exists – and it's not only stigma, it's the premonition of stigma. Quite a few of the directors would've been fine being shown on screen, but I know the stress of having a camera in your face, and I know how distracting that is. So, first of all, I thought that would be unhelpful and invasive. Secondly, though, I was considering the audience: they know that this is a film about psychosis, so they're going to imagine that someone in this scene has got psychosis. Which one is it? Who's got psychosis? Oh, there is the one that's mad. Let's dump everything that we know about psychosis on that person before we've even started.

With only one person on screen, that decision can't be made. It's just not there. It feels like the convention of identification is to substantiate or to debunk your own prejudice. If those decisions are being made constantly, if that's the filter or the technique of identification, that's really unhelpful. That's what I wanted to avoid.

The films were originally shown across five different locations in Pimlico, London, in and around the Churchill Gardens Estate. What did The Directors *gain from being staged here?*

MC: The whole premise of using those spaces like the shop, the flat, the doctor's surgery and vacant restaurant was that I wanted to root it in people's everyday lives. The audience for the films are literally entering someone else's world.

The idea I likened it to was when you're a kid and you go around to someone's house for a play date, and all the rules are different. All the food's weird, water tastes funny, the carpet's weird, the smell – everything's just strange and it takes ages for you to just settle in. I wanted everyone to be confronted with that, to have to adjust and navigate that.

After the first time I visited the psychiatric hospital, I got the bus home. I said to myself, 'My God, I can look out the window and I can look at people on the street and on the bus without fear, they're not all talking about me, they are not all plotting against me or disgusted by me. I have choices about what I believe in. I live in a world I don't fear. I'm really, really lucky to be able to be in the world like this.' I learned not to take my reality for granted and I wanted a similar experience for the audience: leaving one director's reality at the doctor's surgery, crossing the road, seeing people on the street, then entering another director's reality in the film in the second hand shop. This was a lovely thing that happened between the films, that people reflected on their own reality and perception of the world between the venues.

V. A WHOLE DIFFERENT RELATIONSHIP WITH ILLNESS

Do you see what you do as a tool that could be used in clinics? Could it be applied beyond your own specific experiences?

MC: What I find exciting, and I think why I'm interested in it and why I do it, is that what I'm doing engages with play and is guided by play. By play, I mean non-thinking or non-rational thought: embodying fantasy, embodying physicality, and being challenged to let go, being challenged not to be bound by rational frameworks. Within that, it feels like you don't have to be yourself, but you become more available to yourself, if I can say that. I think in lots of therapy contexts this kind of approach is used.

I always find it very difficult when someone says, 'Well, tell me about yourself.' I don't want to tell you about myself. I want us to experience ourselves together, that's how I find out about you. I'm a bit obsessed by this dynamic when you go into the doctor's, I have to say, because I've had years of health issues. And I'm always confronted with the thought, 'Okay, I've been asked here in this consultation to come up with a narrative that describes myself and my situation in the way that you can help me with.' What I really want the doctor to say is, 'Just talk to me', or 'Let's just have a conversation. How do you need to talk to me about this?' and then the relevant narrative and the important needs will emerge from that, though probably not in the language or rational order the doctor needs. There's a kind of territory of experience, or territory of understanding that we need to step into and explore first before we can even enter into anything that's reciprocal or trusted.

Doctors also need to protect themselves, though, don't they? Isn't that part of their motivation?

MC: We all do, at some level in our relationships, need to balance how and in what way we are available to others. I understood, particularly in the secure psychiatric units, why psychiatrists would have a shield, and maybe even in just a normal hospital environment with physical illness, why doctors have the need for self-protection on an emotional level, otherwise it would be exhausting and unsustainable. But I'm also querying what they're protecting themselves from and how this resistance to a porous or available self might be a cultural inhibition. I speak to anthropologists about performance practice, particularly the usefulness of that practice in societies and communities. For instance, in the practice of shamans, where we see the practitioner going into the person or the community that they're healing. They actually want to empathize so much, to go inside the person, see and take hold of that illness and take it out.

That's the utter reverse of conventional Western medicine. Doctors don't want an imagined or anthropomorphized relationship with illness. They don't want to identify with that illness as anything other than a materialistic entity. (I'm not saying this is wrong, just that I would like the culture I'm in to be aware of the wider needs of patients and the potential for addressing them.) I always thought it was interesting that whenever I've been with kids and they're ill, that's the one thing they want to do. You've got this illness, you give it a name, you start to relate to it, start to talk to it. There's a whole different relationship. You create a dialogue even though it's imagined. In many ways this seems particularly useful, even necessary for some. The parallel here is so interesting with psychosis, particularly with audible hallucinations or inner voices and how a form of dialogue with the voices is proving to be beneficial.

Do you think doctors need to impose boundaries because of the scale of what they do?

MC: Well, if they took this role [of engaging in an imaginative dialogue] on with many patients a day – I mean, whenever I've done any work where I've really, really empathized in a radical way with somebody, it's utterly exhausting. It takes so much out of you that you need a day or so just to replenish yourself. It's a kind of losing oneself on purpose. I find that fascinating and intriguing and interesting, and I like to go to that place, but it feels like it's not practical as the medical practitioner's role.

There are elements of these performative processes that can be useful to clinicians, and since *The Directors* I have done many talks and workshops with hospitals and doctors who are keen to learn about different approaches to understanding and relating to psychosis. The films are now part of the NHS trust's psychiatric training and part of the curriculum at King's College, London. The processes I developed with the directors could be a complementary role rather than something we would demand from a physician. I could very well develop it and train others to work with this as a framework for relating. What I was doing with the directors was quite extreme, in a way, but there are subtle elements of these performative processes that could be adopted (if they aren't already) – like the need to create space for a mutual dialogue, to disengage from hierarchical positions, to listen to and respect the rationality and logic that the patient uses to relate to their illness, and the understanding that this a key to their recovery. This requires considerable empathy.

Throughout our conversation, you've suggested some past challenges with your own health. Have those challenges, in some way, brought you into this space?

MC: I think everyone attempts to create a world that they need. As an artist, that's probably what I'm doing, however unconsciously. There are a couple of things I'd identify as motivations for me – as needs, and perhaps skills as well. I think one is that as a young child and as a teenager I had very bad eczema, and asthma, so at times I was physically incapacitated, with my skin dried up and flaking, just falling off me. Lying there, not being able to move because my skin would split or break, I understood, 'Okay, my world needs to be in my imagination. That's where I'm living now.' I think I have always been more immersed in an imagined world but the illness made this conscious to me, like my imagination was a tool.

I'm also fascinated by the question about where will or consciousness is, by the sense that because you are ill there's a delay between decision and movement. How in control of ourselves are we? What role does the conscious thought play, and where do we sit fundamentally as personas or as selves? It's not my thoughts or instructions making me sit up. It's something else directing me and making this happen.

When experiencing asthma attacks or pain from my skin, I disassociated myself from my physical being and told myself, 'This isn't me, the breathing or the pain isn't me. I can just stand away from it and watch the pain.' My relationship with self in these moments had to be reimagined and these multiple selves found, places I could reside in and retain autonomy or agency in, even if it was only in my thoughts. Sometimes this anthropomorphized the pain, giving it a character I could communicate with; sometimes it emptied it of character into a rudimentary materialism that wasn't actually me. I think that disassociation became quite important to me, and in my artwork I can perhaps hold that element of someone for them to be able to see and relate to in a different way.

Marcus Gordon said something really quite profound to me about this and about the shame attached to psychosis, not just because of the stigma, but because you're out of control and so vulnerable. After he watched me play out his experiences, he said he needed to give that guy on the stage (meaning himself) a break. He wanted to say to him, 'You've really been through it.' He felt a powerful need to give that person sympathy, and to take care of him. For the first time in a very long time, he said he cried because he could give himself compassion, and recognized that he needed that from himself.

REFERENCES

Cull, Laura. 'Affect in Deleuze, Hijikata, and Coates: The Politics of Becoming-Animal in Performance'. *Journal of Dramatic Theory and Criticism* 26, no. 2 (2012): 189–203. https://doi.org/10.1353/DTC.2012.0023.

'Marcus Coates'. *Modern Painters* (March 2012): 15.

Martin, Colin. 'Art and Empathy: Five Lived Experiences of Psychosis'. *The Lancet*, 9 October 2022.

'What's Going On?' Artangel Collection. www.whatsgoingon.org.uk/.

PART FOUR

The Pasts of Performative Medicine

When literary critic Anatole Broyard was diagnosed with metastatic prostate cancer, he reached for the language and conventions of theatre and performance to imagine a more convivial model of care. 'To help the doctor reach the patient, and to help the patient reach the doctor, the mood of the hospital might have to be modified', he wrote. 'It ought to be less like a laboratory and more like a theatre, which would be only fitting, since no place contains more drama.'[1] Broyard's observations have been cited many times in the literary health humanities. The 'drama' he means, more than lifesaving heroics and sudden reversals in health, is a comedy of manners, as patients and doctors try (and mostly fail) to recognize what each other needs. Much of what he notices amounts to a litany of performance critiques. Broyard sees everyone in medical care caught up in histories of performing that they unwittingly reiterate, and his stored memory of consultations allows him to compare enactments the way he might compare different actors who have taken on the part of Hamlet. In considering how 'to go past the science into the person', for example, he notices the disconnected ways doctors have of looking at him: 'One doctor I saw had a trick of almost crossing his eyes, so he seemed to be peering warmly, humanistically, into my eyes, but he wasn't seeing me at all', while his psychotherapist avoids eye contact altogether and still others 'give you a generic, unfocused gaze. They look at you panoramically'.[2] Broyard concludes by imagining

[1] Anatole Broyard, 'The Patient Examines the Doctor', in *Intoxicated by My Illness* (Clarkson Potter, 1992), 55.
[2] Ibid., 49, 50.

a better performance, a repetition and reworking of familiar acts that could better sustain everyone in the ensemble. 'If he could gaze directly at the patient, the doctor's work would be more gratifying', Broyard comments. 'Why bother with sick people, why try to save them, if they're not worth acknowledging?'[3] Patients, too, can improve on past acts: 'If a patient expects a doctor to be interested in him, he ought to try to *be interesting*.'[4]

Performances are negotiations with the past: an educational and professionalizing past for doctors that modelled looking indirectly or not at all, as well as a whole life as a patient with its attendant frustrations and longings. One task of performative medicine is to sensitize patients and caregivers to the influence of historical embodiment on the present – as standards and norms, but also as what Diana Taylor has called 'vital acts of transfer, transmitting social knowledge, memory, and a sense of identity'.[5] Performing with someone is also a way of getting to know who they are and what they have been. In a larger sense, performances also convey the structures of thought and feeling that have conditioned them. Marvin Carlson influentially described theatre, a place where performances are specially marked out for scrutiny, as a 'memory machine' that fundamentally relies on repetition, presenting 'the identical thing [audiences] have encountered before, although now in a somewhat different context' – an operation he calls 'ghosting'.[6] In Carlson's analysis, theatre becomes a vehicle for circulating cultural memory; an actor's previous performances will haunt how audiences receive her subsequent performances, much as spectators compare the details of one production of a play or one recitation of a famous speech with another.

The chapters in this section approach theatre as a container for historical medical performances and ideologies that continue to ghost medical practices. They reveal that medicine and theatre are similarly haunted. Broyard, for example, speculates sardonically that modern-day treatment is ghosted by a historical avoidance of contagion, which has seeped into how medical personnel construe all interpersonal contact: 'Originally, the patient was protected by the sterility of the hospital. Only the sterility went too far: it sterilized the doctor's thinking.'[7] Arthur Frank similarly rehearses how the emergence of the 'sick person' as a social type in the eighteenth century was conditioned by the 'clinical reduction' of their symptoms to the generality of a diagnosis that

---

[3] Ibid.

[4] Ibid., 45, emphasis in original.

[5] Diana Taylor, 'Translating Performance', in *The Performance Studies Reader*, 2nd edition, ed. Henry Bial (Routledge, 2007), 381.

[6] Marvin Carlson, *The Haunted Stage: Theatre as Memory Machine* (Michigan University Press, 2001), 7.

[7] Broyard, 'The Patient Examines the Doctor', 55.

alienated them from their particular experience of illness – a form of typecasting that continues to this day, and that performative medicine, like narrative medicine, seeks to redress.[8] As caregivers have long recognized, bodies articulate personal medical histories even if those histories are often difficult to interpret. Performance theorists have likewise attended to how embodied practices record and transmit institutional, cultural and political histories; what seem like ephemeral acts, as Rebecca Schneider has argued, are, in fact, re-enactments that remain and persist through 'body-to-body transmission'.[9]

Chapter 10 investigates both disciplinary and medical histories that have moulded modern drama and its interpretation, as well as the ways that modern drama has shaped and reinforced medical ideologies. It begins with an interview with Stanton B. Garner, Jr, discussing the scholarly acts that dismissed and then returned the medicalized body to the study of theatre since the late nineteenth century. His seminal essay, 'Is There a Doctor in the House? Medicine and the Making of Modern Drama', republished here, then explores how medical assumptions about accessing bodily interiors conditioned both dramatic and medical ways of seeing in realist drama and that continue to inform dramatic representations. Both disciplines instilled an 'ideology of the visible' about the somatic body that prioritized visible signs of illness above medical imaging and a patient's subjective experiences. Garner's chapter invites readers to consider how this earlier intermingling of theatre and medicine ghosts what sociologist Alison Pugh has referred to as the 'cultural ascendancy of data as authority' in twenty-first-century medical care.[10] Medicine's overreliance on information rather than inviting patients' active co-performances makes modern medicine the heir to what Garner names the 'containment' manoeuvers of stage doctors a century ago, attempts to regulate which senses, experiences and forms of evidence were pertinent to understanding illness.

In Chapter 11, Kirsten E. Shepherd recovers a largely forgotten set of performances that influenced avant-garde theatre and dance in the mid-twentieth century and that, she argues, offers a still potent model for promoting structural medical reform. In her analysis, the Federal Theatre Project's (FTP) exuberantly spectacular *Medicine Show*, a Living Newspaper that worked to empower patients and caregivers, as well as actors and audiences, to act together to heal institutions and formulate public policy. In *Medicine Show*, statistics projected on screens and stylized movement 'keep the audience's attention on the forces

[8] Arthur Frank, *The Wounded Storyteller: Body, Illness & Ethics* (University of Chicago Press, 2013), 11.

[9] Rebecca Schneider, *Performance Remains: Art and War in Times of Theatrical Reenactment* (Routledge, 2014), 104.

[10] Alison Pugh, *The Last Human Job: The Work of Connecting in a Disconnected World* (Princeton University Press, 2024), 6.

(economic, political, social, historical) that underpin what they are viewing' and involves them as 'stakeholders in the potential outcomes'. By refusing the individuated personalities and melodrama of prior medical theatre, the FTP instead poses the collective task of bringing structures into being that are difficult to perceive visually: policies and facilities that will affect the well-being of millions of patients.

As these authors suggest, we need to be mindful about the uses we make of history and memory. Performance theorists Soyica Diggs Colbert, Douglas A. Jones, Jr, and Shane Vogel encourage us to see at least two possibilities within the repetitions and dislocations that characterize performance: one that 'has the capacity to perpetuate the familiar and dominant through repetitions that have consolidated into a seemingly consistent state of being or state of nature' and another that 'has the capacity to warp or subvert the familiar and dominant through restorations – as repair or mending – of what has been forgotten, overlooked, misremembered, suppressed, dormant, or denied'.[11] Garner and Shepherd call our attention to repetitions (primarily of realist ideology and aesthetics) within medicine and theatre that can be unsettled through reconsiderations, restorations and resistances to the past.

The final chapter in this section calls attention to a more insidious form of ghosting, sounding an urgent cautionary note about how and why medicine has historically collaborated with theatre. In their essay on 'Performance and Medical Education', Marlis Schweitzer and Sara Masciotra-Milstein demonstrate that while theatre can publicize medical developments, 'democratize scientific knowledge' and incite collaborations and debate, it can also lend populist appeal to scientific racism. The lecture performances of George Combe in the early nineteenth century, dramaturged and assisted by his wife, Cecilia, the daughter of celebrity actor Sarah Siddons, contributed to the 'rapid uptake in Britain and North America' by middle-class audiences of phrenology, a 'science of the mind' that claimed to explain mental ability by measuring the shape and size of skulls. While the pairing of theatre and medicine gave women like Cecilia opportunities to participate in medical discourses that would have otherwise been closed to them, Schweitzer and Masciotra-Milstein encourage us to resist 'utopian' accounts of what theatre can bring to medical practice. They trace a link from the Combes to present-day celebrity doctors who use social media and television to promote their dubious products and lifestyle regimens, many of which draw on both the tacit racism of historical science and the legacy of nineteenth-century medical spectacle.

[11] Soyica Diggs Colbert, Douglas A. Jones and Shane Vogel, 'Tidying Up After Repetition', in *Race and Performance After Repetition*, ed. Colbert, Jones and Vogel (Duke University Press, 2020), 8.

While theatre and performance can introduce complexity, historical breadth and ambiguity into medicine, they can also, as this section shows, abet harmful science with charisma and the seductions of familiar plots and characters. Through their restoration of a theatrical past, these chapters unearth a performance tradition that needs to be questioned rather than uncritically reproduced. Performative medicine can be most effective when it considers the histories that shape and suffuse healing actions as well as when it looks to past performances as a repertoire of models, cautions and still-vital proposals.

REFERENCES

Broyard, Anatole. *Intoxicated by My Illness*. Clarkson Potter, 1992.

Carlson, Marvin. *The Haunted Stage: Theatre as Memory Machine*. Michigan University Press, 2001.

Colbert, Soyica Diggs, Douglas A. Jones, and Shane Vogel. 'Tidying Up After Repetition'. In *Race and Performance After Repetition*, edited by Colbert, Jones and Vogel. Duke University Press, 2020.

Frank, Arthur. *The Wounded Storyteller: Body, Illness & Ethics*. University of Chicago Press, 2013.

Pugh, Alison. *The Last Human Job: The Work of Connecting in a Disconnected World*. Princeton University Press, 2024.

Schneider, Rebecca. *Performance Remains: Art and War in Times of Theatrical Reenactment*. Routledge, 2014.

Taylor, Diana. 'Translating Performance'. In *The Performance Studies Reader*, 2nd edition, edited by Henry Bial. Routledge, 2007.

10

Medical influences on modern theatre and theatrical influences on modern medicine

AN INTERVIEW WITH STANTON B. GARNER, JR

Stanton B. Garner, Jr, James Douglas Bruce Professor of English and Theatre at the University of Tennessee, is a pioneer in the field of medicine and theatre. In addition to his 2023 book *Theatre & Medicine*, he has published articles on literary naturalism and physiology, reconstructive surgery and the avant garde of the First World War, theories of contagion and the French writer Antonin Artaud, theatre and medical science, performances about dementia, and theatre and vaccine resistance. He has also published books on the phenomenology of theatre. This interview was conducted to reflect on Garner's seminal essay reprinted below, 'Is There a Doctor in the House? Medicine and the Making of Modern Drama',[1] and on how the field has developed since its publication in 2008.

[1] This essay was originally published in *Modern Drama* 51, no. 3 (2008): 311–28, and is reprinted with permission.

I. THE GENESIS OF A SCHOLARLY FIELD

You are a pioneer in the field of medicine and theatre, and well positioned to explain how the field has developed since the publication of 'Is There a Doctor in the House?' Can you tell us how and why you began researching this field?

Stanton B. Garner, Jr (SG): I became interested in the connections between theatre and medicine when I was exploring the intersections of phenomenology, embodiment and performance in the mid–late 1980s. I felt that the body had vanished somehow from the theoretical discourse around theatre and I wanted to bring it back. Some of the best work being done on the subject, I found, was by medical and other phenomenologists. Their descriptions of illness, the phenomenology of illness and how a body becomes an object to itself in states of pain and illness really resonated with the kind of research that I wanted to do.

Were there any playwrights whose work resonated with your nascent interests?

SG: At the time, I was working closely with Samuel Beckett's plays. I was struck by the similarities between the bodily experiences of Beckett's characters and neurological descriptions of non-normative phenomena – medical conditions such as phantom limbs, schizophrenia and Parkinson's disease, which Beckett's mother suffered from. In his plays – particularly the late ones – it was as if I were reading the theatrical equivalents of phenomenologically informed medical descriptions in the displaced, decentred characters whose bodies there and not there. His work persuaded me that he and his fellow dramatists were attuned to the medical concerns of the day.

I was also influenced by Tony Kushner's *Angels in America* (1991), by Margaret Edson's *W;t* (1995) and by the earlier work of British writers in the 1980s including Sarah Daniel's *Byrthrite* (1986). While exploring a broader historical terrain, I became fascinated thinking about the connection between experimental physiology – particularly, the work of Claude Bernard in France – and the role it played in novelist and playwright Emile Zola's theory of naturalism in both the theatre and the novel.[2]

[2] Once I put medicine and theatre next to each other during the period that I was interested in, all kinds of things started to flash. My research led to an article on Tristan Tzara's *Gas Heart* and reconstructive surgery during the First World War, specifically, the subject of facial disfigurement ('*The Gas Heart*: Disfigurement and the Dada Body', *Modern Drama* 50, no. 4 (2007): 500–16). I also wrote an article on Antonin Artaud's essay 'Theater and the Plague' about germ theory and contagion ('Artaud, Germ Theory, and the Theatre of Contagion', *Theatre Journal* 58, no. 1 (2006): 1–14).

How did you move from exploring a personal research interest to meeting like-minded scholars and collaboratively developing the field?

SG: In 2000 I delivered a paper on Zola, experimental medicine and the naturalist stage at a conference. Selected proceedings from the conference were published by the editors of *Modern Drama* in 2000. A number of people who read the collection shared my sense that there were important intersections between modern medicine and theatre. Meeting researchers in this emerging interdisciplinary field inspired me to research other connections. I subsequently met scholars working in related areas when I organized a working group on theatre and medicine for the 2006 American Society for Theatre Research conference.

Due to its humoral basis of characterization, early modern theatre demonstrated that how we explain bodies medically influences how we think of them theatrically. Although scholars of early modern theatre addressed this connection, very little research of this kind focused on modern drama – particularly the period that I was interested in, from 1880 to 1945, when so much was happening in the fields of medicine and theatre. During that time, in my view, medicine and theatre simultaneously explored their own modernity in intersecting ways. I was struck by the number of people who attempted to go to medical school but ended up dropping out and becoming dramatists. Reading about these overlaps, at the time, I said to myself, 'There's a story here that needs to be told.'

In fall 2008, I guest-edited a special issue of *Modern Drama* on the topic of Theatre and Medicine. The essay reprinted here was the introduction to the special issue. It lays the framework for understanding the medical influence on modern theatre, and the theatrical influences on modern medicine. Broadly speaking, the essay argues for the historical intersection of these two fields. Theatre and medicine, after all, are both discourses and technologies of the body. That insight helped frame not only my thinking, but other people's thinking about the intersection as well.

Why do you focus on the figure of the doctor?

SG: The first half of the essay's title, 'Is There a Doctor in the House', was quite deliberate. When I investigated who else was writing about medicine and modern drama during this period, I kept coming up with discussions of doctors. My contribution to the field entailed reappropriating the figure by presenting doctors not as plot devices or thematic signposts, but as threshold figures who mediate the body's somatic disclosure, particularly in realist and naturalist drama.

II. BRIDGING HEALTHCARE AND THEATRE

Did you have a sense that there were also medical practitioners picking up that excitement or sharing it? Or was it more one-sided?

SG: The essay I wrote for the introduction was directed primarily at theatre scholars. From the start, however, I was aware of the medical side of the interdisciplinary questions I was asking. I suspected it was going to be a big ask to get health professionals engaged. Traditionally, the field of medical humanities has tended to marginalize theatre and performance in favour of literature and other arts. When it comes to theatre, I attribute this oversight to theatre's ambivalent place in the humanities generally. Drama is a literary art, but it's also a practical art. Implicitly, then, my audience included medical practitioners, since medical humanities programmes operate not just in universities, but also in hospitals. It seemed to me that my work would potentially be useful to conversations in the medical humanities.

Do you think that theatre enables medical practitioners to recognize philosophical approaches that implicitly or explicitly influence the structure and scope of their practice?

SG: In the United States, an important example of what practitioners can learn is evident from what happened with Margaret Edson's play about a terminal cancer patient, *W;t* (1995). The play was staged in New York with talkbacks including cancer patients, medical professionals, actors and the director. The play opened up a dialogue. I saw it in New York and sat through the talkback at the end. The play was subsequently incorporated into the *W;t* Educational Initiative, which was brought to medical centres in the form of local theatre productions. Later, after the film adaptation came out, they screened it as well.

In the discussions after the performance of *W;t*, theatre was used therapeutically to vent emotions and reflect on people's experiences in the healthcare system. But it was also useful for medical education. After witnessing these possibilities, I became much more interested in the institutional connections between theatre and medicine. I researched a number of plays about dementia, autism and other neuro-atypical conditions in Britain that played to medical audiences as well as theatrical audiences. Powerful and vital exchanges between theatre and medicine were emerging, especially with *W;t*. I know less about other countries, but that was a big one in the United States.

Your reference to W;t *clarifies how drama can operate as a therapeutic space, as a space for education and pedagogy, or even simply to open up a dialogue. Can you talk about the impact of Tony Kushner's play about the AIDS crisis,* Angels in America *(1991), in that regard?*

SG: It had a huge impact. When it opened in New York, I took a drama class to see it. Its medical realism – Prior Walter's body on stage with the lesions on his body, completely naked – was more troubling for many of the students I brought than its explicit sexuality. There were other plays about AIDs, but Kushner's was singular in the way it took the disease and portrayed it in the context of contesting ideas of America. It linked Prior Walter with AIDS to his ancestors grappling with the Bubonic Plague and the Great Plague of London as a way of linking AIDS with earlier epidemics.

Recently you wrote about the use of theatre in vaccination campaigns in Nigeria and Bangladesh. This kind of collaboration strikes us as a powerful example of a dialogue between medicine and theatre.

SG: I'm fascinated by collaborations between theatre and pharmaceutical companies. I wrote about George Bernard Shaw and the anti-vaccination campaigns of the nineteenth century, which were often quite performative affairs, owing to the rallies that occurred. I also wrote about Jonathan Spector's play, *Eureka Day* (2019), that was written before the pandemic, which is about vaccination panic in a progressive school. But the part I really enjoyed most was researching community theatre-based vaccination campaigns. This type of theatre – the use of community theatre, specifically, participatory theatre – to overcome fears, preconceptions that people have about vaccinations goes way back.

I researched a 1994 vaccination campaign in Nigeria and a 2019 one with the Rohingya refugee population in Bangladesh to understand how theatre could be used in this way. In Nigeria, the playwright Jimi Solanke wrote a number of plays to be performed in villages in Nigeria as part of vaccination and other public health campaigns. Previous campaigns had been conducted using television and radio, but many people living in villages did not have access to those media. In response to this, a team of performers and health workers travelled to these villages. After meeting with members of the village beforehand to learn about each village and the issues it faced, they incorporated the information into the play. People from the village also participated in the plays.

III. CHANGING TERMS: FROM THEATRE TO PERFORMANCE

Your discussion of your research brings us to the current moment. What are some of the most interesting and exciting contemporary directions in the field?

SG: That's a big question. For me, a key moment was the publication of Alex Mermikides and Gianna Bouchard's edited collection *Performance and the Medical Body* in 2016. That book instigated a shift from theatre to performance, a category that includes theatre along with a number of other things that theatre and medicine do. The term 'performance', of course, means different things in these two fields. The medical meanings of performance include things that are not exactly theatrical, but it opens a space where practitioners, medical educators and scholars in the humanities and arts can discover how they're approaching medical issues from different directions.

I recently read Roberta Barker's book *Symptoms of the Self: Tuberculosis and the Modern Stage*. The article you're reprinting here focused heavily on physiology, which I saw as a master trope in theatre in the late nineteenth century just as humoral theory was in the early modern period. I raised questions about the body's interiorities and scientific frames for understanding this. After reading Barker's book on tuberculosis, I realized the story that I didn't tell, which is the impact of the sentimental tradition, and particularly consumption drama such as Alexandre Dumas fils's *Camille* (1852), on the medical consciousness of the late nineteenth and early twentieth centuries.

Even as physiology was mapping a research-based notion of the body as an internal system, consumption plays were employing medical realism and graphic depictions of what it does to the body, but doing it in highly theatrical ways. I realized that even as dramatists might have been influenced by the scientific writings of physiology and other medical sciences, they were borrowing the tropes of consumption performance to portray illness. That insight complicates how we view the relationship between theatre and medicine in interesting ways.

Can you comment on the frustration occasionally articulated in modern drama about patients' unwillingness to perform, or resistance to making their interior experience legible? For example, in Lisa Kron's Well *(2006) the daughter enlists an entire spectacular apparatus to integrate the mother's experience into the daughter's drama of healing and wellness, but the mother insists on following her own inscrutable and, to her daughter, illegible journey. On a meta-theatrical level, the mother interferes with the play: her illness remains inscrutable to the end.*

SG: *Well* demonstrated that illness is on the surface, but it's also inside. One of the preoccupations of what we think of as modern medicine has to do with ways of measuring and accessing the interior. That impulse to sound the depths seemingly entails turning away from the performative. The idea begins with the X-ray, a technology that brings the interior into view. But no matter how well you do that, the subjective register of disease remains elusive. Like everything else that's internal, illness must be disclosed using external means, and performance is a good model for doing that.

Of course, performance brings its own issues of verifiability. I'm fascinated by Munchausen's syndrome, the psychological disorder where someone pretends to be ill and even produces the symptoms of illness, and by the question of when an illness is real and when it is faked. There's no clear answer to that, but the fact that we would ask that question points to the slipperiness of performing illness in theatrical and other contexts.

IV. THEATRICAL DISRUPTIONS

What do you see disability studies adding to the consideration of the intersection between medicine and theatre?

SG: Disability is such a contested term, particularly its relation to the medical model. Contemporary disability theory and disability activism counterpoints the social with the medical notion of disability. The loss in that, I think, is the recognition that in many cases (not necessarily all) there are medical aspects to many disabilities.

I have found disability studies useful for thinking about embodiment and human difference. When we talk about the body in medicine, what body are we uncritically assuming? And if what we say about how people experience illness is not true for all people, then what are our responsibilities for including non-normative forms of embodiment? Do we need to think of experience not as single things, but as fields of variability? In addition, because disability is fundamentally about agency, it raises questions that can be brought back into the analyses of medical and theatrical performances in ways that make our thinking more nuanced and responsive.

I wrote a book, for example, on spectatorship and movement – in the sense of how performers move on stage and, more specifically, how spectators kinaesthetically process the movements they observe by vicariously inhabiting them. Most of the accounts that I drew on from phenomenology and cognitive science posited an able body. Using the insights of disability studies, I wanted to write that book without that presupposition and to seek in phenomenological accounts and in descriptions for people who move with disabilities, what the variables are for that.

As part of this project, I wrote about the 2017 Sam Gold production of Tennessee Williams's *The Glass Menagerie*, which cast Madison Ferris, an actor with muscular dystrophy, as Laura Wingfield. Playing Laura with a differently abled body in this way thrilled and also upset people. There is a history of disability with *Glass Menagerie*; Williams's stage directions indicates that Laura is disabled – 'crippled' is the word he uses – but also specifies that this 'defect' need only be suggested. It's as if he wants to have physical disability in the play but also disown it. In the end, of course, whatever physical disability Laura has serves as a metaphor or a symbol of psychological and emotional disability. Casting an actor in a wheelchair who moves across the stage on her own with an elaborate, but beautiful, arched crawling was a powerful portrayal of what disability is and what it isn't.

One topic you address in your work that has influenced subsequent scholarship is how theatre contests the totalizing nature of the medical gaze. As you explain, by its very nature, theatre offers us so many different observational positions. Has that foundational observation continued to inform your work?

SG: Theatre is the medium that looks back. To give voice on stage to someone with an illness is to bring into an objectifying field of vision a perspective and agency that can never be contained by anyone's gaze. *W;t* is the classic example of this dynamic. Vivien Bearing, the central character who is dying of cancer, talks to the audience. A John Donne scholar, she describes being read by the clinical staff as though she were a text. While lecturing in her hospital gown, a slide of John Donne's poetry is projected over her body. 'Now I know how poems feel', she says at one point. But in saying that – in recognizing the experience of objectification – she simultaneously reclaims her voice in the depersonalization of the hospital encounter. And the clinicians and students all come in; they have their rounds; they talk about her like she's not there. We all know that kind of thing. It seems to me that *W;t* highlights that in any performance of illness, there is always implicitly or overtly a speaking-back, a co-opting of the gaze. That's one of the reasons why I've always had an issue with applying totalizing interpretations of 'the gaze' to the theatre – the kind of thing Michel Foucault writes about, and that film theorist Laura Mulvey describes.[3] Theatre and performance don't indulge that gaze; instead, they challenge it from a position of subjectivity.

[3] Michel Foucault, *Naissance de la clinique: une archéologie du regard médical* (Presses universitaires de France, 1963, English translation, 1973); Laura Mulvey, 'Visual Pleasure and Narrative Cinema', *Screen* 16, no. 3 (1975): 6–18.

REFERENCES

Barker, Roberta. *Symptoms of the Self: Tuberculosis and the Modern Stage*. University of Iowa Press, 2022.

Foucault, Michel. *Naissance de la clinique: une archéologie du regard medical*. Presses universitaires de France, 1963.

Garner, Stanton B., Jr. 'Artaud, Germ Theory, and the Theatre of Contagion'. *Theatre Journal* 58, no. 1 (2006): 1–14.

Garner, Stanton B., Jr. '*The Gas Heart*: Disfigurement and the Dada Body'. *Modern Drama* 50, no. 4 (2007): 500–16.

Mermikides, Alex, and Gianna Bouchard, eds. *Performance and the Medical Body*. Bloomsbury Methuen Drama, 2016.

Mulvey, Laura. 'Visual Pleasure and Narrative Cinema'. *Screen* 16, no. 3 (1975): 6–18.

'Is there a doctor in the house? Medicine and the making of modern drama' (2008)

STANTON B. GARNER, JR

I. MEDICINE AND THE MODERN STAGE

In July 2005, the British theatre company Sound and Fury, in collaboration with artists from a performance collective named Shunt, presented a theatre piece entitled *Ether Frolics*. Performed in an underground vault beneath London Bridge Station, the work explored the history and contemporary practice of anaesthesia. Modern anaesthetics originated in the 1840s, when the surgical use of nitrous oxide, ether, and chloroform was pioneered by dentists and doctors in the United States and Europe. *Ether Frolics* – its title refers to gatherings that were organized around recreational use of the chemical in the 1830s and 1840s – explored the boundaries between consciousness and unconsciousness and the shifting somatic experiences that these developments opened to awareness. The production's spectator/participants were seated in a room that was closed off by hospital screens and illuminated by bright lights. One of the performers delivered a monologue to the audience, in which he compared their position as spectators to that of medical patients. When the lights were suddenly extinguished, the resulting darkness created a visceral experience of sensory disorientation. Sounds arose in the darkness – far-off tinkling bells, grinding, groaning – and the performance area was illuminated by brief, dream-like images and scenes. Geometric shapes emerged from the darkness; a woman in evening clothes responded to disembodied heads in boxes on the floor. The concluding sequence reproduced the experience of awakening from anaesthesia. Michael Billington of the *Guardian* described this sequence and its effect: 'The moment of recovering consciousness, with distant voices slowly acquiring sharper definition as one re-enters the real world, will stay with me for some time.'

In its interdisciplinary genesis, *Ether Frolics* demonstrates the deepening connections between theatre, performance, and the field of medicine in recent[1] decades. Co-commissioned by the Battersea Arts Centre and the Warwick Arts Centre, Coventry, the production was funded by Arts Council England and the Wellcome Trust, which funds biomedical research, research in medical history, and interdisciplinary projects in the arts and humanities that address issues of medical science. Additional support was provided by BOC Medical, one of Britain's leading providers of medical gas products. David Rosenberg, one of the cofounders of Shunt and a performer in *Ether Frolics*, is a trained anaesthesiologist, and a trio of medical researchers acted as scientific advisors to the project ('Sound and Fury: *Ether Frolics*'). Similar collaborations between theatre artists and medical practitioners have proliferated over the past twenty years, and these have concerned themselves with a range of medical and public health issues: medical technology, AIDS education, vaccination, trauma therapy, public health policy, disability activism, and medical training.[2]

The relationship between theatre and medicine is a long-standing one. Aristotle's notion of tragic *katharsis* as 'purgation' and 'purification' reflects the word's medical origins, and the term *cathartic* is still used in medicine to refer to a laxative or other agent used to purge the bowels. The humoral system of health, illness, and personality that formed the cornerstone of Galen's medical theory influenced dramatic characterization on the Greek, Roman, and Elizabethan and Jacobean stages. The practice of anatomy during the sixteenth and seventeenth centuries, which acquired intellectual and cultural prestige from the publication of Andreas Vesalius's *De humani corporis fabrica*

---

[1] Note that as this essay is reprinted in its original form, relative time expressions here and throughout refer to the original publication date of 2008.

[2] In another example of such collaboration, the theatre/performance company Clod Ensemble, founded in 1995, has developed a programme of courses and workshops entitled the Performing Medicine Project that uses theatre and the arts in the training of doctors and other health professionals; current collaborators on this project include Lois Weaver and Peggy Shaw of the New York-based performance group Split Britches. See www.clodensemble.com/ and https://performingmedicine.com/.

(On the Workings of the Human Body) in 1543, was deeply theatricalized, and spectators attended public demonstrations by surgeons and physicians in specially built anatomical theatres. The English architect and stage designer Inigo Jones, who collaborated with Ben Jonson on Stuart court masques, was commissioned in 1636 to design an anatomical theatre for the Barber-Surgeon Company, which was licensed to perform four public anatomies a year. While anatomical demonstrations were designed to disseminate knowledge of the human body and were attended by medical practitioners, they also served – like the public executions that provided bodies for dissection – as festive occasions and forms of popular entertainment. In Bologna, public anatomies were linked to carnival and a wider field of performance forms; indeed, members of the audience sometimes attended these demonstrations wearing carnival masks.[3]

Following the publication of Jonathan Sawday's groundbreaking study *The Body Emblazoned: Dissection and the Human Body in Renaissance Culture* in 1995, and in keeping with a growing interest in the medical within literary studies since 1990,[4] the role of medicine in early modern society and culture has received extensive attention from literary and theatre scholars over the past ten years. Not surprisingly – given the prevalence of disease, bodily violence, remedies, poisons, pregnancy, fits, and possessions and the presence of doctors, healers, and charlatans on the Elizabethan and Jacobean stage – a majority of the most recent work in this area has been devoted to early modern drama in England. In *Sick Economies: Drama, Mercantilism, and Disease in Shakespeare's England* (2004), Jonathan Gil Harris examines the ways in which dramatic and mercantilist writers used the newly developed language of infectious disease to articulate an emerging national economy and a foreign economic sphere increasingly viewed as pathological. In *Drugs and Theater in Early Modern England* (2005), Tanya Pollard explores the representations of drugs in Elizabethan and Jacobean drama in the context of the changing field of early modern pharmacology. And in *Beyond the Body: The Boundaries of Medicine and English Renaissance Drama* (2005), William Kerwin considers the role played by the influence of non-medical controversies, economic factors, and historical trends in the meanings of medical culture, medical practice and their representation in early modern drama. Hillary M. Nunn, Maurizio Calbi, Ken Jackson, Todd H. J. Pettigrew, and others have extended this study of the relationship between early modern English theatre and the

[3] Hillary M. Nunn, *Staging Anatomies: Dissection and Spectacle in Early Stuart Tragedy* (Ashgate, 2005), 9.

[4] See Rothfield, Davis, Archimedes and Kickel for examples of this critical movement.

practices, discourses, institutions, and contesting professions of early modern medicine.[5]

Compared to the expanding and productive work that has been done in this area by early modern scholars, it is surprising how little attention has been paid to the intersections of theatre and medicine in modern drama. The histories of medicine and theatre during the last hundred-and-fifty years certainly encourage such attention. The second half of the nineteenth century and the first quarter of the twentieth witnessed innovations in both fields, as a self-styled 'modern' theatre asserted itself against the conventions of an earlier period and medical science claimed new authority – and cultural prestige – within the emerging network of modern disciplines. In the medical field, this period saw revolutionary advances in medical technologies for penetrating, measuring, and representing the body; for reconstructing and extending it prosthetically; and for treating its states of disease. The development of germ theory ushered in the heroic age of microbiology, in which Louis Pasteur, Robert Koch, and other medical researchers conquered such ancient scourges as typhoid fever, rabies, cholera, diphtheria, tetanus, bubonic plague, and syphilis. Parallel accomplishments in the areas of sanitation and public health addressed the relationship between disease and environment. As earlier nineteenth-century developments in anaesthesiology transformed the practice of surgery, they also raised medical, cultural, and literary interest in the relationship between consciousness and pain. Finally, the expansion of colonial (or tropical) medicine as a discipline underscored the medical face of European and American imperialism, while the research of Jean-Martin Charcot, Sigmund Freud, and others on the nature of hysteria propelled the development of neurology and a modern science of mind along a distinctively gendered trajectory. All of these medical developments were influenced by – and, in turn, influenced – a broader social concern with such issues as social degeneracy, physical culture, race, and the changing relationship between workers' bodies and the mechanisms of production in early twentieth-century capitalism.

The biographical and other circumstantial connections among theatre, drama, and medicine are well known. Henrik Ibsen served six years as a pharmacist's apprentice in Grimstad before failing his matriculation exams at the University of Christiana and abandoning his plans to study medicine. August Strindberg, who, as a young man, tutored the children of two prominent physicians, studied medicine for two years before failing a qualifying exam in chemistry. Although both men abandoned careers in medicine, they retained an interest in medicine and medical observation throughout their subsequent careers as writers. Not all of the modern playwrights who expressed an interest

[5] This scholarly list includes the contributors to Moss and Peterson.

in medicine, of course, were frustrated in this way. Even as he was establishing himself as a writer of comic sketches, parodies, dialogues, and short stories in small-press periodicals, Anton Chekhov earned a medical degree from the Moscow University School of Medicine, and while he soon gave up private practice in order to pursue his career as a writer, his medical training remained an essential part of his personal and professional identity. In 1888 Chekhov wrote to his friend and publisher Alexei Suvorin, 'Medicine is my lawful wedded wife, and literature is my mistress. When one gets on my nerves, I spend the night with the other.'[6] He continued to treat patients, often for free, and he demonstrated a life-long interest in matters of public health. During the famine and cholera epidemic of 1892–93, he served as head of a district sanitary committee and treated many of the epidemic's poorest victims. George Bernard Shaw served on the Health Committee of the St. Pancras Vestry Committee, while Bertolt Brecht served as a medical orderly in Augsburg during the closing months of World War I.

The discipline of medicine, in other words, is written into the biographical history of early modern drama to an extent that other non-literary disciplines (law, for instance) are not. But while the staging of medical issues has received some scholarly treatment – one thinks of Roger Boxhill's 1969 study of Shaw and the medical profession, for example, or Daryl Ogden's more recent 'immuno/virological' analysis of *Angels in America* – the important role of the medical in modern drama has, for the most part, gone unremarked. An apparent exception is recent work on the body in performance in the field of disability studies.[7] While this work addresses such medical issues and conditions as Alzheimer's disease, depression, and cancer, it does so in deliberately non-medical terms. Because disability studies focuses on the cultural construction of bodily difference in terms of oppositional categories – ableness and disability, normality and freakishness – it is strategically opposed to the 'medical model' that identifies and pathologizes extraordinary bodies in biological terms. The benefits of this critical movement for drama, theatre, and performance studies, all of which deal with the body's personal and social performances, are obvious; indeed, no approach has yielded greater fruits in these fields in recent years. But the emphasis of disability studies on cultural construction is often at odds with a study of the somatic body, its conditions of ease and dis-ease, and the biosphere to which it belongs, while the suspicion of the medical on the part of disability theorists limits their interest in broader developments in medical discourses, practices and technologies. The difficulty presented by a

---

[6] *Anton Chekhov's Life and Thought: Selected Letters and Commentary*, trans. Michael Henry Heim with Simon Karlinsky (University of California Press, 1975), 107.

[7] See Fahy and King; Kuppers; Sandahl and Auslander.

narrow application of this approach to the study of theatre and medicine is evident with a figure such as Samuel Beckett, whose drama and fiction are rife with medical terminology and with characters marked by bodily impairment and illness. The medicalized *mise en scène* of Beckett's plays resonates with the work of contemporary neurology, medical phenomenology, and medical ethics, but because Beckett's work does not foreground the social meanings of impairment, it has been received little attention from disability theorists. Those who consider it, such as Ato Quayson, inevitably confront the question of whether one can speak of disability at all in Beckett's dramatic and fictional universe.[8]

One reason for the relative neglect of medical history in the study of modern and contemporary drama lies, no doubt, in the changing nature of medical theory and practice over the past two-hundred years. The connections between medicine and theatre in the early modern period have rewarded scholarly attention, in part, because illness and its various forms of treatment were so deeply implicated in the theatrical. The theory of the humours – positing, as it did, that health and illness resulted from an imbalance of bodily fluids – was an acutely performative understanding of somatic conditions and psychological temperaments. Individuals performed their physical and mental states, and these performances – which involved appearance, expressions, bodily disposition, movements, and behaviours – had recognizable types or personalities: sanguine, phlegmatic, choleric, melancholic. Disordered dispositions, such as those caricatured in Ben Jonson's humours comedies, existed on a performance continuum with disease, which had its own forms of display in early modern Europe: the discolorations and grotesque swelling of bubonic plague, the facial disfigurements of syphilis, which was introduced to Europe in the sixteenth century (or reintroduced, according to some theories) as a result of contact with the New World. Disease treatment was often in keeping with this external emphasis, with bleedings and purgings designed to release substances and fluids from the body's interior. To an extent less true in later periods, in other words, illness was a public affair in early modern Europe; anatomy theatres and the popular exhibitions of the insane in Bethlem ('Bedlam') hospital were the most overt manifestations of disease's social face. The scenes of Jonson's *Volpone*, in this sense, reflect the theatricalized medical landscape within which they were

[8] 'Since the complicated and multifaceted structures of Beckett's texts resist any assumption of mimesis, we are bound to ask whether we can ultimately claim him for disability studies. The elusive status of impairment in his work makes no straightforward answer available' (Ato Quayson, *Aesthetic Nervousness: Disability and the Crisis of Representation* (Columbia University Press, 2007), 85). Approaching this issue from a different critical perspective, Ruby Cohn raises a similar question: 'Although Beckett probably stages more handicapped or fragmented characters than do other playwrights, he provides no social context for their afflictions' ('"It Hurts?" Afflicted Bodies in Beckett's Drama', in *Peering behind the Curtain: Disability, Illness, and the Extraordinary Body in Contemporary Theater*, ed. Thomas Fahy and Kimball King (Routledge, 2002), 53).

written: a mountebank hawking his wares in the marketplace of remedies; a lawyer falling to the floor in a feigned seizure; a dying man whose drawn face and runny eyes are the hottest ticket in town.

While modern medicine has not abandoned the theatrical in its presentation and treatment of disease – the experiments of Louis Pasteur and others in the development of modern microbiology were often highly staged events, and Charcot's lectures on hysteria and other disorders at the Hôpital de la Salpêtrière became fashionable public spectacles – its dominant institutional and theoretical developments have been in less performative directions. Germ theory defines the genesis, progression, and transmission of disease in terms of microbial agents invisible to the naked eye. With developments such as this and the advent of physiological anatomy – which focused attention on the body's internal workings as an organic system – in the work of Claude Bernard and others, illness and disease became increasingly the business of the medical laboratory, the clinic with its technologies for measuring the body's internal states, and the epidemiological study. In his well-known discussion of the birth of the modern clinic, Michel Foucault describes the late eighteenth and early nineteenth centuries as

> one of those periods that mark an ineradicable chronological threshold: the period in which illness, counter-nature, death, in short, the whole dark underside of disease came to light, at the same time illuminating and eliminating itself like night, in the deep, visible, solid, enclosed, but accessible space of the human body.[9]

There is dramatic interest, to be sure, in medical discovery, clinical treatment, and the disclosure of bodily tissues to radiological and other technologies of micro-imaging. But the drama of the somatic body under the regime of modern medicine does not lend itself as easily to theatrical forms of enactment as it does (say) to the emerging medium of film, which was an important component of modern medicine's early technologies.[10] What would a drama of germ theory, for one, look like? To appreciate the challenges facing such a drama, one need only look at the opening of Shaw's 1932 play *Too True to Be Good*. Shaw, who

---

[9] Michel Foucault, *The Birth of the Clinic: An Archaeology of Medical Perception*, trans. A. M. Sheridan Smith (Random, [1975] 1994), 195.

[10] 'The history of cinema is, from its beginning, bound up with medical cinematography. Étienne-Jules Marey, whose "photographic gun" was an immediate technological precursor to the cinema camera, was one of the most important physiologists of his era, and the Lumière brothers, who are credited (along with Edison) with inventing motion pictures, used their devices to study human movement' (T. Hugh Crawford, 'Visual Knowledge in Medicine and Popular Film', *Literature and Medicine* 17, no. 1 (1998): 24). For a fuller discussion of this connection, see Cartwright, Screening the Body.

rejected germ theory and opposed the practice of vaccination, opens his play in a sickroom where a woman lies asleep, her medicine table covered with bottle, pills, and thermometer. Near her, in an easy chair, sits a Monster – '*made of a luminous jelly with a visible skeleton of short black rods*'[11] – who subsequently identifies himself (if such identification were needed) as a microbe. In Shaw's playful inversion of disease aetiology, the microbe laments the doctor's claim that the patient caught measles as the result of a germ, insisting that she, in fact, passed the disease on to him. An actor costumed as a microbe makes for a strikingly comic effect, but its very absurdity underscores a discrepancy between the theatre's externalizing spectacle and the interior of the body where microbial disease takes its course. In the absence of Shaw's animated microbe, the play's opening consists of nothing more than a woman lying ill in bed. In terms of traditional notions of dramatic action, the model of illness as defined by microbiology is, for the most part, untheatrical. As Sigmund Freud famously observed in his essay 'Psychopathic Characters on the Stage',

> a person who is physically ill can only figure on the stage as a piece of stage-property and not as a hero, unless, indeed, some peculiar physical aspects of his [*sic*] illness make psychical activity possible – such, for instance, as the sick man's forlorn state in the Philoctetes or the hopelessness of the sufferers in the class of plays that centre round consumptives.[12]

An additional impediment to recognizing the role of the medical in modern drama has been the prominence of realism – the most under-appreciated and easily dismissed of theatrical aesthetics – within this tradition. The representational limitations of this aesthetic are readily apparent. Because of realism's investment in the ideology of the visible, the interior landscape of disease is consigned to one of its many offstage realms, while the technological devices by which this realm might be disclosed to the audience – image and sound projection, X-ray imaging, and so on – are precluded from strictly illusionistic theatre. While medical settings have made their way into modern and contemporary plays – Sidney Kingsley's *Men in White* (1933), Tony Kushner's *Angels in America* (1991), and Margaret Edson's *Wit* (1995), for example – the most successful of these plays interrupt the realistic *mise en scène* with explicitly presentational techniques. Caryl Churchill's *Vinegar Tom* (1976), which includes the emerging medical profession in its critique of seventeenth-century institutions, stages the procedures of bleeding and 'pricking' with gestic boldness.

---

[11] George Bernard Shaw, *Too True to Be Good: A Political Extravaganza*, in *Plays Extravagant* (Penguin, 1981), 37.

[12] Sigmund Freud, 'Psychopathic Characters on the Stage', in *The Complete Psychological Works of Sigmund Freud*, vol. 7, trans. James Strachey (Hogarth, [1942 (1905 or 1906)] 1953), 307.

Even here, though, representational limits remain. Many theatre artists have overcome these aesthetic boundaries by rejecting not just realism but dramatic representation itself. Antonin Artaud's 'plague' theatre rejected dramatic form as decisively as it did the narrow definitions of contagion offered by microbiology, while the responses of Dada artists and performers to the facial disfigurements of World War I often took the form of non-dramatic 'manifestations' (Garner, 'Artaud'; '*The Gas Heart*'). And, as the example of *Ether Frolics* makes clear, later theatrical and performance artists have carried the theatrical exploration of medicine into new fusions of technology, performance, and spectatorship. Some of the most striking of these explorations have happened at the margins of theatre as a medium and institution. Anna Furse's ART (Advanced Reproductive Technology) performances use ultrasound and other technologically mediated images to explore the internal landscapes of infertility, while Annie Sprinkle famously staged a cervical examination using a speculum on her exposed body. Compared to these and similar performances, the dramatizations of medicine and medical issues by Chekhov, Ibsen, and later modern playwrights can feel narrow and conventional.

II. REALISM'S DOCTORS

But what about those doctors – aspiring, established, conservative, forward looking – whose presence around and inside individual plays hovers over the early history of modern drama? Ibsen's Dr Rank (*A Doll House*), Strindberg's Doctor (*The Father*), Chekhov's Astrov (*Uncle Vanya*), the doctors in Maeterlinck, Hauptmann, Shaw, Wedekind, O'Neill – the presence of these and other medical figures underscores how centrally the idea of medicine functions in the emergence of modern drama in Europe. That the majority of the plays featuring doctors are written in the mode of realism suggests that the representational limitations mentioned above mask a more fundamental centrality of this movement – and of naturalism, its putatively scientific relative – to the theatrical examination of medicine and the somatic body on the modern stage. Lawrence Rothfield has argued for the connection between clinical medicine and the nineteenth-century realist novel in what he calls the aesthetic of 'medical realism'. Pointing to the importance of Gustave Flaubert in establishing this connection, he writes,

> *Madame Bovary* marks the emergence of a mode of writing in which the real has become medical, in which the relation between author and text is modelled on medical precepts, with the author viewing characters and situations as a doctor views patients and cases.[13]

[13] Lawrence Rothfield, *Vital Signs: Medical Realism in Nineteenth-Century Fiction* (Princeton University Press, 1992), 37.

Realist and (particularly) naturalist drama reflect a similar interest in medical modes of embodiment and observation, though the 'real' they offer to theatrical attention is medicalized in different ways than the textual 'real' that animates and limits the novel. These differences derive from the body's actual staging in dramatic representation – in contrast to the body's being linguistically constructed in literary fiction – and from the theoretical instabilities that characterize realism as a dramatic and theatrical aesthetic.

Emile Zola is an important figure for understanding these differences, not only because he sought to articulate a medicalized aesthetic for both the novel and drama but also because his vision of theatrical naturalism highlights the conflicting aspirations driving realism and naturalism as dramatic movements. Inspired by the experimental physiology of Claude Bernard (author of *An Introduction to the Study of Experimental Medicine* (1865) and himself a failed playwright), Zola sought to apply the scientific method to the literary and dramatic study of the human organism in its natural environment. Central to Zola's formulation of naturalism is the body as an organic entity: 'The great naturalistic evolution ... involves the gradual substitution of physiological for metaphysical man.'[14] As Zola writes elsewhere, 'If the terrain of the experimental physician is the body of man as it manifests itself through its organs, both in their normal and pathological condition, our terrain is equally the body of man in its cerebral and sensory manifestations, both in their healthy and morbid condition.'[15] The theatre presents a special challenge to the achievement of this medicalized presentation of character because of its historical reliance on artifice, rhetoric, and convention. Zola describes this 'counterfeiting of nature' and the inevitable triumph of naturalism using the imagery of clothing: 'Today the naturalist thinkers are telling us that truth has no need of clothing; it must walk naked. This, I repeat, is the quarrel.'[16]

Zola's ideal of transparent actuality is an intensification of the realist project of bringing theatre closer to life and thereby abolishing the artifice of convention. In imagining his theatre of truth walking naked, Zola envisions a dramatist of genius 'smashing the imposed patterns, remaking the stage until it is on equal footing with the auditorium, giving the shiver of life to the painted

[14] Emile Zola, *Le Naturalisme au théâtre*, vol. 29 of *Oeuvres complètes* (50 vols) (Bernouard, 1927–9), 92. Translations from Zola's French are my own; for *Le Naturalisme au théâtre*, I have consulted Albert Bermel's translation 'From *Naturalism in the Theatre*' (in *The Theory of the Modern Stage: An Introduction to Modern Theatre and Drama*, ed. Eric Bentley (Penguin, 1968).) For further discussion of Zola's debt to experimental medicine, see Stanton B. Garner, Jr, 'Physiologies of the Modern: Zola, Experimental Medicine, and the Naturalist Stage', *Modern Drama* 43, no. 4 (Winter 2000): 529–42.

[15] Emile Zola, *Le Roman expérimentale*, vol. 36 of *Oeuvres completes* (50 vols) (Bernouard, 1927–9), 33.

[16] Zola, *Naturalisme au théâtre*, 23.

tress on the wings, letting in through the backcloth the great, free air of real life'.[17] In nineteenth-century and more recent productions, realism has sought to accomplish this objective through an actualizing of the stage: increasingly life-like production elements (set, lighting, sound design) and the frequent importation of objects from real life. As the term 'life-like' indicates, though, the truth that realism seeks also hinges on the contrasting ideal of illusionism, the principle that what theatre gives us is not the actualities of life but the arrangement of theatrical elements in such a way that a self-contained illusion of reality is created. According to this notion of realism (expressed, for instance, in Strindberg's well-known preface to *Miss Julie*), the 'real' is achieved through the separation of the dramatic world from the auditorium and its non-illusionistic actuality. The contradiction between these principles – between disclosure and containment, actuality and representation – underscores the competing imperatives driving realism as a theatrical aesthetic: a mandate to bring the offstage world onstage and a mandate, equally strong, to insulate dramatic representation from the actuality that grounds it. Much of the pleasure of realist theatre comes from the inevitable oscillation between these ontological and epistemological levels.[18]

To the extent that such a theatre is grounded in the physiological and medicalized body, realist acting, stagecraft, and dramatic writing play out the tension between an ideal liberation of the organic body and its pathologies and their containment within representational practices. The body in theatre, of course, is always caught between a radical actuality – it is alive and physically present to itself and its spectators – and its subordination to fictional otherness. But the realist dramatic tradition presents this dialectic in particularly interesting ways. The medical subjects it deals with are explored within specific dramatic worlds, and the reality they convey depends on the counter-actual fact that the actor playing Osvald in Ibsen's *Ghosts*, for instance, does not descend into blindness and dementia at the end of every performance. At the same time, the actuality upon which dramatic enactment is built – that it 'ingests', to quote Bert States[19] – involves a field of organic individuals in proximity to one another in ways that disregard the containment of illusionistic representation. As Artaud understood, theatre is a contagious space, in which actual organisms influence each other directly. When outbreaks such as bubonic plague occur, theatres are among the first gathering-places to be closed. Though realism may

[17] Ibid., 11.

[18] For a fuller discussion of this, see Stanton B. Garner, Jr, 'Sensing Realism: Illusionism, Actuality, and the Theatrical Sensorium', in *The Senses in Performance*, ed. Sally Banes and André Lepecki (Routledge, 2007).

[19] Bert O. States, *Great Reckonings in Little Rooms: On the Phenomenology of Theater* (University of California Press, 1985) 37.

seek to bracket this space in the interests of its fictionality, the field of somatic co-presence makes itself known at every turn. The intermittent (or non-intermittent) coughing that accompanies every theatrical performance is an unavoidable feature of this medium where performers and spectators, artwork and consumers, share the same air.

The somatic body that Zola championed, in other words, threatens the displacement of representation with the claims of a radical, inter-corporeal actuality. The forcefulness of this threat is evident in realism's historical uneasiness with the undisguised physicality of illness. Zola's fantasy of truth walking naked is countered by the resistance of early realism and naturalism to the direct presentation of illness in the theatre. There are cultural conventions and taboos governing this resistance, of course. When *Ghosts* addressed hereditary syphilis through an onstage protagonist, its playwright was accused of turning the theatre into a hospital: 'We see the patient before us. His symptoms are described with revolting minuteness.'[20] But propriety in this and other cases disguises a more aesthetic fear of the uncontained body in dramatic representation. The body's ability to assert itself against realism's containments is evident in contemporary stagings of illness. Kushner's *Angels in America* portrays the ravages of AIDS with uncompromising directness, and this portrayal involves direct representation of the human body in distress. In Part One, Act Two, Prior Walter shits blood, and in a later scene he takes off his clothes in an outpatient clinic, his body covered in lesions. Although the symptoms are performed in both scenes, the body that is disclosed and eventually disrobed in Kushner's play is the actor's actual body, vulnerable beneath the audience's gaze, its privacy invaded by machineries of theatre and medical treatment. Like the body in pain (Shakespeare's blinded Gloucester, for example, or the mutilation of characters in Jacobean revenge tragedy), its somatic reality challenges the protectiveness of theatrical make-believe.

The doctors who appear throughout modern drama, then, can be seen as threshold figures who represent the medicalized reality that realism both embraces and seeks to disown. To understand them as containing agents is to recognize their role in realism's frequent attempt to keep illness from disrupting the regimes of representation. For every doctor who makes an appearance in modern drama, another exists offstage, and the scenes of illness and medical treatment with which most onstage doctors are engaged are never shown to the audience. At the same time, doctors are often the theatrical devices through which the medicalized body and the issues attendant upon it are introduced and framed on the modern stage. From Ibsen to the present, doctors and medical

[20] Review of *Ghosts* by William Archer, 'Ghosts and Gibberings', *Pall Mall Gazette*, 8 April 1891, in *Henrik Ibsen: The Critical Heritage*, ed. Michael Egan (Routledge, 1972), 212.

scientists negotiate the social visibility of illness, demarcate the line between normal and pathological, and often represent theories and disciplinary ideologies that construct the human in medical terms. The Baron Docteur in Suzan-Lori Parks's *Venus*, for example, is the principle spokesperson for a European anatomical tradition that was complicit in the colonial 'othering' of African populations. Doctors also serve as focal points for ethical questions concerning responsibility, empathy and care. Some of these are thematized within the plays themselves: dehumanizing medical treatment in Margaret Edson's *Wit* and the ethics of non-socialized medicine in Clifford Odets's *Waiting for Lefty*. Others, less explicit, are embedded within the field of relationships that constitute individual plays.

Chekhov's Astrov, for instance, introduces the medical face of such issues as social and interpersonal commitment, knowledge and responsibility, and care of the self and others that confront *Uncle Vanya*'s broader ensemble of characters. In the play's opening dialogue, Astrov speaks of the numbing, exhausting work of caring for patients, including those he treated in a recent outbreak of spotted typhus: 'In the huts the peasants were packed side by side ... Mud, stench, smoke, bull calves on the floor right next to the sick ... Piglets too.'[21] The life he describes was a familiar one to rural Russian physicians in the late nineteenth century, particularly those who worked in zemstvo medicine, a free health program pioneered in the 1870s and 1880s to serve the medical needs of a rural population traditionally underserved in terms of medical care.[22] What Astrov faces in light of these incessant demands is a detachment from emotional involvement that leaves his commitment to the betterment of humanity largely disengaged from the affective claims of others. 'I don't believe I could form an attachment to anyone any more',[23] he explains to Sonya at one point during several-month period in which he neglects his medical duties in order to visit the Serebryakov estate. In *Platonov* (Chekhov's unpublished early play), Astrov's counterpart – the young doctor Triletsky – is blatant in his professional neglect and the condescension he displays toward those he treats.[24] Astrov's disengagement and weary idealism, rooted in a life spent dealing with illness and disease, provide a more nuanced portrayal of the psychological costs of the public health mission to which he has devoted himself and his career. His presence in *Uncle Vanya* also calls attention to the body and its needs, an

[21] Anton Chekov, *Uncle Vanya*, in *The Complete Plays*, trans. and ed. Laurence Senelick (Norton, 2006), 820, ellipses in original.
[22] See Nancy Mandelker Frieden, *Russian Physicians in an Era of Reform and Revolution, 1856–1905* (Princeton University Press, 1981), 77–104.
[23] Chekov, *Uncle Vanya*, 842.
[24] The merchant Bugrov says to Triletsky, 'When it comes to treating patients, you don't treat 'em, but you do take your fee' (Chekov, *Untitled Play*, in *The Complete Plays*, 60).

experiential stratum that hovers in the background of Chekhov's drama and is largely repressed by the characters in their social and familial interactions.

Doctors are important to the interpretive field of modern drama for a final, equally important reason. As diagnosticians trained in an increasingly scientific body of knowledge for examining, interpreting, and treating the body, doctors occupy a privileged position in the observational field within which the embodied subject is apprehended onstage. Dramatic spectatorship, after all, is never a solitary activity, nor is it restricted to the experience of audience members watching a play. Instead, spectatorship is an interactive process in which audience points of view and modes of reception interact with those of characters, performers, directors, and designers. By representing and enacting medical forms of observation within the dramatic world, doctors and other medical workers can highlight the dramatic world and its inhabitants in terms of disciplinary ways of seeing. Georg Büchner's *Woyzeck*, a precursor to later nineteenth-century drama in its medicalized conception of character and dramatic action, offers a striking example of this process. The play's doctor conducts a scientific experiment involving the unfortunate Woyzeck (and a diet of peas) and perceives his symptoms and behaviours through the language of physiological anatomy ('Woyzeck, you've got a marvelous *aberratio mentalis partialis*, second species, beautifully developed'[25]). This perspective serves a dual function in Büchner's play. On the one hand, as his exchange with Woyzeck makes clear, the Doctor's narrowly medical view of character forms part of a larger contrast between the institutional regimentation of Woyzeck and the other poor and the contrary demands of nature. On the other hand, while the Doctor appears in only two of the play's scenes, the objectifying perspective he embodies parallels the play's own dramaturgical strategy, in which the dramatized world is presented in discrete snapshots, like specimens in a scientific laboratory. Büchner – who studied medicine, wrote a dissertation on the nervous system of a European freshwater fish, and held a position as lecturer in comparative anatomy at the University of Zurich – models his own dramatic anatomy on the observational procedures of medical science.

It has been common practice over the past twenty years for literary and other critics addressing issues of medical observation and its social institutionalization to employ Foucault's notion of the 'medical gaze'. According to Foucault's earliest formulation of this concept in *The Birth of the Clinic* (1963; trans. 1973), modern clinical experience involves a non-reciprocal relationship between an institutionally supported 'sovereign' eye that isolates, classifies, calculates, and governs and a patient conceived as an object of knowledge and

---

[25] George Büchner, *Woyzeck*, in *The Complete Collected Works*, trans. and ed. Henry J. Schmidt (Avon, 1977), 190.

intervention.[26] In his later study *Discipline and Punish* (1975; trans. 1977), professional medicine forms one of the disciplinary institutions that, emerging in the eighteenth century, subjected the human body to individual and collective forms of coercion. Like prisons, military camps, schools, factories, and workshops, the modern hospital was organized in terms of surveillance and visibility in what was, essentially, an optical exercise of power. Foucault writes,

> Side by side with the major technology of the telescope, the lens and the light beam, which were an integral part of the new physics and cosmology, there were the minor techniques of multiple and intersecting observations, of eyes that must see without being seen; using techniques of subjection and methods of exploitation, an obscure art of light and the visible was secretly preparing a new knowledge of man.[27]

The notion of the 'medical gaze' has proved useful to literary and cultural scholars interested in the history of subjectivity and its relation to modern discourses and technologies of the individual. But the critics who use this term – influenced by its association with panopticism in *Discipline and Punish* – have often presented medical observation as a totalizing mechanism of surveillance and control. This tendency may also result from the term 'gaze' – Alan Sheridan's idiosyncratic translation of Foucault's *le regard* – which suggests a continuous, vaguely disembodied perceptual state instead of the more nuanced, embodied field of encounters evident in Foucault's early discussions of medicine. This totalizing model proves particularly resistant to the study of drama and theatre, which employ 'multiple and intersecting observations' in decidedly non-totalizing ways. When institutional and disciplinary perspectives operate within modern drama, they are countered and often contested by other observational positions. This is true even in those plays – such as *Wit* – that are set within the confines of the modern hospital. Edson's play shifts scenes through theatrical flashback, represents a range of attitudes toward medical science and treatment, and centres on a cancer patient whose body, emotions, and lively intellect resist the objectifying operations to which she is subjected. By speaking her illness to an audience that shares her performance present, Vivian Bearing insists on a subjective space within the hospital's medicalizing environment. That the end of Edson's play tends to sentimentalize its opposition to dehumanizing medical study does not take away from the fact that its acts of resistance draw upon – and are enabled by – the theatre's decentred operations.

---

[26] Foucault, *The Birth of the Clinic*, 89.

[27] Michel Foucault, *Discipline and Punish: The Birth of the Prison*, trans. Alan Sheridan (Random, 1979), 171.

In the context of Foucauldian surveillance, the doctors of realist modern drama are figures of considerably limited omniscience and diminished powers of intervention. While their appearance in late nineteenth-century drama coincided with a period during which medical science enjoyed unprecedented cultural authority, such characters as Rank and Astrov participate in the larger epistemological challenges of theatrical spectatorship: seeking the evidence of internal experience in external behaviour, 'reading' the body for the signs and symptoms that are given to observation. That their concern is for the somatic body (and the somatic roots of psychological states) grounds spectatorship in the living body that theatre takes as its own. The institutionalized medical setting of *Wit* might be compared to the elusive figure of Doctor Hardy in Eugene O'Neill's *Long Day's Journey into Night*. Hardy, who never appears onstage, is the 'cheap' doctor who treats Mary Tyrone's morphine addiction by lecturing her when she's 'in agony and half insane'.[28] Along with the quack who earlier prescribed morphine after her son Edmund's birth without telling her what it was, Hardy represents non-benign therapeutic intervention, an abuse of medical authority marked by complacency, insensitivity, and irresponsibility. Characterized in this way, he stands in contrast to the more qualified – and more expensive – doctors for whom James Tyrone is unwilling to pay.

At the same time, Hardy's presence – and that of the sanatorium workers and other medical personnel who people the play's offstage world – is fundamental to O'Neill's play in ways that go beyond the economics and ethics of medical care. Connected to the Tyrones through years of medical observation and treatment, Hardy focuses the play's broader concern with reading appearance and behaviour for the signs of interior somatic conditions. The four Tyrones observe each other obsessively, and, in the scrutinizing of Mary and Edmund for signs of morphine use and the feared tuberculosis, this observation assumes a medicalized form. A nervous tic, glassy eyes, a cough – these provide the objects of a diagnostic vigilance that defines and modulates the characters' onstage relationships. The psychological, of course, is deeply embedded in the somatic in this play where illness and health are one means by which characters express and interpret their emotions and those of others.[29] To approach *Long Day's Journey into Night* in terms of somatic observation, in other words, is to negotiate the often complex symptomology of modern drama, in which the boundary between the body's surface and interior becomes the site of spectatorial interpretive operations. That this reading of somatic states occurs most

[28] Eugene O'Neill, *Long Day's Journey into Night*, corrected ed. (Yale University Press, 1989), 74.

[29] Reproaching herself for leaving her baby Eugene with her mother while she joined her husband on the road, Mary refers to Jamie's entering the baby's room while sick with the measles: 'I've always believed Jamie did it on purpose. He was jealous of the baby. He hated him' (O'Neill, *Long Day's Journey into Night*, 87). Illness, in this assertion, becomes a literal acting on others.

regularly in realist drama and its offshoots indicates the centrality of this tradition to the theatre's medical explorations.

The tightly particularized realism of *Long Day's Journey into Night* may seem a long way from the immersive, highly technologized performance field of *Ether Frolics*. But the distance between the two is less complete than this way of describing them suggests. The experiential landscapes of the somatic body shadow, intrude upon, and threaten to eclipse O'Neill's realism, particularly in the fourth and final act. Edmund's description of walking in the fog establishes a verbal image of the body's retreat from contact with the world around it, and this anaesthetizing movement is reinforced by the wall of fog outside the window and the fog horn's recurrent drone. When Mary appears in the play's closing sequence – her eyes 'enormous', glistening 'like polished black jewels'[30] – she presides over a *mise en scène* that mirrors her morphine-induced enclosure. For its part, Ether Frolics never loses touch with the referential world that grounds O'Neill's play. Its elliptical scenes evoke the world of human interaction even as this world is bracketed and estranged by anaesthesia's deforming operation. Just as fundamentally, the two theatre pieces are linked by their use of living, breathing performers whose somatic presence onstage underwrites the theatre's focus on illness, health, and their many manifestations. While the tradition of theatrical anti-realism has often sought mechanical replacements for the somatic body – one thinks of Edward Gordon Craig's theatre of the *Über-Marionette*, which sought to banish 'the weakness and the tremors of the flesh'[31] – the medium's reliance on the human body ensures that realist and anti-realist theatre alike admit the somatic to their explorations of representation and embodiment. From Ibsen to Brecht, Chekhov to Foreman, Strindberg to Sound and Fury, the body's physiological claims to attention have preoccupied – and continue to preoccupy – the modern stage.

REFERENCES

Archer, William. 'Ghosts and Gibberings'. *Pall Mall Gazette*, 8 April 1891. In *Henrik Ibsen: The Critical Heritage*, edited by Michael Egan. Routledge, 1972.
Archimedes, Sondra M. *Gendered Pathologies: The Female Body and Biomedical Discourse in the Nineteenth-Century English Novel*. Routledge, 2005.
Billington, Michael. 'Ether Frolics'. *The Guardian*, 21 July 2005. *Theatre Record* 25, no. 15 (16 August 2005): 981.
Boxhill, Roger. *Shaw and the Doctors*. Basic, 1969.
Büchner, George. *Woyzeck*. In *The Complete Collected Works*, translated and edited by Henry J. Schmidt. Avon Books, 1977.

[30] O'Neill, *Long Day's Journey into Night*, 170.
[31] Edward Gordon Craig, *On the Art of the Theatre* (Theatre Arts, [1911] 1956), 80.

Calbi, Maurizio. *Approximate Bodies: Gender and Power in Early Modern Drama and Anatomy*. Routledge, 2005.

Cartwright, Lisa. *Screening the Body: Tracing Medicine's Visual Culture*. University of Minnesota Press, 1995.

Chekhov, Anton. *Anton Chekhov's Life and Thought: Selected Letters and Commentary*. Translated by Michael Henry Heim with Simon Karlinsky. University of California Press, 1975.

Chekhov, Anton. *The Complete Plays*. Translated and edited by Laurence Senelick. Norton, 2006.

Churchill, Caryl. *Vinegar Tom*. 1976. French, 1982.

Cohn, Ruby. '"It Hurts?" Afflicted Bodies in Beckett's Drama'. In *Peering behind the Curtain: Disability, Illness, and the Extraordinary Body in Contemporary Theater*, edited by Thomas Fahy and Kimball King. Routledge, 2002.

Craig, Edward Gordon. *On the Art of the Theatre*. 1911. Theatre Arts, 1956.

Crawford, T. Hugh. 'Visual Knowledge in Medicine and Popular Film'. *Literature and Medicine* 17, no. 1 (1998): 24–44.

Davis, Cynthia J. *Bodily and Narrative Forms: The Influence of Medicine on American Literature, 1845–1915*. Stanford University Press, 2000.

Edson, Margaret. *Wit*. Faber, 1999.

Ether Frolics. Created by Sound and Fury in collaboration with Shunt Collective. London Bridge Station, July 2005.

Fahy, Thomas, and Kimball King, eds. *Peering behind the Curtain: Disability, Illness, and the Extraordinary Body in Contemporary Theater*. Routledge, 2002.

Foucault, Michel. *The Birth of the Clinic: An Archaeology of Medical Perception*. Translated by A. M. Sheridan Smith. Random, [1975] 1994.

Foucault, Michel. *Discipline and Punish: The Birth of the Prison*. Translated by Alan Sheridan. Random, [1975] 1979.

Freud, Sigmund. 'Psychopathic Characters on the Stage'. In *The Complete Psychological Works of Sigmund Freud*, vol. 7, translated by James Strachey. Hogarth, [1942 (1905 or 1906)] 1953.

Frieden, Nancy Mandelker. *Russian Physicians in an Era of Reform and Revolution, 1856–1905*. Princeton University Press, 1981.

Garner, Stanton B., Jr. 'Artaud, Germ Theory, and the Theater of Contagion'. *Theatre Journal* 58, no. 1 (March 2006): 1–14.

Garner, Stanton B., Jr. 'The Gas Heart: Disfigurement and the Dada Body'. *Modern Drama* 50, no. 4 (Winter 2007): 502–20.

Garner, Stanton B., Jr. 'Physiologies of the Modern: Zola, Experimental Medicine, and the Naturalist Stage'. *Modern Drama* 43, no. 4 (Winter 2000): 529–42.

Garner, Stanton B., Jr. 'Sensing Realism: Illusionism, Actuality, and the Theatrical Sensorium'. In *The Senses in Performance*, edited by Sally Banes and André Lepecki. Routledge, 2007.

Harris, Jonathan Gil. *Sick Economies: Drama, Mercantilism, and Disease in Shakespeare's England*. University of Pennsylvania Press, 2004.

Jackson, Ken. *Separate Theaters: Bethlem ('Bedlam') Hospital and the Shakespearean Stage*. University of Delaware Press, 2005.

Kerwin, William. *Beyond the Body: The Boundaries of Medicine and English Renaissance Drama*. University of Massachusetts Press, 2005.

Kickel, Katherine E. *Novel Notions: Medical Discourse and the Mapping of the Imagination in Eighteenth-Century English Fiction*. Routledge, 2007.

Kuppers, Petra. *Disability and Contemporary Performance: Bodies on Edge*. Routledge, 2003.
Kushner, Tony. *Angels in America: A Gay Fantasia on American Themes. Part One: Millennium Approaches*. Hern, 1992.
Moss, Stephanie, and Kaara L. Peterson, eds. *Disease, Diagnosis, and Cure on the Early Modern Stage*. Ashgate, 2004.
Nunn, Hillary M. *Staging Anatomies: Dissection and Spectacle in Early Stuart Tragedy*. Ashgate, 2005.
Odets, Clifford. *Waiting for Lefty*. In *Six Plays of Clifford Odets*. Random, 1939.
Ogden, Daryl. 'Cold War Science and the Body Politic: An Immuno/Virological Approach to Angels in America'. *Literature and Medicine* 19, no. 2 (Fall 2000): 241–61.
O'Neill, Eugene. *Long Day's Journey into Night*. Corrected ed. Yale University Press, 1989.
Parks, Suzan-Lori. *Venus: A Play*. Theatre Communications Group, 1997.
Pettigrew, Todd H. J. *Shakespeare and the Practice of Physic: Medical Narratives on the Early Modern English Stage*. University of Delaware Press, 2007.
Pollard, Tanya. *Drugs and Theater in Early Modern England*. Oxford University Press, 2005.
Quayson, Ato. *Aesthetic Nervousness: Disability and the Crisis of Representation*. Columbia University Press, 2007.
Rothfield, Lawrence. *Vital Signs: Medical Realism in Nineteenth-Century Fiction*. Princeton University Press, 1992.
Sandahl, Carrie, and Philip Auslander, eds. *Bodies in Commotion: Disability and Performance*. University of Michigan Press, 2005.
Sawday, Jonathan. *The Body Emblazoned: Dissection and the Human Body in Renaissance Culture*. Routledge, 1995.
Shaw, George Bernard. *Too True to Be Good: A Political Extravaganza*. In *Plays Extravagant*. Penguin, 1981.
'Sound and Fury: Ether Frolics'. *Fuel*, 12 December 2007. www.fueltheatre.com/sound&fury/ether/index.html.
States, Bert O. *Great Reckonings in Little Rooms: On the Phenomenology of Theater*. University of California Press, 1985.
Zola, Emile. 'From *Naturalism in the Theatre*' (trans. Albert Bermel). In *The Theory of the Modern Stage: An Introduction to Modern Theatre and Drama*, edited by Eric Bentley. Penguin, 1968.
Zola, Emile. *Le Naturalisme au théâtre* (Naturalism in the Theatre). Vol. 29 of *Oeuvres complètes* (Complete Works). 50 vols. Bernouard, 1927–9.
Zola, Emile. *Le Roman expérimentale* (The Experimental Novel). Vol. 36 of *Oeuvres completes* (Complete Works). 50 vols. Bernouard, 1927–9.

11

'250,000 unnecessary deaths': Theatricalizing the national healthcare debate in Broadway's *Medicine Show* (1940)

KIRSTEN E. SHEPHERD

In the spring of 1940, a play called *Medicine Show* opened on Broadway at the New Yorker Theatre and brought medicine to the stage as never before. It ran for thirty-five performances over the course of three months and ushered a debate about healthcare directly into the theatre precisely when this issue was at the forefront of politics, with Roosevelt's National Health Care Bill then making its way through Congress. With a script created from real-life sources and statistics and with a strong, starry cast, *Medicine Show* made a powerful intervention in this healthcare debate, and its great innovation was its departure from increasingly realistic depictions of medicine and hospitals in drama, film and TV. The play modelled how theatre could galvanize medical reform through deliberate anti-realism and exuberant theatricality, making spectacularly available aspects of medical care that had previously eluded (modern) theatrical representation.

Medicine Show started life as a 'Living Newspaper', a form of documentary theatre pioneered by the Federal Theatre Project (FTP) that drew almost entirely on real-life source material such as newspaper articles, academic books, court proceedings and transcripts of Congressional hearings. Yet in its move to Broadway the script of *Medicine Show* became even *more* focused, not less, on what might seem like dry statistics and facts about healthcare. My chapter argues that *Medicine Show* showed how theatre can make statistics, bureaucratic impasses and other 'undramatic' (or para-theatrical) aspects of medical care into compelling drama to motivate change – and that these are discoveries that theatre makers and medical practitioners who are still operating in a primarily 'realist' mode can learn from and harness.

FROM LIVING NEWSPAPER TO BROADWAY SHOW

'Living Newspapers' were a form of documentary theatre that emerged from the FTP, part of Roosevelt's Works Progress Administration, the cornerstone of his New Deal. The FTP ran from 1935 to 1939 and put thousands of unemployed theatre workers to work. Its stage productions reached millions of people, with plays often opening in multiple cities across the United States simultaneously, as well as radio drama ('the Federal Theatre of the Air') reaching 10 million listeners per week.[1] As James Shapiro notes, in its short lifetime the FTP managed to stage, 'for a pittance, over a thousand productions in twenty-nine states seen by thirty million, or roughly one in four Americans, two thirds of whom (according to audience surveys) had never seen a play before'.[2] Among the FTP's many notable Living Newspapers were *Triple A Plowed Under* (1936, on agriculture); *Power* (1937, on the need for public ownership of utilities); *One Third of a Nation* (1938, on poor housing for a vast number of citizens); and *Spirochete* (1938–9, on the need for medical testing to control and prevent the spread of syphilis). *Spirochete* promoted the adoption of screening for syphilis through blood tests, which the play directly helped make mandatory through legislation passed only a month after the Seattle performances[3] (see Figure 11.1).

The FTP's director, Hallie Flanagan Davis (a theatre professor at Vassar College), created the Living Newspaper form from her first-hand experience of European and Russian avant garde, experimental theatre and workers' theatre

[1] Studies of the FTP include Barry B. Witham, *The Federal Theatre Project: A Case Study* (Cambridge University Press, 2003); Bonnie Nelson Schwartz, ed., *Voices from the Federal Theatre* (University of Wisconsin, 2003); and James Shapiro, *The Playbook: A Story of Theatre, Democracy and the Making of a Culture War* (Faber & Faber, 2024).

[2] Shapiro, *The Playbook*, xvi.

[3] Susan Duffy and Bernard K. Duffy, 'Theatrical Responses to Technology During the Depression: Three Federal Theatre Project Plays', *Theatre History Studies* 6 (January 1986): 155.

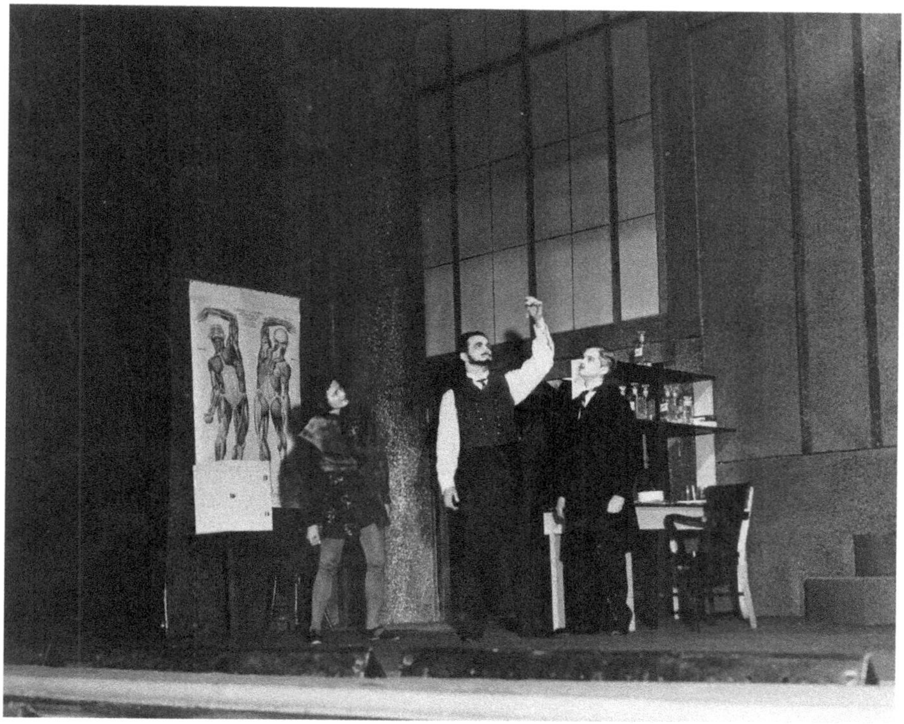

FIGURE 11.1 *Spirochete*, by Alfred Sundgaard, Federal Theatre Project Seattle Unit, 1939 (*Spirochete* premiered in Chicago in 1938). University of Washington Libraries, Special Collections, UW41559.

by Erwin Piscator, Bertolt Brecht, Vsevolod Meyerhold and others. Scripts were didactic, entertaining and topical – the idea was to update and adapt them for each new venue and in light of new information. The typical Living Newspaper followed a simple format: Act 1 educates the audience about the background to a pressing contemporary social problem; Act 2 shows how that new knowledge might be activated by illustrating possible routes to a solution. The ending is left open; it is up to the audience, newly enlightened, to make the right decision about what path to take. This form and method could accommodate seemingly any pressing topic of the day. The original typescript of *Medicine Show* in the Library of Congress opens with a lengthy bibliography, the standard *modus operandum* for Living Newspapers and a method that makes them an early form of verbatim theatre.[4] But when the FTP was

[4] Duffy and Duffy, 'Theatrical Responses'; Barbara Melosh, 'The New Deal's Federal Theatre Project', *Medical Heritage* 2, no. 1 (1986): 36–47.

shut down by Congress in 1939, plans to produce *Medicine Show* had to be shelved.[5]

In addition to building on the success of *Spirochete*, *Medicine Show* was at least indirectly indebted to George Bernard Shaw's three polemical 'doctor' plays, *The Doctor's Dilemma* (1906), *Too True to Be Good* (1932) and *The Millionairess* (1936). These pioneered a more combative, critical tone in depicting doctors and medical practice on stage. In this regard, *Medicine Show* was the true inheritor of the 'Progressive Era' label, much more than its splashy, successful predecessor in depicting hospital life, *Men in White* (1933) by Sidney Kingsley. *Men in White* established its twenty-seven-year-old author as 'a major force in the new American realism', revealing (and generating) an appetite for medical drama that increased throughout the 1930s, becoming hugely popular and lucrative entertainment.[6] *Medicine Show* capitalized on this development, but for consciousness-raising purposes rather than financial gain. With ticket prices capped at $1.65 (the show was privately backed by the producer Carly Wharton and Martin Gabel, who played the leading role), the production strongly signalled its FTP origins. As reviews indicate, audiences were drawn not by affordability alone but by the powerful combination of topicality and theatricality that they associated with FTP productions. My discussion explores and analyses what makes *Medicine Show* distinct in its engagement of theatre and medicine, and an exception to the ways in which theatre, cinema and TV more broadly were depicting medicine in the period.

Where *Medicine Show* differed most strikingly was in its mode: deliberately and unabashedly non-realistic, bearing the hallmarks of its roots in the FTP. That choice is arguably the lynchpin of its success and why the play still matters today, because it challenged the way medicine could be depicted on stage and shifted the focus from personalities and melodramas to real issues and problems directly affecting audiences. *Medicine Show* boldly used Living Newspaper techniques when the form itself was being killed off by politicians; it turned away from the high drama of doctors in operating rooms and their personal lives at a time when these were becoming increasingly popular; and it shifted the focus of the drama to the economics, statistics and politics of medicine – the forces dictating the delivery of healthcare, both then and now. The production was rare in foregrounding these forces as the main subject of the drama, and

---

[5] See Shapiro, *The Playbook*. In his otherwise riveting account of the FTP, Shapiro erroneously refers to *Medicine Show* as '*Medicine*', and then only in passing.

[6] Evangeline Morphos, 'Sidney Kingsley's "Men in White"', *TDR (The Drama Review)* 28, no. 4 (1984): 13. A blockbuster hit on Broadway during the bottom of the Depression, *Men in White* won the Pulitzer Prize for drama in 1933 and was made into a Hollywood film in 1934 starring Clark Gable and Myrna Loy while the play was still running on Broadway.

the show clearly touched a nerve. Critics noted that 'the American Medical Association appears as villain and was roundly hissed by an excited first night audience' and there was 'passionate applause' at the mention of the unbalanced budget.[7]

Despite the highly engaged responses of those audiences, history seems to have forgotten *Medicine Show*, as it has Roosevelt's failed National Health Bill. Although it did not change national policy directly, the play staged a national debate about how the United States should care for the health of its citizens, a question that continues to haunt us.[8]

REINVENTING THE LIVING NEWSPAPER FOR BROADWAY

Many of the facts and statistics in the Broadway version of *Medicine Show* focus on New York City, which is typical of the show's FTP origins – suiting the script to the location in which it will be performed. By contrast, the 1939 version was more general and meant to be edited according to the various cities across the United States in which it would be produced. *Medicine Show* had regional appeal already embedded in its text in the device of a group of archetypal patients from key cities across the country and from representative walks of life in terms of key demographics (occupation, race, gender, class).[9] The Broadway version retains the standard structure of a Living Newspaper (Act 1 educates the public about a social problem, Act 2 lays the groundwork to a solution), despite the complete rewriting of the text; this suggests widespread familiarity with the formula and a degree of popularity, hardly surprising given the freshness of the FTP's shows in recent memory. In his review of *Medicine Show* for the *New York Post*, John Mason Brown paid glowing tribute to the Living Newspapers for their skilful writing and theatricality and for their 'ability to achieve pulverizing emotional effects', wherein lay their 'almost terrifying strength'.[10] This strength derived at least in part from the sheer size of the

---

[7] Brooks Atkinson, 'The Play', *New York Times*, 13 April 1940.

[8] *Medicine Show* joins the ranks of political plays that have engaged directly with policy-making, such as the British examples of *The Golden Rump* (unknown author, 1737), which prompted the institution of theatrical censorship; John Galsworthy's *Justice* (1910), which helped bring about a change in the law regarding solitary confinement; *Hang Down Your Head and Die* (premiered 1964 Oxford Playhouse, transferred to London's Comedy Theatre 1964), which helped end capital punishment; and Edward Bond's *Saved* (1968), which hastened the demise of theatrical censorship.

[9] While the word 'Show' carries a sense of revealing as well as performing, and of promising to display and entertain, the phrase 'medicine show' perhaps unintentionally aligns Native American medicine men with the quackery shows that toured the United States in the nineteenth and early twentieth centuries.

[10] John Mason Brown, 'Two on the Aisle', *New York Post*, 13 April 1940.

company: the purpose of the FTP was to put as many theatre professionals to work as possible during the Depression, so shows typically employed hundreds of people and opened simultaneously in dozens of cities across the country. For Broadway, *Medicine Show* had to become much more streamlined. The Broadway playbill illustrates the shift from a large ensemble production to a star-led show with a smaller cast. But the 'pulverizing effects' and 'terrifying strength' of the drama were not diminished, as they were also a function of formal and scenographic innovations. All that needed updating was the medical knowledge and the politics: the debates and issues at the play's core around the state of the nation's healthcare and people's attitudes toward socialized medicine.

The creative team behind *Medicine Show*, from its FTP origins through to the Broadway production, was remarkable in both its artistry and its commitment to the play's political ideals.[11] Carly Wharton was 'the only woman producer active on Broadway' at the time and a visionary innovator who had created the first colour film in Hollywood.[12] In 1939 she and Martin Gabel made a fortune with the hit play *Life with Father*, enabling them to finance *Medicine Show* at such a low ticket price in order to get its message on stage. 'She worked 18 hours a day seven days a week on *Medicine Show*', reported the *World-Telegram*.[13] It was a labour of love that could afford to lose money in the service of an urgent political argument.

TURNING THE MEDICAL GAZE ON ITSELF

The idea that 'illness is an ensemble drama', as the editors of the current volume put it, is particularly apt in the cases of *Medicine Show* and its forerunner *Men in White*. Although with sharply different agendas and political orientations, the plays shared a focus on what doctors and nurses actually do and how they treat patients – both medically and as fellow citizens. Both plays relied on finely tuned ensemble acting whose careful choreography was almost 'balletic' (a word used by a reviewer at the time). *Men in White* was the first hit of the Group Theatre, formed in 1931 by Harold Clurman, Cheryl Crawford and Lee Strasberg (it is notable that both *Medicine Show* and *Men in White* were largely driven by woman producers). It had a melodramatic plot but was notable for its ground-breaking realism in depicting surgery and hospital activity on stage, drawing on extensive research by Strasberg, Clurman and Crawford

[11] The play was staged on Broadway by Jules Dassin, with scenic design by Samuel Leve.
[12] The 1935 short *La Cucaracha*.
[13] Helen Worden, 'Woman Producer of Medicine Show Made Hollywood Take Up Colored Films', *New York World-Telegram*, unknown date, 1940.

in shadowing surgeons, doctors and nurses in hospitals and bringing what they witnessed directly into their staging.[14]

The role that scenography played in conveying its political message is what interests me most about *Medicine Show*, which is evident when we compare the original FTP typescript (1939) with the promptbook for the Broadway production (1940). The original version of the show involves some extraordinary feats of staging, including simulating a working hospital using a complex interplay of mime and projections; this did not make it into the Broadway version, which is intriguing given how popular the previous hospital drama, *Men in White*, had been. Likewise, music was to have been prominent in the original version of *Medicine Show*, but no score survives. Nor do we know precisely what audiences would have seen in the way of projections that were meant to be used throughout the FTP production.

What is certain is that in the move from FTP to Broadway, the show got less theatrical and more text-centred, and much less interested in staging the inner workings of a hospital than in its first iteration.[15] Although this development might seem counter-intuitive – one might expect more theatricality, not less, in the move to Broadway – it suggests that there was a context that predisposed audiences to receive a talky play about healthcare. American theatre had been engaging for decades with medicine and, more broadly, with scientific ideas, putting science at the heart of much of the theatre of the time, whether overtly or obliquely.[16] Questions of how diseases were transmitted or how hereditary traits were passed on, for example, dominated many plays of the era. *Men in White* focuses squarely on doctors as absolute heroes in the operating room, if sometimes morally weak outside it. Most importantly, their heroic surgical deeds redeem their personal failings.

Men in White's stance towards doctors can be gleaned from reviews and from the text itself, which highlight the staging as innovative and gripping in its

[14]An important precursor to *Men in White* was Wallace Thurman's gritty naturalistic novel *The Interne* (1932), which he adapted from a play he had written, exposing the appalling conditions of an inner-city hospital. See *African American Literature Beyond Race: An Alternative Reader*, ed. Gene Andrew Jarrett (New York University Press, 2006), 175.

[15]See Kirsten E. Shepherd, 'Staging a "Vast Human Dustbowl" of Disease: The Federal Theatre Project's *Medicine Show* in its 1939 (Pre-Broadway) Version', in *Microscopic Life in 20th- and 21st-Century Literature and Performance*, ed. Sarah Bouttier, Liliane Campos, François-Joseph Lapointe and Sarah Montin (Open Book Publishers, 2026).

[16]Tamsen Wolff, *Mendel's Theatre: Heredity, Eugenics, and Early Twentieth-Century American Drama* (Palgrave, 2009); Kirsten E. Shepherd-Barr, *Theatre and Evolution from Ibsen to Beckett* (Columbia University Press, 2015) and '"Golden Dust" in the Wind: Genetics, Contagion, and Early Twentieth-Century American Theatre', in *The Palgrave Handbook of Twentieth and Twenty-First Century Literature and Science*, ed. Neel Ahuja et al. (Palgrave Macmillan, 2020); Max Shulman and J. Chris Westgate, eds, *Performing the Progressive Era: Immigration, Urban Life, and Nationalism on Stage* (University of Iowa Press, 2019).

simulation of hospital life: 'One of the most memorable aspects of the original production was a precisely choreographed and brilliantly lit pantomime of surgeons scrubbing, gowning, gloving, and operating.'[17] The British production of the play in London the following year noted its 'authentic hospital background' which was done 'brilliantly'.[18] Perhaps with this recent model of hospital drama in mind, *Medicine Show* was likewise originally meant to present the interior of a hospital, though depicting archetypes rather than individuals. Both versions of *Medicine Show* depict a group of patients who collectively represent the problems with healthcare across the United States. By contrast, *Men in White* focuses on the story arc of psychologically drawn characters – a young doctor, his boss, his fiancé, his lover and her botched abortion – especially showing the pressures on him from his boss, senior surgeon Dr Hochberg. *Men in White*'s most dramatic scene, set in a tense operating room where a male doctor barks 'scalpel!' as he races to save a patient's life, might barely raise an eyebrow now. But 'in 1933, this stunning scene made theatrical history as it introduced large audiences to a sanctum sanctorum once accessible only to surgeons and nurses'.[19]

CHALLENGING REALISM

Notably absent from the critical response to *Medicine Show* is any reference to *Men in White*, accentuating the vast differences between their theatrical modes. But these plays both helped to shape public interest and receptivity to medical drama and the 'behind the scenes' realities of healthcare and hospitals on radio (*Dr Kildare*), TV (*Medic*, 1954–6), and film as well as theatre, and their longer-term legacy can be seen in shows such as *ER*, *House*, *Chicago Hope* and *New Amsterdam*, and spoofs like *Scrubs*, as well as the bestselling book by Adam Kay, *This is Going to Hurt*, and the TV series it spawned.[20] A strong tendency

[17] Howard Markel, '*Men in White*: The Operating Room's Debut into Popular American Culture', *JAMA* 302, no. 21 (2009): 2376–8.

[18] Russell Gregory, 'Review of Men in White', *Saturday Review*, 7 July 1934.

[19] Markel, 'Men in White', 2378. Even The Three Stooges caught the medicine-on-film bug, capitalizing on the popularity of *Men in White* by making a spoof called *Men in Black* in 1934 (which garnered their only Academy Award nomination, for Best Short Comedy Subject) and a few years later another short film about medicine and hospitals, called *Dizzy Doctors* (1937).

[20] In Britain, there has been a steady succession of NHS-themed plays that echo the debate staged by *Medicine Show*: *The National Health* by Peter Nichols (1969); Nina Raine's *Tiger Country* (2011); Alan Bennett's *Allelujah!* (2018); and, though it only partly deals with the NHS, David Hare's *I'm Not Running* (2018). At the time of writing, three new NHS dramas were premiering in Britain: Lucy Kirkwood's *The Human Body* (Donmar Warehouse, 2024); *Nye* by Tim Price (National Theatre, 2024); and Sophia Chetin-Leuner's *This Might Not Be It* (Bush Theatre, 2024). On film, see Eelco Wijdicks, *Cinema, M.D.: A History of Medicine on Screen* (Oxford University Press, 2020).

in many of these works is their dedication to the realistic portrayal of doctors and their technical skill and expertise, simulating all kinds of situations from emergency medicine to routine medical care. The more realistic such scenes are, the more they seem to attract viewers.

Realism, as Stanton B. Garner, Jr points out, plays a powerful yet vexed role in the relationship between theatre and medicine, invested as it is in 'the ideology of the visible'.[21] What we see and what we do not see are carefully arbitrated in ways that most audiences are not aware of. Prior to the 1930s, medical dramas often left the 'interior landscape of disease' off stage, out of sight; and the technological means by which audiences might access that realm – through projections, X-ray images and other effects – do not figure in 'strictly illusionistic' theatre.[22] So the doctor takes on particular significance within realist and naturalist plays, acting as a 'threshold figure' who helps the audience understand the medical body and the situations they are seeing: are these 'normal', or 'pathological'? How conscious will an audience be of the ideologies that lie behind such medical situations and states?

Medicine Show seems to defy these norms of medical drama in its deliberate embrace of non-illusionistic methods, becoming instead unabashedly *un*realistic, relying on projections, simulation, mime and other stylized techniques that were typical of the Living Newspaper mode. For example, the original FTP version (1939) of *Medicine Show* included the staging of a busy hospital. But where *Men in White* had simulated a working hospital realistically, *Medicine Show* went for deliberate stylization. If a nurse attended a patient, there was no actor lying on the operating table, she simply mimed the interaction. If a doctor used an instrument like a scalpel, it was not in his hand but projected onto a screen. This defamiliarizing technique prevents emotionalism and keeps the audience's attention on the forces (economic, political, historical, social) that underpin what they are viewing.

American playwriting had long been experimenting with non-realistic forms – from the innovative plays of Susan Glaspell in the teens and twenties through the expressionism of Treadwell and Rice in the 1920s to Thornton Wilder's *Our Town* (1938), which bore strong resemblance to the techniques of the FTP, such as in its use of the Stage Manager and in having actors come on stage seemingly spontaneously from the audience. Theatre audiences were well trained in non-realist performance tactics, for example flocking to see the zany *Hellzapoppin'* which ran on Broadway from 1938 to 1941 and brilliantly combined elements of vaudeville, musical comedy and complex and sophisticated

[21] Stanton B. Garner, Jr, 'Introduction: Is There a Doctor in the House? Medicine and the Making of Modern Drama', *Modern Drama* 51, no. 3 (2008): abstract.
[22] Ibid.

narrative strategies. Living Newspapers had raised awareness of pressing economic and political concerns affecting millions of people by harnessing methods that eschewed realism in order to activate audiences through education and entertainment. The creators of *Medicine Show* presented their production in this tradition, rejecting the encroaching realism of hospital drama as encapsulated by *Men in White* and its encouragement of a passive diagnostic gaze, in favour of an overt theatricality that spoke directly to the onlooker, addressed their concerns head-on and involved them as stakeholders in the potential outcomes.

Sound and music played a role in minimizing or disrupting realism. The sound of a heartbeat recurred throughout the play, an expressionist device reminiscent of Eugene O'Neill's 1920 *The Emperor Jones* (a production in living memory for *Medicine Show*'s audience). In O'Neill's play, the beating heart signalled the psychological state of the protagonist; in *Medicine Show*, its function was 'responding to scenes, surrounding the audience with its rhythmical pumping, responding to the action on stage, speeding up when agitated and finally ceasing dramatically in the final act'.[23] The beating heart was part of the wider soundscape of the intended FTP production of *Medicine Show*, and it would be illuminating to know the songs and incidental music that Hanns Eisler provided.[24] Eisler's involvement suggests that *Medicine Show* fused the Living Newspaper approach (itself derived from Russian and German models) with German avant-garde theatre and music to create a unique hybrid – and one that was distinctly 'un-American'. There is a delightful irony here: Wharton and Gabel managed to take a show to Broadway that had been shut down by the very government committee that would soon be targeting and blacklisting alleged Communists for their un-American behaviour. In this regard, too, the salvaging of *Medicine Show* was a triumph.

Yet the production's non-realistic methods and especially its harnessing of scenography to suggest medical themes and settings can be found in other performance domains during this period, such as opera and dance. For instance,

[23] Duffy and Duffy, 'Theatrical Responses', 157.

[24] Something of their character may be inferred by knowing Eisler's background and style. He was a distinguished composer who was known throughout Europe for his avant-garde work. He had been the first student of Schoenberg to implement his twelve-tone system (although it apparently irritated Schoenberg that Eisler brought in elements of jazz and cabaret). Eisler wrote a hit song in Germany in 1932 that made fun of Hitler and fled when the Nazis came to power ('Eisler Score in New Play', unnamed newspaper clipping in NYPL archives on *Medicine Show*, T-cpl. Medicine Show (Saul and Hays) 1940). An exact contemporary of Bertolt Brecht, they both went to Hollywood where they worked on film scores, sometimes together (in addition, Eisler composed the songs for Brecht's 1947 *Life of Galileo*), and they were both blacklisted. Eisler was pursued for more than six years with obsessive zeal by Herbert Hoover; the FBI file on him amounts to nearly 700 pages.

an opera called *The Medium* (1947) by Gian Carlo Menotti with stage design by Jean Rosenthal and Horace Armistead scenically evoked the interior of a brain.[25] The phantasmagoric, non-realistic staging meant that 'you never really knew what was happening', which was precisely its magic.[26] The production used a scrim, a diaphanous cloth membrane between audience and actors that can achieve extraordinary scenic effects when lit from behind; this marvellously versatile bit of set design kit was to have been used extensively in the 1939 *Medicine Show*. Rosenthal later designed a ballet with George Balanchine based on Schoenberg's *Opus 34* in 1954 that involved physiological depiction and dramatizing doctors at work – and required precisely the kind of effort by the spectator that Garner, Jr describes. Schoenberg's music was 'eighteen dismal minutes long' and was repeated in its entirety. The second time around it was accompanied by 'a grisly surgery in pantomime, [in which] dancers were costumed in bandages and as cadavers',[27] wearing charts of nerves and muscles:

> In a *pas de deux* the dancers were overcome with pain. Doctors rushed in with an operating table. And so it went, with dancers appearing and disappearing, and ended with a battery of lights upstage focused meticulously so that everyone in the audience was blinded … The critics were pretty flabbergasted – but it turned out to be a very popular number in the repertory.[28]

What unifies these disparate productions is the use of pantomime, dance and music; scrims; and the fact that they do not come from so-called avant-garde or Modernist theatre but from the realms of dance and opera, a reminder that we need to cast our research nets very widely when it comes to the performance of medical scenarios and material (see Figure 11.2). Scenographers and lighting designers, as well as directors, composers, costume designers and more, habitually worked across different performance modes. Letting these domains lead scholarship, rather than playtexts or authors, can be extraordinarily liberating and can uncover performances that otherwise would have gone unnoticed by scholars from other disciplines by remaining within artificially separate generic categories.

---

[25] Jean Rosenthal with Lael Wertenbaker, *The Magic of Light: The Craft and Career of Jean Rosenthal, Pioneer in Lighting for the Modern Stage* (Little, Brown, 1972), 99. It was presented along with *The Telephone*, also by Menotti, at the Heckscher Theatre on 18 February 1947 and then at the Ethel Barrymore, 1 May–1 November 1947, for 212 performances.

[26] Ibid.

[27] '301. Opus 34 1954', *Balanchine Catalogue*, https://balanchine.org/balanchine-catalogue/catalogue-of-works/301-opus-34-1954/.

[28] Rosenthal and Wertenbaker, *The Magic of Light*, 124.

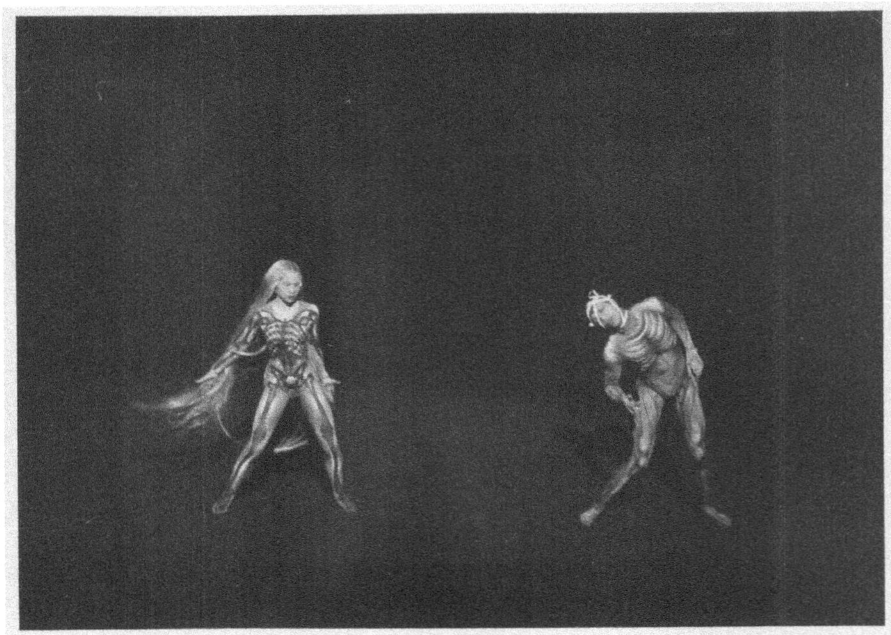

FIGURE 11.2 Schoenberg, *Opus 34* (1954), choreographed by George Balanchine, designed by Jean Rosenthal, photo by Fred Fehl. Fred Fehl Dance Collection, copyright Harry Ransom Center, The University of Texas at Austin.

CONTENTS OF *MEDICINE SHOW*

Comparing the FTP script of 1939 and the revised version for Broadway in 1940 reveals some significant changes.[29] I summarize these in what follows to

[29]The script exists in various versions: the typescript that was created for the FTP (two copies held at the Library of Congress, one of them dated 26 April 1939 that represents the first full version of the play and the other, nearly identical one dated 29 February 1940 and used for copyright deposit) and the typescript promptbook used for Wharton and Gabel's Broadway production and held in the New York Public Library. The latter version differs markedly from those in the Library of Congress and shows that, as one critic at the time noted, the play was 'completely rewritten' in the transition from FTP to Broadway (Wilella Waldorf, 'Medicine Show', *New York Post*, date unknown, 1940).

I do not, however, treat the 1940 script as definitive, because it does not seem entirely consistent with descriptions of the play in reviews, for example bearing no trace of the *Alice in Wonderland* spoof to which many critics refer and that is present in the 1939 script but not the 1940 version. (In this scene, Alice gets more and more ill and the Mad Hatter, her employer, coldly refuses her time off, the Queen of Hearts driving home the cruel irony that the sicker Alice gets, the more she needs a hospital but the less she can afford it.) According to several of the reviews of the 1940 production, this scene was jarring and less successful than other parts of the play; most reviewers deplored it as ill-fitting and 'infantile', with Atkinson calling it 'intolerably precious' and 'an artistic solecism, to say the least' (Atkinson, 'The Play') and Brown finding that the show 'falters badly in

provide readers with as clear a sense of the key changes to the play as it evolved, as far as it is possible to gauge.[30]

Both versions have an overarching figure who controls the action. In the 1939 script it is Loudspeaker, a standard device used in all of the FTP's Living Newspapers. The fact that we never see but only hear him underscores hiddenness and emphasizes the need to rely on all our senses, not just the visual. In the Broadway version, Loudspeaker is replaced by Statistician, a role created for Martin Gabel as the star of the show. This MC-type character never leaves the stage and drives the show forward, serving also as its narrator and moral centre. The other main character in the 1939 version was to have been Mr Average Citizen, to whom Loudspeaker would explain and show key developments and statistics. In the Broadway version this figure becomes a group of people plucked apparently at random from the audience by Statistician, with deliberately ordinary names and occupations ('Dora', 'Joe', Taxi driver, Sharecropper, Mother and so on).

Another key change is the structure of the show. The original version is episodic in nature, with scenes set in vastly different time periods. Such transtemporal movements define the 1939 version, in contrast to the sustained contemporary setting and single narrative line of the Broadway show with its fast-paced, fact-strewn speech, a punchy and raw route to the intellects and emotions of the audience.

The scenographic high point of the 1939 version was to have been the staging of a modern hospital, reminiscent of *Men in White*. In the Broadway version all that remains of this spectacularly planned hospital scene is a brief interlude, off to one side of the stage and using a single bed to signify a hospital and to illustrate further statistics that should outrage the audience, such as the number of empty hospital beds despite an apparent shortage and the attendant financial waste, along with the revelation that it costs just as much to keep hospital beds empty as full. But it is illuminating to read the stage directions of the 1939 version, which show that the representation of the hospital was suggestive and done in pantomime, relying on the imagination of the audience. This new hospital was focused on sterilization of environment – actors are scrubbing floors, cleaning, wearing gauze facial masks, washing hands, all at the forefront, not in the background of the action. The hospital is a modern marvel with its spacious

its unfortunate digression' in this scene (Brown, 'Two on the Aisle'). Yet the spoof is not present in the promptbook for the Broadway production, suggesting that we still do not have that production's final script.

[30]For discussion of the 1939 script, see Shepherd, 'Staging a "Vast Human Dustbowl of Disease"'.

and well-organized layout, spotlessly sterile environment and state-of-the-art equipment run by well-trained medical professionals. Even the microscope is imaginary.

There is an interesting navigation of mimesis here, a deliberate choice as to what to show realistically and what to convey only in mime, engaging what Garner, Jr calls 'spectatorial interpretive operations'.[31] The 1939 script purports to make visible the unseen or the previously hidden, yet only goes so far. Why? The reason becomes brilliantly clear in the climax of the hospital scene, when it is revealed that this wonderful, 'free' hospital does not actually exist. But, as Loudspeaker explains, it could come into being with government funding, namely through supporting the National Health Care bill. Audiences at the time would have been aware of this context. Yet reading the play now creates some cognitive dissonance, as it feels as if these problems have remained just as acute.

Both versions of *Medicine Show* hinge on a single statistic, gravely intoned throughout: that there were over 250,000 preventable deaths in the United States at that time. The gap between this appalling fact and the evidence of what modern medicine has achieved and can potentially provide for everyone is the focal point of both plays, although their ways of conveying this content varies so much. Most striking in comparing the 1939 version with the Broadway script (1940) is the briskness of the latter. The staging is also streamlined so that it just features an enormous door, signifying decisions that must be made in the course of the show in order to open it to a better future.

THE MAZE

This enormous door visualizes the central conceit of the Broadway version: the idea of the 'medical maze' that we must find our way out of. This maze is the paradox flagged up in the opening lines: in a society that has some of the most advanced healthcare on earth, so many people die unnecessarily from illnesses and conditions that could have been treated and cured. The outsized door, coupled with the heartbeat in the background and the archetypal figures (Statistician and the groups of representative characters), set the anti-realistic, interactive and sometimes Expressionist-inflected tone of the Broadway version.

Statistician explains to the group: 'You are in the medical maze every day of your lives. You can't escape the figures' (Act 1, page 6).[32] The only way out is to change the maze itself. 'I did not create the maze. The maze conjures me

[31] Garner, Jr, 'Is There a Doctor in the House?', abstract.

[32] H. R. Hays and Oscar Saul, *Medicine Show* (The New York Theatre, 1940); all quotations from this version will be cited in text by act and page number.

up. Solve it and you defeat me. Change the figures and the books will be kept accordingly', says the Statistician. In other words, for the rest of the play they will learn what needs to be done to alter that alarming statistic of 250,000 preventable deaths.

The maze motif also introduces an element of competition, heightening the stakes for the participants and evoking the game shows that were popular on radio and that were just starting to be launched on TV. The idea of the medical maze reconfigures the realist visible/invisible framing that had dominated medical dramas, attesting to *Medicine Show*'s investment in revising that passive audience role of watching/spectating/consuming and instead seeking to engage them more actively through a sense of competitiveness. This aligns *Medicine Show* with Brecht's notion that watching a play should resemble watching a boxing match – at once intensely involved yet detached, more focused on the sport itself than the personalities and characters and their stories.

It truly is a maze because no matter where you turn there is no way out. There is more than a whiff of the storyline and setting of *The Wizard of Oz* (1939) in all of this – the wandering of Dora (like Oz's Dorothy) and coming across a farm, the motley but doughty group of companions, the maze-like yellow brick road, the need to find a way out, the constant obstacles, the sense of an overarching force (the Statistician and the Wizard) and the clear-cut villain wrecking everyone's welfare (the American Medical Association (AMA) and the Wicked Witch of the West). No reviewers at the time noted this parallel, yet the film was released just a year before *Medicine Show* (indeed, the FTP version of the play was being written during *Oz*'s release).

An added twist to the maze conceit is that as the group wends their way through it, they each learn their own medical fates. These are signalled starkly in the 1939 version: the characters simply vanish into the darkness as the cause of death is announced, a tragic variation on the play's theme of invisibility and of being 'unseen'. This vanishing is preserved intact in the 1940 version but is more protracted and didactic, as the Statistician addresses each one, telling them their fate and watching them go to their deaths.

HIGHLIGHTING THE REALITIES OF MEDICAL CARE THROUGH NON-REALISM

Just as the role of the Statistician became far more prominent in the Broadway version, so too does the role of the Quack, played by star actor Norman Lloyd. This role was much extended from the funny and entertaining song for radio about quack medicine that features in the 1939 version, touting quackery as the last resort of the poor whose desperation these sham doctors exploit. Judging by the attention given to this episode of quackery (and the fact that the title of play satirically foregrounds such 'medicine shows'), reviewers found it to be a highlight of the play.[33] The Quack is both charming and sinister. He brings on 'witnesses' to attest to the veracity of the miracle cure he peddles – two scantily clad 'girls' who sing and dance their testimony to what is, no doubt, a very catchy song written by Eisler. But the quack medicine fails to open the big door hulking over the characters; the maze is still impassable.

Another similarity between the two versions, although handled differently, is that they both feature groups of representative characters. In the Broadway version, Statistician introduces what the stage directions call 'a group of people standing together uncertainly in a spot', representing America – black and white, city and country, immigrants, southerners, northerners, 'they come from all over the country, from every industry and occupation' (Act 1, 36). The idea is that this group can potentially help the wandering characters escape the maze by learning about this second group's medical experiences so that wrongs can be righted in the future. Each one of this second group tells their story in turn. For example, Eli, a black sharecropper from Arkansas, relates a dismal tale of deprivation, concluding 'If it's bad with white folks, you can bet your life it's twice as bad with us' (Act 1, 39). We sympathize, but stop short of identification because each tale of woe is brief, representative and framed by non-illusionist methods. When we are told, along with the characters, how they will die of treatable causes, the emphasis is on the need to change these circumstances through political action, not weep over the tragedies.

In line with Living Newspaper structure, Act 2 of *Medicine Show* shifts from education to solutions. Various scenarios moot possible ways forward: more money being set aside in state and federal budgets, doctors pooling their expertise and resources as Group Plans, and so on. But each one is defeated: budgets get cut, and neither hospitals nor specialist doctors are willing to work with physicians in Group Plans because it is 'against the rules' of the AMA, and therefore 'unethical'. Statistician states the central argument of the play: there must be 'a plan for all the people'. We almost had one, he reminds us:

> The President's Committee presented a plan calling for the expenditure of 850 million dollars a year, to bring medical care, preventive medicine, and health education to all the people, to bring adequate hospital facilities to the 1300 counties in the United States that have none, to bring patients to the doctors and doctors to the needy patients. (Act 2, 10)

[33] It is likely that Norman Lloyd was going to be in the original FTP show, as he was 'virtually a living newspaper fixture, having played important roles in three previous editions [shows]', as reported by one article devoted solely to Lloyd's appearance in the production, which hails his 'merry quizzical phiz' (unknown source, in newspaper clippings file on *Medicine Show* at the New York Public Library, New York).

But its fate was sealed by a single word: 'Taxes'.

The play then becomes a political hearing, featuring the group of ordinary citizens confronting a smug older medic representing the AMA (and therefore the villain of the show) before an imaginary panel and in the presence of the Statistician, who accuses the doctor of using dirty tactics such as intimidation, confusion, 'pressure, slander, and whispering campaigns ... By fighting every progressive move in American medicine, you are condemning these innocent men and women to die as surely as if you were the executioner' (Act 2, 19). Debate ensues. One character says that it is impossible to save everyone, and no single bit of legislation could do that, so why not just enjoy life and be grateful for being one of the lucky, healthy ones? But this attitude only works if everyone can enjoy life, not just the lucky few. A younger doctor then bravely drives home the key message of the show: political change. 'I can tell you what lies on the other side of that door. Outside that door is change ... Outside that door is an idea "The Health of the people is the direct concern of the government!"' (Act 2, 22). This powerful notion is threatened by economic worries about US industry being 'bankrupt' and budget cuts being necessary, tax hikes, unemployment – thus overwhelming the medical issues that have been debated. Although this final section reads effectively in showing how quickly ideals can get subsumed by realities, it disappointed some critics who found this conclusion 'bogged down by statistics'.[34]

RESPONSES TO THE SHOW

Reviews of the production ranged from the lukewarm to the rave, and they are our most reliable evidence of how it was performed and received. 'A rather boring illustrated lecture', complained Sidney B. Whipple of the New York *World-Telegram*, while Richard Watts, Jr pronounced it 'one of the most dramatic shows in its theatrical season', likening its power to that of *One-Third of a Nation* and saying that it 'pulsates with life and fury'.[35] Brooks Atkinson of the *New York Times*, probably the critic with the greatest authority, declared it 'profoundly impressive':

> Although it is generally a little presumptuous for a drama reviewer to urge readers to see a specific play, perhaps the occasion is sufficiently unusual to warrant an exception this morning. For 'Medicine Show' is original as theatre and vital in its material ... incontrovertible and far-seeing.[36]

---

[34] Brown, 'Two on the Aisle'.

[35] Sidney B. Whipple, 'Review of Medicine Show', *New York World-Telegram*, 13 April 1940; Richard Watts, Jr, 'Socialised Medicine', *New York Herald Tribune*, 13 April 1940.

[36] Atkinson, 'The Play'.

It is striking to see Atkinson baldly exhorting audiences to see the show. One critic went even further, deeming it a 'public service' in laying bare the 'vast human dustbowl of disease' that is emerging through lack of proper national healthcare: 'If "Medicine Show" has aroused us even slightly to the danger it will have accomplished a public service all out of proportion to its lamentably short run.'[37] Critics especially drew attention to the show's combination of education and entertainment. Richard Lockridge wrote that it had 'the vitality of good polemic. It is vigorous debate, with little beating about the bush and many statistics beating about the head'.[38] Most agreed that the show was uneven, generally favouring the first half, which John Mason Brown of the *New York Post* found 'as fascinating as it is appalling', while John Anderson felt that the second half was 'lopsided and unconvincing'.[39]

Scenography also received attention. An illustration from an unnamed newspaper shows brilliantly how the staging worked, with multiple points of action and groups of actors, the Statistician in the centre in front of the enormous doors, and the representation of the hospital, much curtailed from the more intricate and extended 1939 script. The *New Yorker* shed valuable light on the show's staging techniques: 'Greenish faces materialize high on the walls, rapidly delivering the Hippocratic oath; actors appear and disappear through enormous gates of doubtful symbolism; Mr Gabel's factual comments on the situation are delivered in somewhat the manner of a train announcer'; and the production crowds 'an almost unlimited number of episodes onto the stage in a very brief time, which is a great help when you are trying to present all the aspects of a large and intricate problem'.[40] Unless this last comment is well-disguised sarcasm, it suggests that despite the fully fledged rewriting of the script, it retained its episodic flavour and harnessed it to good effect.

This critical response attests to the significance of *Medicine Show* as pioneering in the way it staged a complex layering of medical facts, statistics and situations (and, at least in its original 1939 script, portrayed a working hospital), patients representing different regions and walks of life, and in the way it shifted the diagnostic gaze from the ailing human body to the collective people suffering under the lack of equal access to healthcare and, most importantly, a government system to deliver it to everyone. This marked a distinct change from the way medicine on stage had often been depicted in realist and naturalist modes, which invoked the body and its mysterious inner workings as the

---

[37] Ernest L. Meyer, 'As the Crow Flies', *The Progressive*, 10 April 1940.
[38] Richard Lockridge, unknown source, in newspaper clippings file on *Medicine Show* at the New York Public Library, New York.
[39] Brown, 'Two on the Aisle'; John Anderson, 'Medicine Show', *N.Y. Journal-American*, 13 April 1940.
[40] Wolcott Gibbs, 'The Theatre', *New Yorker*, 20 April 1940.

passive recipient of the heroic interventions of the doctor. The radical step of *Medicine Show* was to rethink the body as both individualized and collective, as something that we all share and have a stake in protecting and, when necessary, healing.

A MEDICAL SHOW FOR THE TWENTY-FIRST CENTURY

Medicine Show followed a period often known as the 'New' Era (1920s–30s) that grew out of the Progressive Era at the turn of the century (*c.*1900–20). The show revealed the deeper history behind the delivery of modern medicine and was openly critical of the AMA's refusal to support the national healthcare bill. As the *New York Post* noted on its opening, *Medicine Show* was 'especially timely right now with the American Medical Association facing anti-trust charges in Washington, and a good deal of discussion going on about public health'.[41] *Medicine Show* made it into Burns Mantle's *The Best Plays of 1939–40*, one of a long-running series of volumes that were reliable markers of esteem. Yet *Medicine Show* remains unpublished and obscure, despite its success on Broadway and its continued relevance as we face the same problems in healthcare today in the United States that the play grappled with in its time. *Medicine Show* was a play of the past that depicted a contemporary problem, analysed how it came about and offered clear solutions going forward, projecting a future that had not yet been attained but was tantalizingly within reach.

This chapter has illuminated some of the scenographic inventiveness in portraying the human body and its inner workings in the mid-twentieth-century United States. These various medical performances both tap into and help to generate audience curiosity about the inner workings of the body, of hospitals, of healthcare itself. Although we may think of this pervasive interest in all things medical as a contemporary phenomenon, aided by the internet and social media in addition to film and TV, *Medicine Show* and the other examples I have discussed suggest that it has always been there.[42] What *Medicine Show* uniquely demonstrated was that theatre could engage with medicine in a much broader way than it had ever done before, going beyond the realistic drama of doctors, nurses and emergencies to present the unseen yet vital issues that shape healthcare delivery and modelling how to debate and resolve them.

---

[41] Waldorf, 'Medicine Show'.

[42] Alex Mermikides and Gianna Bouchard, eds, *Performance and the Medical Body* (Bloomsbury, 2016), 1.

REFERENCES

'301. Opus 34 1954'. *Balanchine Catalogue*. https://balanchine.org/balanchine-catalogue/catalogue-of-works/301-opus-34-1954/.

Armstrong, Patrick. *Microscopy, Magnification and Modernist Fiction: Micro-Modernism from Hardy to Beckett*. Bloomsbury Academic, 2024.

Bold, Christine. *'Vaudeville Indians' on Global Circuits, 1880s–1930s*. Yale University Press, 2022.

Duffy, Susan, and Bernard K. Duffy. 'Theatrical Responses to Technology During the Depression: Three Federal Theatre Project Plays'. *Theatre History Studies* 6 (January 1986): 143–64.

Garner, Stanton B., Jr. 'Introduction: Is There a Doctor in the House? Medicine and the Making of Modern Drama'. *Modern Drama* 51, no. 3 (Fall 2008): 311–28.

Garner, Stanton B., Jr. *Theatre & Medicine*. Methuen Drama, 2023.

Hays, H. R., and Oscar Saul. *Medicine Show*. The New York Theatre, 1940.

Jarrett, Gene Andrew, ed. *African American Literature Beyond Race: An Alternative Reader*. New York University Press, 2006.

Markel, Howard. 'Men in White: The Operating Room's Debut into Popular American Culture'. *JAMA* 302, no. 21 (2009): 2376–8.

Melosh, Barbara. 'The New Deal's Federal Theatre Project'. *Medical Heritage* 2, no. 1 (1986): 36–47.

Mermikides, Alex, and Gianna Bouchard, eds. *Performance and the Medical Body*. Bloomsbury, 2016.

Morphos, Evangeline. 'Sidney Kingsley's "Men in White"'. *TDR (The Drama Review)* 28, no. 4 (1984): 13–22.

Rosenthal, Jean, with Lael Wertenbaker. *The Magic of Light: The Craft and Career of Jean Rosenthal, Pioneer in Lighting for the Modern Stage*. Little, Brown, 1972.

Shapiro, James. *The Playbook: A Story of Theatre, Democracy and the Making of a Culture War*. Faber and Faber, 2024.

Shepherd-Barr, Kirsten E. '"Golden Dust" in the Wind: Genetics, Contagion, and Early Twentieth-Century American Theatre'. In *The Palgrave Handbook of Twentieth and Twenty-First Century Literature and Science*, edited by the Triangle Collective. Palgrave Macmillan, 2020.

Shepherd-Barr, Kirsten E. *Theatre and Evolution from Ibsen to Beckett*. Columbia University Press, 2015.

Shepherd-Barr, Kirsten E. 'Staging a "Vast Human Dustbowl of Disease": The Federal Theatre Project's *Medicine Show* in its 1939 (Pre-Broadway) Version'. In *Microscopic Life in 20th- and 21st-Century Literature and Performance*, edited by Sarah Bouttier, Liliane Campos, François-Joseph Lapointe and Sarah Montin. Open Book Publishers, 2026.

Shulman, Max, and J. Chris Westgate, eds. *Performing the Progressive Era: Immigration, Urban Life, and Nationalism on Stage*. University of Iowa Press, 2019.

Wijdicks, Eelco. *Cinema, M.D.: A History of Medicine on Screen*. Oxford University Press, 2020.

Wolff, Tamsen. *Mendel's Theatre: Heredity, Eugenics, and Early Twentieth-Century American Drama*. Palgrave, 2009.

12

Performance and medical education: Bridging the gap between public and private phrenology

MARLIS SCHWEITZER AND SARA MASCIOTRA-MILSTEIN

This essay asks how interactions between medical professionals and theatre artists shaped the development and dissemination of phrenology, the wildly popular 'science of the mind', which remains one of the more troubling examples of scientific racism as it materialized in the nineteenth century. Through detailed measurement of the brain's distinct 'faculties', phrenologists believed they could develop a fairly accurate reading of an individual's behavioural tendencies. This essay considers the extent to which theatrical techniques contributed to phrenology's rapid uptake in Britain and North America by focusing on two of its most influential advocates, George and Cecilia Combe. Though medical practitioners and health humanities scholars today may wonder how – or indeed if – a historical case study at this distance can impact their working lives, we maintain that an examination of the relationship between theatre and medicine in the past can deepen understanding of how theatre continues to support the uptake of medical science in the present. This essay argues that the dramaturgical structures within Combe's lectures popularized phrenology – and therefore scientific racism – paving the way for the entanglement of these theories into both medical and popular society, the effects of which we still see to this day. In addition to harnessing theatrical techniques to disseminate emerging medical ideas in public settings, George and Cecilia Combe gave shape to the smaller scale parlour theatre of the nineteenth century, where clinical encounters between doctors (i.e. as phrenology lecturers) and their patients (audience) resembled mini performances.

George Combe, a Scottish lawyer turned medical scientist, was one of the more recognizable figures of the nineteenth century. Tall, thin, with sharp facial features and a distinctive mane of curly white hair, he lectured on public stages throughout Great Britain, Europe and North America proselytizing on behalf of phrenology, the new science of the mind that promised to explain the internal workings of the brain. As his reputation grew, authorized and unauthorized images of Combe appeared in book frontispieces, caricature prints and academic journals. Strolling down Chambers Street in Edinburgh today, you might encounter his portrait bust mounted on the front exterior of the building that once housed the Edinburgh Phrenological Society. Such images helped to secure his celebrity akin to that enjoyed by some of the era's greatest stage stars. Indeed, Combe was a regular theatregoer, a fan of the celebrated actress Sarah Siddons, and a friend of her niece, the actress turned abolitionist, Fanny Kemble. In 1833, Combe concretized his ties to the Siddons family by marrying Cecilia Siddons, Sarah Siddon's youngest daughter. In many ways, the popularization of Combe through his lectures, and furthered by his marriage into the theatre world, blurred the distinction between the man as a performer and as a physician. Essentially, he performed the role of lecturer as he disseminated his phrenological theories, gaining celebrity status for himself while popularizing the science. Through his embrace of spectacle, Combe offered the average man and woman access to phrenology's self-assessment tools, anticipating the deployment of television and social media platforms by such celebrity figures as Dr Oz and Dr Phil.

Despite her close ties to theatrical royalty, surprisingly few images remain of Cecilia Combe, known to her friends and family as Cecy.[1] Unlike her mother, whose image proliferated widely throughout Britain via paintings, engravings and figurines,[2] or her cousin, Fanny Kemble, who likewise sat for dozens of portraits and was acknowledged as one of the most beautiful women of the era,[3] Cecy seems to have avoided the artist's studio. This isn't to suggest that Cecy

[1] Throughout this chapter, the authors use 'Cecy' in cases of domesticity and familial settings. 'Cecilia' is reserved for academic and more professional contexts.

[2] Heather McPherson, 'Sculpting Her Image: Sarah Siddons and the Art of Self-Fashioning', in *Women and Portraits in Early Modern Europe*, ed. Andrea Pearson (Routledge, 2008); Claudia Corti, 'Poses and Pauses: Sarah Siddons and the Romantic Theatrical Portrait', in *Women's Romantic Theatre and Drama*, ed. Lilla Maria Crisafulli and Keir Elam (Routledge, 2010).

[3] Deidre David, *Fanny Kemble: A Performed Life* (University of Pennsylvania Press, 2007).

avoided images altogether. The artist Thomas Lawrence, a man with a complicated relationship to the Siddons family, created a chalk drawing of a grumpy-looking Cecy when she was a toddler as part of a family portrait series.[4] Two decades later she sat for the artist George Clint, where her resemblance to both Fanny Kemble and her mother is undeniable.[5] Yet unlike so many of her family members – uncles, aunts, cousins, siblings – Cecilia Siddons Combe did not pursue a life on the theatrical stage, nor did she follow her husband onto the lecture stage. Rather, she seems to have preferred (or accepted) a life of service to those in the limelight – a life lived in the wings, if you will.

Though she avoided the attention lavished on those around her, Cecy was hardly a passive observer or a voiceless helpmeet in the Victorian mould of the 'angel in the house'.[6] While her husband embraced his role as the public face of phrenology, a status aided by the growing popularity of his 1828 publication *The Constitution of Man*, Cecy laboured behind the scenes to support the wider phrenological project. In addition to tracing phrenology's dynamic relationship with the theatre, this essay considers how Cecilia Combe used her knowledge of acting, dramaturgy and theatrical staging to enhance her husband's lecture performances. It further argues that she contributed to the advancement of her husband's work by writing a closet drama that explains the principles of phrenology for young readers.

In her unpublished *Fictitious dialogue*, Cecy imagines a dramatic conversation between a young boy and a woman well versed in the intricacies of phrenological science. The manuscript, now held in the Combe Papers at the National Library of Scotland, points to her efforts to bring phrenology from the masculinized realm of the lecture hall into the feminized domestic sphere. Whereas her husband engaged adult middle-class audiences in intensive six-week lecture courses, promising to help them unlock phrenology's secrets for self-assessment, Cecilia Combe proposed a different educational approach, one more closely aligned with Socratic methods, adjusted for the attention span of prepubescent children. One could even argue that this *Fictitious dialogue* works as a prescription (or script) for clinical encounters between doctor-phrenologists and their patient-audiences.

---

4 Shearer West, 'The Professional and Personal Worlds of Artists and Actors: Thomas Lawrence and the Siddons Family', *Nineteenth Century Theatre & Film* 39, no. 1 (2012): 1–25; Laura Engel, *Women, Performance and the Material of Memory: The Archival Tourist* (Palgrave Macmillan, 2019), 53–79; David Stack, *Queen Victoria's Skull: George Combe and the Mid-Victorian Mind* (Continuum Books, 2008), 123.

5 George Clint, *Miss Cecilia Siddons (1794–1868)*, Dundee Art Galleries and Museums Collection (Dundee City Council), Art UK, https://artuk.org/discover/artworks/miss-ceciliasiddons-17941 868-92268.

6 The phrase 'angel in the house' was made popular by the poem of that name by Coventry Patmore, published in 1854.

Cecy's labours in the wings as Combe's pseudo-dramaturg, and as a writer herself, show how nineteenth-century medicine relied on theatre – in essence, became theatre – and, by virtue of her efforts, was disseminated widely to middle-class audiences both publicly and privately. Through its examination of Cecy's hidden or previously unacknowledged labour on behalf of phrenology, this essay extends feminist scholarship on nineteenth-century women's negotiations of the public and private spheres and contributes to existing conversations about phrenology's democratic promise. We aim to highlight the often-elided role women played in transmitting and educating the public about medical models – a historical oversight that underscores the prevailing tendency in medicine and the sciences to relegate women's contribution to the 'back-of-the-house' or 'in the wings', where they are all too often forgotten. More specifically, we extend historian Carla Bittel's work on phrenology's appeal to women as 'readers, consumers, proselytizers and practitioners of this knowledge system' in the mid-nineteenth century.[7] We seek to contextualize Cecy's contributions as a dramaturg, legacy caretaker and advocate of phrenology in her own right.

At the same time, this essay remains attentive to phrenology's damaging legacy, most obviously its founders' aggressive quest for 'unique' and 'distinctive' human remains to add to their collections, which were subsequently used by white, Anglo-American lecturers like Combe to prop up hierarchies of race, gender, class and ability. Like many other nineteenth-century sciences, phrenology benefited from and enhanced white supremacist goals and ideals, spreading racist ideas about human difference that linger today. This essay does not excuse or aim to whitewash phrenology's contribution to the perpetuation of racial stereotypes. To the contrary, it furthers Marlis's previous writing on phrenology's entanglement with theatrical spectacle and demonstrates how educated, well-connected women like Cecilia Combe aided its wider pedagogical goals, for better *and* worse.[8] Indeed, we hasten to emphasize that the theatrical dissemination of phrenological principles offers a corrective to those who view of the stage as a utopian space for therapeutic witnessing, catharsis and social transformation. While theatre can serve as a useful tool for democratizing scientific knowledge, its potential for populist appeal carries with it an obvious danger, as

---

[7] Carla Bittel, 'Woman, Know Thyself: Producing and Using Phrenological Knowledge in 19th-Century America', *Centaurus* 55 (2013): 105.

[8] See Marlis Schweitzer, 'Casting Clara Fisher: Phrenology, Protean Farce, and the "Astonishing" Career of a Child Actress', *Theatre Journal* 68, no. 2 (2016): 167–90; *Bloody Tyrants and Little Pickles: Stage Roles of Anglo-American Girls in the Nineteenth Century* (University of Iowa Press, 2020); 'The Curious Case of the Infant Sappho', *Lady Science*, 10 December 2020, www.ladyscience.com/features/curious-case-of-the-infant-sappho-2020?rq=schweitzer; 'Lecture on Heads and Lectures with Skulls – Performance Transmutations', in *Identity, Culture, and the Science Performance, vol. 1: From the Lab to the Street*, ed. Vivian Appler and Meredith Conti (Methuen Drama, 2023).

seen in the racist connotations of phrenology in the nineteenth century, as well as in today's 'fake news' and medical theories with deeply entrenched racism. For this reason, we maintain, it is critical for medical practitioners and health humanities scholars to pay heed to the past even as they advocate for justice in the present.

A FEW WORDS ON PHRENOLOGY

Phrenology was founded in the late eighteenth century by Franz Joseph Gall, a Viennese physician who later lived in Paris, and Gall's student, J. G. Spurzheim, who toured widely through Europe and the United States. Through the dissection of human and animal brains, the study and measurement of human skulls and analysis of the heads of living human subjects, Gall and Spurzheim developed a method for 'compar[ing] cerebral development with the manifestations of mental power, for the purpose of discovering the functions of the brain, and the organs of the mind'.[9] They proposed that the size of an individual's brain and constitutive organs affected their behaviour; thus, for example, an individual's ability to 'experienc[e] the emotion of beauty [was] in proportion to the perfection of the organ of Ideality', just as an individual with an enlarged 'Destructiveness' organ would feel a greater desire for revenge.[10] Working from this premise, phrenologists grouped each of the brain's faculties into two Orders and six Genera for a total of thirty-three (later thirty-five) separate faculties, each tied to a specific organ. These ranged from Order 1 feelings of Philoprogenitiveness (love of offspring), Self-Esteem and Benevolence to Order 2 intellectual faculties, which included the senses, perceptive faculties and faculties related to external objects (e.g. Time, Tune, Language). Phrenologists argued that understanding the correlation between the size of the brain's organs and the faculties associated with them was critical to understanding individual human behaviour and the broader differences between national groups.

George Combe became convinced of phrenology's promise in 1817 after attending a private demonstration of a brain dissection held in a colleague's drawing room. The dissection was conducted by Spurzheim himself, who had travelled to Edinburgh in response to a recently published article in the *Edinburgh Review* which had dismissed phrenology as mere quackery. During the demonstration before fifteen writers and doctors, Spurzheim laid the offending article beside the brain he was to dissect, challenging his audience to take sides as he took up a scalpel. The provocative demonstration left a deep impression on Combe, whose own lecture demonstrations would later deploy

---

[9] George Combe, *Elements of Phrenology*, 4th American ed. (Marsh, Capen & Lyon, 1835), 30.
[10] Ibid., 31.

similarly theatrical techniques.[11] In 1820 Combe joined with his brother and other prominent men to establish the Edinburgh Phrenological Society. Over the course of fifty years, society members compiled an extensive collection of human remains for study (including skulls of Indigenous peoples) and shared research that ranged from the analysis of historical subjects such as Robert the Bruce to reports on unusual or surprising contemporary human subjects. For example, in 1820, Combe created a cast of the head of the juvenile actress Clara Fisher in order to analyse the source of her creative talent.[12] Combe's findings were published in 1824 as 'Report upon the Cast of Miss Clara Fisher', and he transported a cast of her head, along with an assemblage of other skulls and casts, with him when he toured lecture halls in Europe and North America. In so doing, he encouraged the average man and woman to understand the application of phrenological teachings outside of the realm of a clinical encounter. In other words, Combe's performance as a phrenological lecturer democratized and popularized this 'science of the mind'.

While Combe emphasized the unique characteristics of each phrenological subject, he also believed that humans were capable of change and should strive towards a universal ideal. As he remarked in a paper first delivered to the Edinburgh Phrenological Society in 1822, 'the actual dispositions and talents of individuals, are the result, not of their natural and mental constitution merely, but of this modified in a thousand ways, by education and external circumstances'.[13] Put differently, biology was not (necessarily) destiny. Influenced by the work of Thomas Brown and Bishop Joseph Butler, Combe argued that it was the individual's responsibility to improve him- or herself through a course of study, exercise, healthy eating and related activities. In *The Constitution of Man* (1828), he moved beyond the realm of phrenological analysis to propose a natural and moral philosophy, one that argued for adhering to a set of universally recognizable physical, moral and natural laws. He stressed the potential for all humans to achieve self-knowledge and moral improvement by understanding how their individual faculties functioned. Those who learned to suppress or control lower faculties such as Destructiveness and Acquisitiveness, which contributed to vice, and instead privileged virtuous faculties such as Benevolence and Philoprogenitiveness, would live a superior moral life in keeping with the laws of nature.[14]

Although Combe acknowledged the importance of environmental and cultural factors in the development of individual and national dispositions, his

---

[11] David Stack, *Queen Victoria's Skull: George Combe and the Mid-Victorian Mind* (Continuum Books, 2008), 34–5.

[12] Schweitzer, 'Casting Clara Fisher'.

[13] George Combe, *Elements of Phrenology* (John Anderson, Jr, 1824), 308.

[14] Stack, *Queen Victoria's Skull*, 83.

views were undeniably entangled with white supremacist perspectives. For example, his 1830 book *A System of Phrenology* includes a chapter titled 'National Character and Development of Brain', with a chart comparing the measurements of 'national skulls' from Brazil, Switzerland, the Caribbean, India, Africa and North America. Combe's study of these and other skulls led him to conclude 'that there was a hierarchy among nations'.[15] Like many other (white) scientists of the era, Combe took the superiority of Caucasians over non-white groups as a given and viewed Caucasian brains as the norm against which all other racial or 'national' brains should be measured. This included attributing the 'savage state' of North American Indigenous peoples to deficiencies in cranial development, which became apparent in comparing their measurements to the considerably larger measurements of the ancient Greeks and Egyptians. Thus, while phrenology's emphasis on self-transformation and its democratic leanings, particularly its relative accessibility and its insistence that anyone could learn to practise phrenology, appealed to some African American thinkers, including Henry 'Box' Brown and Frederick Douglass, its claims to radical inclusivity rang false to others.[16] As Afro-American studies scholar Britt Rusert asserts, Combe's friendship with the American craniologist Samuel George Morton who more aggressively promoted racial hierarchies by insisting that cranial size was a distinguishing feature of racial difference and a key indicator of intelligence, 'did much to tether phrenology to craniology, and by association, to the history of scientific racism'.[17] It is therefore impossible to disentangle phrenology from the history of white supremacy; it must be understood as one of a series of sciences that supported the naturalization of racial hierarchies in the nineteenth century. Indeed, to echo a point made above, this history underscores how medical science in general, and the doctor–patient relationship more specifically, carries with it the prejudices of that society, which often linger in unexpected ways.

Outside his Edinburgh circle, Combe promoted phrenology through public lectures that combined scientific show-and-tell with calm, persuasive argumentation. These lectures offer insight into how doctors and medical lecturers like Combe became actors of sorts, performing their lecture theories for large audiences at a time. With this celebrity status, though, came scrutiny, mockery and accusations of quackery. Nowadays, we might associate these risks with celebrity doctors (think Dr Phil or Dr Oz) who offer Ted Talks and popularize their theories on our modern lecture circuit – the Internet and social media. For Combe, we see this backlash to his public persona as medical-actor in the form

---

[15] George Combe, *A System of Phrenology*, 3rd ed. (John Anderson, Jr, 1830), 621.
[16] Britt Rusert, *Fugitive Science: Empiricism and Freedom in Early African American Culture* (New York University Press, 2017), 292.
[17] Ibid., 125.

of caricatures. However, it would be foolish to write off all caricatures as mere mockery; some actually offer historians insight into the dramaturgy of Combe's lectures and parlour theatre. An 1826 caricature of a phrenological lecture by Henry Thomas Aiken (likely a satire of Combe), entitled 'Calves Heads and Brains, or a Phrenological Lecture', offers some indication of how phrenologists engaged their audiences and were viewed by those less convinced of their claims.[18] Surrounded by a large assemblage of casts, skulls and busts, the unidentified lecturer in Aiken's image extends an arm to his rapt audience, which includes men, women and a small boy. Standing authoritatively behind a table, he is surrounded by the tools of his trade, which include busts and casts of notable figures, along with skulls and other human remains. Though clearly satirical, the caricature accurately reflects the broad multigenerational, heterosocial appeal of Combe's lectures. For example, during a lengthy stop in Boston in 1838, Combe noted 'audiences numbering from 500 to 1500 hundred [*sic*] persons of both sexes'.[19] Such lectures were especially attractive to middle-class white women looking to advance their education at a time when women were not yet admitted into colleges; as we discuss further below, Combe's public lectures and corresponding publications enhanced women's knowledge of phrenology and allowed them to bring it into the home.[20] His success as a touring lecturer did not come overnight, though, but rather was enabled by the theatrical knowledge and support of his wife, Cecilia Siddons Combe.

LECTURE PERFORMANCE AND COMBE'S TIES TO THE KEMBLE-SIDDONS FAMILY

Combe's strategic approach to performance is hardly surprising given the flourishing relationship between nineteenth-century science and medicine and the stage, which provides a helpful context for reflecting on how twenty-first-century medical practitioners and others in the health humanities draw on theatre and related performance practices today. As Bernard Lightman observes, 'the boundary between science and theatre was especially porous' in the nineteenth century.[21] Studies such as Tiffany Watt-Smith's *On Flinching: Theatricality and Scientific Looking from Darwin to Shell Shock* and Iwan Rhys Morus's *Frankenstein's Children: Electricity, Exhibition, and Experiment*

[18] Henry Thomas, *Calves Heads and Brains, or a Phrenological Lecture*, 1826. *OnView*, Center for History of Medicine, Harvard University, https://collections.countway.harvard.edu/onview/items/show/6158.

[19] Quoted in Bittel, 'Woman, Know Thyself', 125.

[20] Ibid., 116.

[21] Bernard Lightman, Afterword to *Staging Science: Scientific Performances on Street, Stage, and Screen*, ed. Martin Willis (Palgrave Macmillan, 2016), 128.

in Nineteenth-Century London have brilliantly documented the influence of theatrical ideas and staging practices on scientific experimentation and exhibitions of scientific achievement in the nineteenth century. Actors played scientists onstage in productions ranging from *Doctor Faustus* to dramatizations of *Frankenstein*, while playwrights brought the latest scientific trends to the stage, often inflected by satirical critique; in 1838, for example, August von Kotzebue premiered his comedy *The Organs of the Brain*, a none-too-subtle parody of phrenology. Scientists likewise deployed spectacle to engage audience interest, often competing with other lecturers for the attention of a spectacle-seeking public. These lectures varied widely in their subject matter, covering everything from politics and history to literature and religion; scientific lectures were extremely popular, among both men and women. Indeed, as Carla Bittel remarks in her study of phrenology's uptake in the United States, 'early Victorians, in both Britain and America, experienced science as central to Victorianism itself'.[22]

Like their theatrical counterparts, scientific lecturers deployed spectacle to engage audiences and demonstrate their expertise through the manipulation of objects, animals, other human beings (and human remains) and an emphasis on persuasive performance techniques.[23] During the 1830s, for example, the Royal Polytechnic Institution built up a strong membership among London's middle and upper classes thanks to the inspiring lecture performances of men such as Humphry Davy and Michael Faraday. Davy's early lectures on such topics as electrochemistry were so well attended that traffic jams were a frequent occurrence outside the institution entrance, a challenge London's civic leaders addressed by making Albemarle Street the city's first one-way street.[24] After Davy's retirement, Faraday continued to expand the institution's lecture programming, paying heed to such practical matters as lighting, ventilation and the entrance to the lecture theatre in an effort to keep audiences alert. Faraday was also keenly aware that strong visuals – interesting scientific equipment, illustrations and so forth – and a compelling lecture style were critical for engaging a lay audience. In an 1813 letter to a colleague, he described his approach to lecturing: 'The utterance should not be rapid and hurried and consequently unintelligible but slow and deliberate conveying ideas with ease from the Lecturer and infusing them with clearness and readiness into the minds of the audience.'[25] Faraday's lectures were so popular that he regularly attracted hundreds

[22] Bittel, 'Woman, Know Thyself', 107.
[23] Lightman, 'Afterword', 128–31.
[24] Frank A. J. L. James, '"Never Talk About Science, *Show* It to Them": The Lecture Theatre of the Royal Institution', *ISR* 27, no. 3 (2002): 225.
[25] Quoted in ibid., 226; see also David Knight, 'Scientific Lectures: A History of Performance', *ISR* 27, no. 3 (2002): 217–24.

of eager auditors to the institution, casting what fellow lecturer John Tyndall described as a kind of 'magic on his hearers that sent them away persuaded that they knew all about a subject of which they knew but little'.[26] As historian Frank A. J. L. James observes, Faraday's primary goal was to 'make science a polite entertainment that required the sort of suspension of disbelief that is associated with the theatre'.[27] He wanted to inspire audiences and excite them about science's potential; if they learned something along the way, so much the better.[28]

George Combe similarly sought to appeal to his audience with carefully crafted lecture performances that also paid heed to audience attention spans, incorporating intermissions to allow time for rest and refreshment. Commenting on his lecture style, Andrew Boardman, the recording secretary for the Phrenological Society of New York, remarked that while Combe was not 'splendid', 'brilliant' or 'fascinating', he nevertheless engaged audiences with language that was 'slow and flowing'. Where others dazzled, Combe's style was 'familiar, chaste, earnest, and unambiguous'.[29] Reading between the lines of Boardman's statement, it would appear that Combe was less interested in delighting his audiences than educating them, equipping with the necessary tools to take up the mantle of phrenology themselves.

What further distinguished Combe from other lecturers was his direct connection to the theatre via his close ties to some of the era's leading actors, most notably the members of the Kemble-Siddons family. Combe first gained access to the theatrical family through his brother Andrew, who served as a doctor to Harriet Murray or Mrs Henry Siddons, Sarah Siddons's widowed daughter-in-law.[30] When they met, Mrs Harriet (Henry) Siddons was proprietor of the Theatre Royal in Edinburgh, a position she had assumed in 1815 when her husband Henry died. A strong-willed and savvy businesswoman, she was much beloved by the local community who fondly referred to her as 'Our Mrs Siddons'. Over time, Mrs Henry Siddons came to trust Andrew Combe as a confidante and advisor and welcomed both Combe brothers into her home, where they met the rest of her family, including her niece, the actress Fanny Kemble. The Combes were regulars at the Siddons' home throughout the 1820s

[26] Quoted in James, 'Never Talk About Science, *Show* It to Them', 227.

[27] Ibid.

[28] This paragraph on Faraday and Davy is reworked from Schweitzer, 'The Infant Sappho'.

[29] Andrew Boardman, Introduction to *Lectures on Phrenology* by George Combe (Samuel Colman, 1839), v–vi. For more on twenty-first-century instructions for the ideal physician's performance, see the essays in the Part One of this collection.

[30] A note again on names: This essay uses the name 'Mrs Harriet (Henry) Siddons'. While she was known professionally as 'Mrs Henry Siddons', we believe that her contributions to the theatre industry of the nineteenth century warrant the use of her given name, especially in the context of all that she achieved prior to her marriage to Henry the theatre manager, and after his death upon assuming his role.

and Mrs Siddons's daughters and Fanny Kemble also visited George Combe's home 'for evenings of singing, interspersed with philosophical debate'.[31] Mrs Siddons's cultivation of a circle of friends that included doctors, lawyers and actors calls attention to the importance of the parlour as a site for the intermingling of art and medical science beyond the gendered bounds of the university lecture hall or scientific society. Within the private realm of the parlour, men and women were free to exchange ideas and influence one another. Though neither Fanny Kemble nor Mrs Siddons agreed to study phrenology (much to Combe's chagrin), they remained friends for life and aided Combe in expanding his personal and professional network. Such relationships were common throughout the nineteenth century as travelling actors, musicians, painters and other artists rubbed shoulders with doctors, lawyers and other professionals at public and private gatherings, not just in Scotland, but all across Europe.[32]

Medicine's ties to theatre were furthered strengthened by George and Andrew Combe's growing friendship with the Kemble-Siddons family, which coincided with their establishment of the Edinburgh Phrenological Society in 1820 and the publication of George Combe's first book, *Elements of Phrenology* in 1824, followed by his most celebrated and controversial publication, *The Constitution of Man*, in 1828. One might reasonably conclude that Combe's friendship with the Kemble-Siddons family played some role in the development of his scientific thought. In his 2005 biography of the phrenologist, David Stack traces striking similarities between the moral philosophy Combe presents in *The Constitution of Man* and the neoclassical acting style exhibited by Sarah Siddons. Long before he married her daughter, Combe was a huge fan of Siddons's as an actress, and his writing, both public and private, is peppered with references to seeing her in performance. Understanding Siddons's influences on Combe's thinking, Stack argues, helps 'to resolve the paradox between the *Constitution*'s seemingly Enlightenment-inspired emphasis on universality and phrenology's apparently Romantic concern with particularity'.[33] Like other neo-classicists, Combe and Siddons devoted themselves to the careful study of human nature, with the goal of identifying universal ideals representing the 'higher potentials' of the human mind. But they also realized that each individual possessed unique characteristics and sought to represent these distinctive qualities in their work. Combe and Siddons likewise believed in the importance

---

[31] Stack, *Queen Victoria's Skull*, 104.

[32] See Hacking's discussion of medicine's reliance on art to describe the symptoms of hysteria, which popularized through relationships and gatherings similar to those we see with Combe and his theatrical connections. Ian Hacking, *Travelers: Reflections on the Reality of Transient Mental Illness* (University Press of Virginia, 1998); Roberta Barker, *Symptoms of the Self: Tuberculosis and the Making of the Modern Stage* (University of Iowa Press, 2023).

[33] Stack, *Queen Victoria's Skull*, 101.

of uplift for inspiring change and refrained from overly realistic depictions of human behaviour.

Attending to the specifics of Siddons's acting is therefore critical to understanding Combe's approach to lecturing, as the two responded to shifting cultural and political contexts in similar ways. Yet it would be a mistake to characterize Sarah Siddons's performances as belonging exclusively to the neoclassical school of acting, or that Combe's own ideas about performance, in turn, are likewise restricted to neoclassical thought. As theatre historian Robert Shaughnessey observes:

> Siddons's characteristic performance style is best thought of in terms of the transition from neo-classicism to romanticism – the first aspect becoming visible in a classically inspired, literally statuesque composition of posture, gesture, and costume which rendered her characters as legendary, iconic figures, the second element being found in the focused emotional intensity of her delivery.[34]

Henry Siddons's publication, *Practical Illustrations of Rhetorical Gesture and Action* (1807), a revised translation of the German theorist Johann Jakob Engel's *Ideen zu Einer Mimik*, offers further evidence that his mother's acting style bridged neoclassical and Romantic ideals. Writing about her death scenes, he remarks, 'had she never been present at the bed of a dying person, her acting, under such circumstances, might have lost one of its most natural and affecting traits'.[35] Indeed, the actress made 'the most happy use' of her observations of death, going so far as to incorporate a 'slight convulsion … apparent only at the ends of her fingers' as her characters enter their final moments.[36] Yet while Siddons drew on personal observations and close study to enliven her performances, she avoided representing death in all of its horrors, softening her actions in order to 'give such an idea of death as every man would wish to feel at that crisis'.[37] Thus what made Siddons such a captivating actress, at least in her son's view, was her ability to offer a realistic-enough representation of death while casting a softening glow around it. This account of Siddons's acting complicates Stack's argument by suggesting that it wasn't just a shared interest in neo-classicism that drew Combe to Siddons, but rather the way that both

---

[34] Robert Shaughnessey, 'Sarah Siddons (1755–1831)', in *Oxford Dictionary of National Biography, vol. 50: Sharp-Smiles*, ed. H. C. G. Matthew and Brian Harrison (Oxford University Press, 2004), https://doi.org/10.1093/ref:odnb/25516.

[35] Henry Siddons, *Practical Illustrations of Rhetorical Gesture and Action* (Richard Phillips, 1807), 15.

[36] Ibid., 15.

[37] Ibid., 16.

straddled the shifting philosophical terrain of the period, negotiating neoclassical and Romantic ideas through their work.

Combe's knowledge of acting (and possibly aspects of his theory) may also have come from a direct reading of Henry Siddons's *Practical Illustrations*. Although the phrenologist never met Siddons's son, who died in April 1815, his close friendship with the widowed Mrs Harriet (Henry) Siddons means that he was likely familiar with her husband's work, particularly his application of biological principles to the study of human gesture. In the following passage, for example, Siddons's emphasis on the importance of collecting and classifying 'different physiognomies' resonates with phrenological interest in the collection of specimens:

> We may with reason conclude, that a collection of different physiognomies, collected and classed with the same industry, is a scheme equally possible, and that a new art would result from the attempt not less important in its kind. Why would not a collection of expressive gestures and attitudes be as easy as a collection of drawings, plants, or shells? And if this affair should one day become an object of serious study, why should not technical words be in time found out, as proper for this science as those at present discovered for the facilitation of the study of natural history?[38]

Like Siddons, Combe also acknowledged individual idiosyncrasies yet promoted a universal model of human behaviour, believing that humans should aspire to improve themselves by accentuating their higher faculties and control their baser ones. Although there is no concrete evidence that Combe ever read *Practical Illustrations*, his deep admiration for Sarah Siddons's talents and his ongoing friendship with the Kemble-Siddons family suggests that he was intimate with Henry Siddons's philosophies. This connection is important to consider when examining the interwovenness of medicine and theatre, and the migration of ideas across disciplines, stages, geographies and bodies throughout the nineteenth century.

CECY'S MIRROR: FANNY KEMBLE'S RESERVATIONS

While we may never know if Combe read Henry Siddons's acting theories, we can confidently say that the phrenologist worked hard to recruit to his cause Siddons's cousin, Fanny Kemble, one of the era's most widely celebrated actresses. If anything, Combe's relationship with the Kemble-Siddons family taught him about the value of self-promotion through performance, art and

---

[38] Siddons, *Practical Illustrations*, 25.

writing, and the potential for celebrity endorsements to further popularize phrenology. Combe's relationships with the Kemble-Siddons family show us that in aligning with stars of the stage, he could promote his own scientific philosophy. While Cecy proved a willing student and later promoter of phrenology, her cousin Fanny Kemble had reservations. Although Fanny resisted the lure of phrenology, she remained friends with Combe and observed with interest phrenology's growing popularity in the United States. Indeed, her letters are valuable documents of phrenology's gradual arrival and reception in the United States and its impact on attitudes about public health. Moreover, her letters offer insight into some of the reservations that she, and others, held about phrenology as a practice and the reasons why she resisted Combe's recruitment.

In an 1835 letter to Combe, written during her ill-fated marriage to the wealthy Philadelphian slave owner Pierce Butler following her retirement from the stage, Fanny acknowledges the public's admiration for Combe's books and anticipates that he would be 'heartily received' if he toured North America.[39] Two years later, she teasingly references the 'present phrenological opportunities' she encounters every morning while attending one of her husband's political meetings where she has 'an admirable view of the back of sixty six [*sic*] legislating craniums, & the front of as many more … my husband & myself amuse ourselves sometimes with speculation about the organs of the worthy members which would doubtless make you laugh'.[40]

Though she remained sceptical of phrenology's claims, Fanny acknowledged its potential for improving the overall health and wellbeing of the general population, noting with horror the poor hygiene of so many of the families she encountered. This attention to the plight of others is consistent with her gradual conversion to the abolitionist cause. In an 8 March 1838 letter to Cecy, written soon after the Combes had confirmed their plans for a North American tour, she wrote:

> You know that I have never sufficiently applied my mind to the study of phrenology to form any opinion upon the subject whatever – but with all the phisiological [*sic*] information which I gathered from your husband's books [and] those of his brother [Andrew Combe] & some of Dr Spurzheim's I have been deeply interested & have deplored ever since my residence in this country the absence of anything like general & adequate knowledge which exists here (upon these points).[41]

[39] Quoted in Alice Hiller, '"This Strangest of Countries": Fanny Kemble's Letters from America', *Literary Imagination* 10, no. 3 (2008): 319.
[40] Quoted in ibid., 321.
[41] Quoted in ibid., 322.

Here, Fanny takes a strategic approach in writing to her cousin. She recognizes that they differ in their dedication to phrenology but seeks to find common ground by acknowledging her shared interest in advancing the education of others. Yet George Combe seems to have taken offence at Fanny's more flippant comments about phrenological observation. The following day (9 March 1838), she wrote to Combe to explain her position:

> You say you wish I could have been persuaded to make a serious study of Phrenology – & deprecate my drawing conclusions from any observations I may make in my present state of ignorance – I have a disinclination partly natural & partly acquired to serious study – that is to say the devoting my mind to any particular object of pursuit or contemplation exclusively – & it is necessary to do this to attain competent knowledge of any subject whatever but at the same time that I plead guilty to this, I beg that you will not suspect me of the fault of forming opinions of any sort upon a subject which I have never investigated – my remark with regard to the head of the members of Convention was a mere jest.[42]

Playing up her reluctance to engage in serious study – a curious argument given her earlier success as a professional actress – Fanny politely yet firmly refuses to engage with phrenology yet reaffirms her friendship with Combe.[43] In making this argument, she draws on phrenology's own interest in distinguishing nature from nurture, claiming that her disinclination is 'partly natural & partly acquired', exhibiting (ironically) more than a passing knowledge of phrenological principles. Indeed, the letter itself can be read as a carefully scripted performance wherein Fanny attributes her aversion to 'serious study' to her own mental shortcomings, leaning into gender stereotypes and phrenology's own belief that women possessed smaller intellectual faculties than men, not to phrenological teachings in themselves.

Whether she felt differently is unclear, though she may have wished to avoid damaging her relationship with Combe and her cousin Cecy by speaking her mind more freely. Fanny goes on to express her hope that his North American lecture tour will be well attended, given ongoing public interest in phrenology and Combe's skill as a lecturer, but warns that 'the majority of minds to which you will address yourself both in New York and Philadelphia are I think intent on far other subjects than theories of human intellect and even the theory of

[42] Quoted in ibid., 325.

[43] Kemble also describes her husband's encounter with a man who fraudulently claimed to be a phrenologist and produced an analysis of his head that amounted to a 'miraculous performance ... the *spelling* was by no means the least miraculous part of it' (quoted in ibid., 325).

human health'.[44] She concludes by hoping that her assessment is wrong and that the Combes' journey across the Atlantic will be rewarded. Indeed, Fanny Kemble's fears were unfounded: George Combe's North American lecture tour was a roaring success, due in no small part to Cecilia Combe's backstage labour.

CECILIA COMBE'S DRAMATURGICAL SUPPORT

Unlike her cousin Fanny, Cecilia Siddons embraced Combe's phrenological ideas and became his eager student. The two met in fall 1832 when Cecy travelled to Edinburgh to visit her sister-in-law, Harriet Siddons; their courtship began soon after she enrolled in his lecture course and she proved herself an adept learner.[45] In a letter to Cecy sent the following May, Combe encouraged her to read *Constitution of Man* and continue to immerse herself in the teachings of phrenology:

> I am anxious that its principles should become so familiar to your mind, that they may form the basis of your thinking without your requiring to call them up by an effort … Feel no anxiety, my dear Cecy, about your adventure in knowledge, for it will come in due time; only keep your mind tuned in that direction and pick up an idea when you can.[46]

Here, Combe balances his eagerness for Cecy to become conversant in phrenological terminology and teachings with an understanding of the time needed to develop proficiency in a new field of study. Perhaps he was also concerned that she might be inclined to follow her cousin and sister-in-law in rejecting phrenology altogether. She did not, and in September 1833, at thirty-nine years of age, Cecilia Siddons married the forty-five-year-old phrenological lecturer at a wedding held in Mrs Harriet (Henry) Siddons's home, embarking on a partnership that endured until his death in 1858.[47]

In Cecy, George Combe found a highly capable partner, an intelligent, multilingual woman (she could write and speak in German and French), who understood the complexities of travel, business and performance due in no small part to decades spent travelling with her aging mother. Through her mother and other family members, she had developed impressive connections to artistic and intellectual communities throughout Europe, and enjoyed friendships with women, including her godmother Hester Piozzi, who flouted gender

[44] Quoted in Hiller, 'This Strangest of Countries', 325.
[45] Stack, *Queen Victoria's Skull*, 111.
[46] Quoted in ibid., 281n15.
[47] Ibid., 115.

convention. Historian David Stack acknowledges Cecilia Siddons's role as Combe's helpmeet and intellectual partner and further suggests that she may also have helped refine her husband's lecture presentations and coordinate his international tours.[48] Additional evidence from the Combe Papers in the National Library of Scotland suggests that Cecy coached Combe through lessons in oration – a skill she undoubtedly acquired from years of observing her mother in performance – and translated his lectures and related speeches into German. In so doing, she helped Combe to refine the overall dramaturgy of his lectures, thereby enhancing his ability to communicate effectively with his audience. Cecy's dramaturgical involvement in Combe's lecture performances thus offers a compelling example of the undertheorized interplay that has long existed between doctors and actors in service to the widespread dissemination of medical models such as phrenology.

Moreover, Cecilia Combe's active involvement in her husband's career aligns with phrenology's perspective on gender. Although Combe and other phrenologists claimed that most women's intellectual faculties were smaller than men's, they insisted that women could work to strengthen them. As Bittel writes, 'Combe's focus on reform and self-improvement via phrenology provided evidence that women should be active agents of social change, and could cultivate areas of deficiency.'[49] Women who attended Combe's lectures or read his books were empowered to apply their new understanding to their own lives, their interactions with family members and their approach to child-rearing. 'Phrenology uniquely blurred the categories of analyst and the analysed by inviting consumers to acquire practical and theoretical knowledge, and to investigate themselves', Bittel observes.[50] Later phrenologists reiterated the importance of training women to practise phrenology. 'We must have FEMALE phrenologists', the *American Phrenological Journal* declared in 1849, arguing that training in phrenological analysis was in keeping with women's wider domestic responsibilities. Female phrenologists 'were needed to analyze and counsel mothers and children, offering them vital scientific guidance'.[51] Mid-century artists carried forward this idea in prints; for example, in Figure 12.1, the artist depicts an idyllic parlour setting in which children play with phrenological toys as their mother and father listen attentively to a phrenologist. With her right hand resting lightly on her chest, the mother smiles appreciatively as the doctor analyses her and draws a correlation between her brain and the faculties detailed on the phrenological model head beside him. With this new knowledge, the woman will not only understand her own behavioural

[48] Ibid.
[49] Bittel, 'Woman, Know Thyself', 108.
[50] Ibid.
[51] Quoted in ibid., 110.

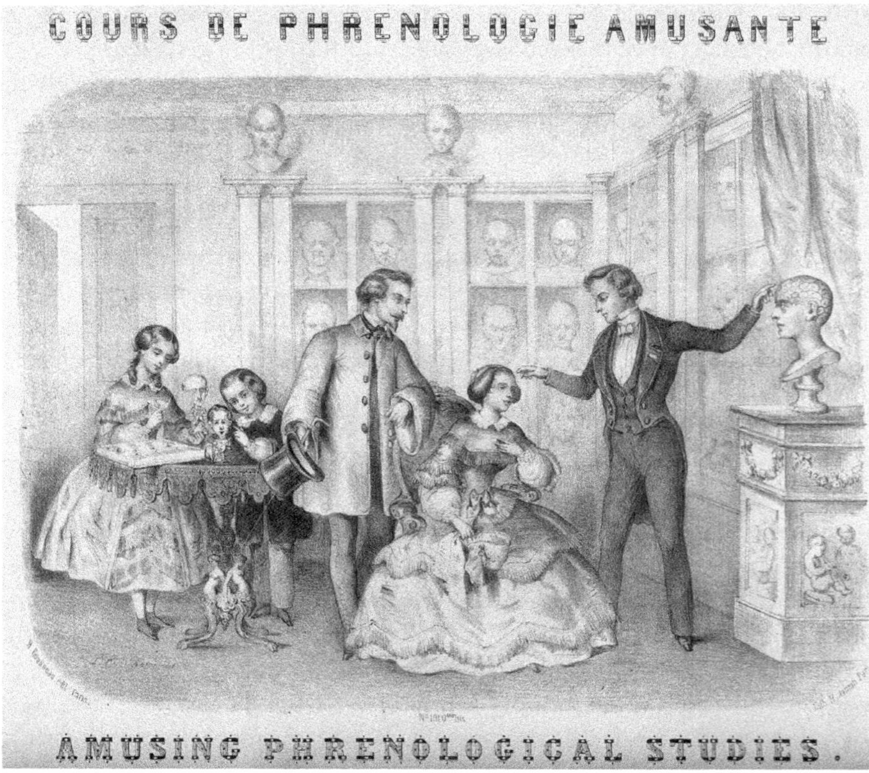

FIGURE 12.1 A phrenologist and some society people in a parlour. Lithograph by H. Jannin after L.C. Bommier (?). Wellcome Collection.

tendencies but be prepared to understand and shape those of her husband and children. For women without access to such an intimate clinical treatment, public lectures, essays and other writing offered an appealing alternative, one that Cecilia Combe sought to utilize.

THE FICTITIOUS DIALOGUE

Though Cecilia Combe never publicly claimed the title of phrenological analyst or clinician, she understood the healing potential of parlour conversations; through writing, she sought to prove useful to the phrenological project and support children's education in the home. She may even have sought her own form of healing through her writing practice, by projecting herself into her fictionalized characters.

The Combes never had children. Combe once stated that his 'only regret' was that he had not met Cecy fifteen years earlier, presumably when they both would have been in their prime reproductive years.[52] Hints of Cecy's feelings about lost motherhood arise from an unpublished and undated novel, wherein the central character of Selina contemplates her childless state and relates her maternal desire to the organ of philoprogenitiveness.[53] So too the character of Aunt Lucy in her *Fictitious dialogue* is childless, and therefore lacking (in Cecy's words) 'an opportunity of becoming useful to others in those points where she had herself felt the evils of early neglect'.[54] This oblique reference to 'early neglect' may point to the trauma Cecy experienced as a young child when her older sisters Maria and Sally, who had played an important caretaking role in her life, died in the same year.[55] While we hesitate to extrapolate too much from this one passage and likewise recognize the limits of comparing Cecy's emotional life with that of her characters, we nevertheless observe that the presence of several childless women in her unpublished works offers evidence that she thought deeply about how such women might contribute meaningfully to society.

Cecilia Combe was especially concerned with improving children's physical and mental development, an interest she shared with her cousin Fanny Kemble and her brother-in-law Andrew Combe, whose advice books on the care of infants were published widely throughout the nineteenth century. In his *Treatise on the Physiological and Moral Management of Infancy* (which reached nine editions by 1870), Combe offers practical advice to parents on such core topics as nursing and weaning, washing and dressing, teething, sleep and exercise. In his final chapter, 'On the Moral Management of Infancy', he draws on his phrenological training to advise parents on the development of the senses and offers 'hints for the exercise of the infant faculties'.[56] He cautions parents about the limits of outside influence on a child, noting that 'the development of the human faculties, and the formation of human character, take place according to fixed laws imposed by the Creator for the regulation of both mind and body'.[57] Although parents might 'modify or improve' the action of the mind 'by fulfilling the conditions under which any organ or function is intended to act', they should not expect to 'alter the nature of the function itself'.[58] Tellingly Combe resists directly referencing phrenology in

[52] Stack, *Queen Victoria's Skull*, 117.
[53] Cecilia Combe, untitled novel, *c.*1825, MS 7457, Combe Papers, National Library of Scotland.
[54] Cecilia Combe, *Fictitious dialogue of Cecilia Combe, Illustrating the Facets of Phrenology*, *c.*1846–50, Combe Papers, MS 7456, National Library of Scotland, 4.
[55] West, 'The Professional and Personal Worlds of Artists and Actors'; Engel, *Women, Performance and the Material of Memory*, 53–79.
[56] Andrew Combe, *Treatise on the Physiological and Moral Management of Infancy*, 4th ed. (Edinburgh: Maclachlan Stewart, 1844), xviii.
[57] Ibid., 377.
[58] Ibid., 378.

his *Treatise* – perhaps aware of growing scepticism about phrenology within the European medical community – though phrenological ideas clearly inform his recommendations.

Cecilia Combe believed that phrenology had a great deal to offer parents, and during a visit with friends in Germany in 1845, she began thinking about how theatre might be used to educate children and inform child-rearing. As she writes in an Introductory statement to her *Fictitious dialogue*: 'The idea of such a little work was first suggested during the summer of 1845, while at a German watering place in company with a widowed friend and her very interesting son then eleven years of age.' According to Cecy, the boy possessed 'an extremely active disposition', which required the adults to 'vary his occupations, and to give exercise to all of his faculties, in order to prevent morbid action in some of them'. His mother was 'a very intelligent woman [who] anxiously sought all means for furthering her son's development', who had previously 'expressed her wish that her son become a disciple of the new philosophy, when old enough'.[59] On hearing this, George Combe apparently responded by saying that 'we are seldom too *young* to begin to learn' and so the mother granted permission for him to speak with her son. The adults were delighted to find that the boy responded with eagerness and intelligence to his phrenological education, demonstrating a readiness to engage with concepts 'generally considered as fitted only for more advanced mental powers'.[60]

Reflecting on the boy's enthusiasm for phrenological ideas, Cecy realized the potential for a publication or text for a younger readership: 'Among all the useful and popular works on Phrenology ... no one, as far as I know, has been addressed to the capacities of the very young, or to the practical attention of those whom nature, affection, and circumstances have tended to make their first Instructors.'[61] This decision to write for a younger audience was also a more acceptable outlet for Cecy as a woman author, because it aligned with the nineteenth century (and arguably present-day) notions of women's role as child-rearer and caretaker. Cecy had already embodied this role of caretaker for her famous actress mother, her famous lecturer husband, and – later – both of their legacies. While she was childless, it follows suit that Cecy would fall into this child-rearing role through her writing, where she could contribute to the field of phrenology within the private sphere. Thus emboldened, Cecy began writing her *Fictitious dialogue*, a dramatic tract of sorts dedicated to 'illustrating the facets of phrenology', with the goal of encouraging parents and other caregivers 'to direct by some such means [i.e. phrenological training] the intelligence

[59] C. Combe, *Fictitious dialogue*, 1.
[60] Ibid., 2.
[61] Ibid.

of young creatures into hundreds of channels, from which it would return with tenfold fruits, to inform, delight and protect, its natural proprietors?'[62] More than writing a play to entertain, Cecilia Combe hoped to shape generations of young people by equipping them with the tools to understand themselves.

The *dialogue* begins with a short narrative introduction to the characters, including an older woman named Lucy – a thinly veiled representation of Cecy herself. Determined to prove useful despite her childless state, she comes to care for her eleven-year-old nephew Willie. In the dialogue that follows, Cecy restages the education of the young boy she and George Combe had encountered in Germany. Willie is curious to learn about phrenology because he sees how happy it makes his Aunt Lucy and how much she loves talking about it. When he expresses confusion about its application, she reassures him that 'it is something that concerns you and everyone very much' and proceeds to teach him the fundamental ideas.[63] The conversation unfolds in a Socratic manner, with Aunt Lucy posing a series of questions. Here is a short excerpt from one of their early lessons:

Aunt L: Well then – come here – close to me. What do you call this Willie?
Willie: Why my head to be sure. –
Aunt L: And do you know what is the use of your head
Willie: That is an odd question
Aunt L: Answer it though – and do not suppose my questions are of no use, or that I shall always ask and never answer – your turn shall come. But now tell me – what do you think is in this head of yours – and [?]
Willie: Why I think there are a great many things – my eyes are in my head – and my ears – and my tongue – and I could not see – nor hear – nor speak nor taste without them –
Aunt L: and they are certainly parts of your head, and very useful ones. But there is more in your head Willie – think a little.
Willie: there are teeth – and there is –
Aunt L: Think again – what do you think with? What was Uncle showing to Mr [Anderson/Spencer?] on that day you talk of? –
Willie: Oh yes – a brain – a brain to think with –

Now, we might question Aunt Lucy's pedagogical strategies, but what is clear from this excerpt is Cecilia Combe's capable use of a dramatic structure to convey complex phrenological ideas. Rather than educate through a lengthy

[62] Ibid., 6.
[63] Ibid., 7.

monologue, she leads the boy to make discoveries for himself, staging his gradual awakening for the delight and edification of her imagined audience. Throughout the *Fictitious dialogue*, she emphasizes the social good that can come from phrenological analysis, especially in terms of community building, while acknowledging some of the criticisms it has faced (e.g. awkward names for organs). She likewise addresses religious concerns that those who practised phrenological analysis were usurping God, emphasizing God's role as the ultimate creator. Through Lucy as her mouthpiece, Cecy also admits that it is difficult to alter people's thinking to accept phrenology if they've been taught something else their whole lives.[64] This last point hints at the growing criticism that phrenologists like Combe were facing in 1840s, as new developments in scientific research cast doubt on its claims.

Unfortunately, the manuscript to the *Fictitious dialogue* is incomplete. The final page ends in the middle of a sentence: 'Now then – we shall begin with the organs of the Propensities. Where do …' – which suggests that Cecy wrote additional pages, though efforts to find these missing pages have (to date) proven unsuccessful. It is likewise unclear when or if Cecy ever presented her *Fictitious dialogue* to an audience or shared it with her husband. What emerges from these pages, however, is Cecilia Combe's passion and her commitment to phrenology and her desire to prove her usefulness as a 'female phrenologist' working in the domestic sphere in support of the children. Her interest in using dramatic techniques to make phrenology appealing for the next generation likewise highlights the entanglement of theatre and phrenology in the first half of the nineteenth century. Yet unlike George Combe, who attracted large audiences to his lecture performances throughout Europe and North America – and whose visage continues to look down upon Edinburgh's urban landscape from atop his perch on Chambers Street – Cecilia Combe brought phrenology into the realm of the home. But in so doing, she demonstrated that incorporating phrenological tools into private education and child-rearing was much more than a domestic affair; it was a way to bridge public and private education.

CONCLUSION: THE DANGERS OF POPULARIZING MEDICINE THROUGH THEATRE

This essay has aimed to bridge the gap between theatre and medicine by highlighting how doctors like Combe were clearly performers, who enhanced their lectures by incorporating dramaturgical techniques learned by attending the theatre, making friends with actors and reading acting theory. In

[64] Ibid., 52.

Combe's case, in addition to moving in an intellectual circle that included Mrs Harriet (Henry) Siddons and Fanny Kemble, his marriage to the daughter of the era's greatest actress gave him access to her deep knowledge of stage practice. While women's roles were circumscribed due to the gender conventions of the age, Cecilia Combe was a highly capable, educated woman who had travelled extensively and spoke multiple languages. Drawing on this knowledge, she endeavoured to perfect her husband's performance and, as a dutiful wife, performed her part as his helpmeet and disciple – going so far as to interpret phrenological ideas for children. Through their collaborative efforts, phrenological ideas and practices successfully moved within and across public and private spheres, including the intimate space of the home and the lecture hall.

Yet, as this essay has also shown, it would be unwise to interpret phrenology's rapid uptake as evidence of the utopian pairing of theatre and medicine. The history of phrenology is heavily intertwined with scientific racism, the effects of which can still be seen today, not just in efforts to repatriate skulls and other human remains that entered phrenological collections in the nineteenth century,[65] but also in lingering associations of brain size with intelligence,[66] and in race-norming practices that inform insurance policies in professional sports like the NFL.[67] Thus while patients can benefit from theatre's potential to democratize medical information by making it easier to understand treatments, knowledge and eventually internalize these learnings (as was Cecy's hope via the *Fictitious dialogue* and her Socratic method), they must continue to be wary of the lure of quippy, easily digestible, popular statements paraded as fact. So too, must doctors ensure that their own practices are not overtaken by theatre's potential for spectacle and their own quest for medical glory. It remains to be seen what actions Dr Mehmet Oz will take as the newly appointed head of the Centers for Medicare and Medicaid Services, though one wonders if he would have received such an appointment had he not followed the playbook laid out by George and Cecilia Combe.[68]

---

[65] The University of Edinburgh, 'A Skull Collection Revisited: From Colonial Resistance to Repatriation', https://exhibitions.ed.ac.uk/exhibitions/mind-shift/colonial-resistance-to-repatriation.

[66] Jonathan Bartlett, 'Phrenology: The Pseudoscience that Just Won't Give Up', *Mind Matters*, 24 May 2021. https://mindmatters.ai/2021/05/phrenology-the-pseudoscience-that-just-wont-give-up/.

[67] Tracie Canada and Chelsea R. Carter, 'The NFL's Racist "Race Norming" Is an Afterlife of Slavery', *Scientific American*, 8 July 2021, www.scientificamerican.com /article/the-nfls-racist-race-norming-is-an-afterlife-of-slavery/.

[68] Fatima Hussein, Amanda Seitz, Collin Binkley and Josh Boak, 'Trump Picks Dr. Oz to Run Medicare and Medicaid, Linda MacMahon for Education, Lutnick for Commerce', *AP News*, 19 November 2024, https://apnews.com/article/trump-commerce-lutnick-elections-transition-cabinet-79cdda378e2affb85722323160306b30.

REFERENCES

Aiken, Henry Thomas. *Calves Heads and Brains, or a Phrenological Lecture*. 1826. *OnView*, Center for History of Medicine, Harvard University. https://collections.countway.harvard.edu/onview/items/show/6158.

Barker, Roberta. *Symptoms of the Self: Tuberculosis and the Making of the Modern Stage*. University of Iowa Press, 2023.

Bartlett, Jonathan. 'Phrenology: The Pseudoscience that Just Won't Give Up'. *Mind Matters*, 24 May 2021. https://mindmatters.ai/2021/05/phrenology-the-pseudoscience-that-just-wont-give-up/.

Bittel, Carla. 'Woman, Know Thyself: Producing and Using Phrenological Knowledge in 19th-Century America'. *Centaurus* 55 (2013): 104–30.

Boardman, Andrew. Introduction to *Lectures on Phrenology* by George Combe. Samuel Colman, 1839.

Canada, Tracie, and Chelsea R. Carter. 'The NFL's Racist "Race Norming" Is an Afterlife of Slavery'. *Scientific American*, 8 July 2021. www.scientificamerican.com/article/the-nfls-racist-race-norming-is-an-afterlife-of-slavery/.

Clint, George. *Miss Cecilia Siddons (1794–1868)*. Dundee Art Galleries and Museums Collection (Dundee City Council), Art UK. https://artuk.org/discover/artworks/miss-cecilia-siddons-17941868–92268.

Combe, Andrew. *Treatise on the Physiological and Moral Management of Infancy*. Fourth edition. Maclachlan Stewart, 1844.

Combe, Cecilia. *Combe Papers*. National Library of Scotland.

Combe, George. *Elements of Phrenology*. Fourth American edition. Marsh, Capen & Lyon, 1835.

Combe, George. *Lectures on Phrenology*. Samuel Colman, 1839.

Combe, George. 'On Inferring Natural Dispositions and Talents from Development of Brain'. In *Transactions of the Phrenological Society*, vol. 1. John Anderson, Jr, 1824.

Combe, George. *A System of Phrenology*. Third edition. John Anderson Jr, 1830.

Corti, Claudia. 'Poses and Pauses: Sarah Siddons and the Romantic Theatrical Portrait'. In *Women's Romantic Theatre and Drama*, edited by Lilla Maria Crisafulli and Keir Elam. Routledge, 2010.

David, Deirdre. *Fanny Kemble: A Performed Life*. University of Pennsylvania Press, 2007.

Engel, Laura. *Women, Performance and the Material of Memory: The Archival Tourist*. Palgrave Macmillan, 2019.

Hacking, Ian. *Travelers: Reflections on the Reality of Transient Mental Illness*. University Press of Virginia, 1998.

Hiller, Alice. '"This Strangest of Countries": Fanny Kemble's Letters from America'. *Literary Imagination* 10, no. 3 (2008): 304–18.

Hussein, Fatima, Amanda Seitz, Collin Binkley and Josh Boak. 'Trump Picks Dr. Oz to Run Medicare and Medicaid, Linda MacMahon for Education, Lutnick for Commerce'. *AP News*, 19 November 2024. https://apnews.com/article/trump-commerce-lutnick-elections-transition-cabinet-79cdda378e2affb85722323160306b30.

James, Frank A. J. L. '"Never Talk About Science, *Show* It to Them": The Lecture Theatre of the Royal Institution'. *ISR* 27, no. 3 (2002): 225–9.

Knight, David. 'Scientific Lectures: A History of Performance'. *ISR* 27, no. 3 (2002): 217–24.

Lightman, Bernard. Afterword to *Staging Science: Scientific Performances on Street, Stage, and Screen*. Edited by Martin Willis. Palgrave Macmillan, 2016.

McPherson, Heather. 'Sculpting Her Image: Sarah Siddons and the Art of Self-Fashioning'. In *Women and Portraits in Early Modern Europe*, edited by Andrea Pearson. Routledge, 2008.

Morus, Iwan Rhys. *Frankenstein's Children: Electricity, Exhibition, and Experiment in Nineteenth-Century London*. Princeton University Press, 2016.

Rusert, Britt. *Fugitive Science: Empiricism and Freedom in Early African American Culture*. New York University Press, 2017.

Rusert, Britt. 'The Science of Freedom: Counterarchives of Racial Science on the Antebellum Stage'. *African American Review* 45, no. 3 (2012): 291–308.

Schweitzer, Marlis. *Bloody Tyrants and Little Pickles: Stage Roles of Anglo-American Girls in the Nineteenth Century*. University of Iowa Press, 2020.

Schweitzer, Marlis. 'Casting Clara Fisher: Phrenology, Protean Farce, and the "Astonishing" Career of a Child Actress'. *Theatre Journal* 68, no. 2 (2016): 167–90.

Schweitzer, Marlis. 'The Curious Case of the Infant Sappho'. *Lady Science*, 10 December 2020. www.ladyscience.com/features/curious-case-of-the-infant-sappho-2020?rq=schweitzer.

Schweitzer, Marlis. '*Lecture on Heads* and Lectures with Skulls – Performance Transmutations'. In *Identity, Culture, and the Science Performance, vol. 1: From the Lab to the Street*, edited by Vivian Appler and Meredith Conti. Methuen Drama, 2023.

Shaughnessey, Robert. 'Sarah Siddons (1755–1831)'. In *Oxford Dictionary of National Biography. Volume 50: Sharp-Smiles*, edited by H. C. G. Matthew and Brian Harrison. Oxford University Press, 2004. https://doi.org/10.1093/ref:odnb/25516

Siddons, Henry. *Practical Illustrations of Rhetorical Gesture and Action*. Richard Phillips, 1807.

Stack, David. *Queen Victoria's Skull: George Combe and the Mid-Victorian Mind*. Continuum Books, 2008.

The University of Edinburgh. 'A Skull Collection Revisited: From Colonial Resistance to Repatriation'. https://exhibitions.ed.ac.uk/exhibitions/mind-shift/colonial-resistance-to-repatriation.

Von Kotzebue, August. *The Organs of the Brain*. Translated by Lieut. Col. Capadose. Edward Bull, 1838.

Watt-Smith, Tiffany. *On Flinching: Theatricality and Scientific Looking from Darwin to Shell Shock*. Oxford University Press, 2014.

West, Shearer. 'The Professional and Personal Worlds of Artists and Actors: Thomas Lawrence and the Siddons Family'. *Nineteenth Century Theatre & Film* 39, no. 1 (2012): 1–25.

PART FIVE

Performative Medicine in Contemporary Theatre and Drama

Bertolt Brecht once described ineffective theatre this way: 'You were what you were; the world stayed as it was.'[1] As we've been arguing throughout this book, medicine and theatre are intrinsically relational arts that put caregivers and patients into scenarios of collaboration, collision and reciprocal transformation; no participant in these ensemble acts stays as they were.

Theatre, etymologically a place of beholding (from the Greek *theatron*), can assist medicine by making perceptible the lattice of relationships that comprises both arts but often goes unnoticed. One prominent recent example of this theatrical capability, Amy Herzog's play *Mary Jane* (2018), features a single mother caring for her two-year-old son, Alex, who was born with cerebral palsy and other chronic conditions. Partly inspired by her own responsibilities as a caregiver for a daughter who died of a rare inherited neuromuscular disorder, Herzog's play is, among other things, about the patience, creativity and shared needs that enliven medical relationships. Mary Jane continually forges small conspiracies with the cast of other women (physicians, mothers, therapists, nurses, social workers) who help her son. These intimacies are survival strategies within a dizzying system: they grant emotional ballast as well as workarounds for systemic constraints that threaten Alex's emotional and physical well-being.

[1] Bertolt Brecht, *The Messingkauf Dialogues*, trans. and ed. John Willett (Methuen, 2002), 18.

Many of the relationships that emerge in the play are self-consciously theatrical, conscripting the bodies of all the participants to work out solutions that cannot – sometimes must not – be spoken. The superintendent of Mary Jane's apartment building in Queens, Ruthie, is obligated to install a window guard to adhere to municipal codes, but Mary Jane has removed them because Alex 'loves looking out the windows, especially when he's sick and I can't take him outside'.[2] To accommodate a dehumanizing law, they rescript Ruthie's performance, awkwardly negotiating an alternative scene in which Ruthie never glimpsed the violation that she then acts out: '*(Ruthie adjusts her body not to see out the window)*' (14). When Alex is brought to the hospital for a lengthy stay in Act 2, Mary Jane stages a similar conspiracy with his attending physician, Dr Toros, that will allow them to chat and eat in the 'parents' room' of the hospital without disturbing Alex as he rests after a difficult night. Even though doctors are 'technically not supposed to discuss patients in public areas' (52), their informal arrangement allows the exhausted clinician and mother to support each other through a repertoire of half-spoken but fully communicated concerns:

Mary Jane: I just want to get through this and take my little guy home.
(Dr Toros nods. Pause.)
Dr Toros: Well ... we want to help you do that. Um ...
(Mary Jane sees that Dr Toros isn't quite sure how to proceed.)
Mary Jane: Should I go ahead with my questions?
Dr. Toros: Yup.
(Mary Jane brings up her questions on her phone.) (53)

Herzog's play attends to the relationships between medical caregivers with the precision of experience refined by dramatic art. By showing how these sudden performative connections enable her characters to endure the demands and uncertainty of illness, Herzog asks us to recognize how medicine is made up of sustaining theatrical acts – and encourages us to seek out, encourage and reproduce them. Like other recent drama and theatre, *Mary Jane* attempts to transcribe (and to behold) the small but powerful signals that provision everyone involved in medical care: what performance theorist Dwight Conquergood has called 'the whole realm of complex, finely nuanced meaning' that exists within and alongside language and narrative, 'embodied, tacit,

[2] Amy Herzog, *Mary Jane* (Theatre Communications Group, 2018), 13. All subsequent quotations cite this edition.

intoned, gestured, improvised, coexperienced, [and] covert – and all the more deeply meaningful because of its refusal to be spelled out'.[3]

The chapters in this section, all of which offer instances of contemporary theatre and performance intervening in medical practice, also explore how interrelationship structures both theatre and medicine. In some cases, medicine is buoyed by theatre's tolerance for uncertainty and playfulness; in others, the medicalized body challenges taken-for-granted conventions and sedimented commercial imperatives in theatre. In Chapter 13, filmmaker Corinne Botz takes readers inside the making of her short film, *Bedside Manner*, which explores the 'ambiguities of playing sick' from the perspectives of standardized patients, the doctors who train with them, and her own lived experiences of treatment. Botz employs photography, film and theatre as defamiliarizing lenses for assumptions about looking within medical care, many of which seek to enable performances but instead disrupt relationships. *Bedside Manner* invites doctors, patients and film viewers to consider how changing one's position of viewing can 'change the way we construct reality'. By asking doctors to take on the role of patients, Botz identifies techniques to suspend other oppositions in medical performance based on hard and fast distinctions between the viewer and the viewed, including clinicians' suspicions that a patient might be 'faking' symptoms. Instead, Botz encourages us to see that medicine, like acting, is constituted by ambiguities that both doctors and patients can learn to inhabit: 'Acting can give birth to feeling, and artifice can expose the real.'

Botz's chapter brings particularly acute attention to the unconscious biases in looking that have shaped medical performances involving women. Chapter 14, 'Theatre for Social Change in the Dementia Context', focuses on another vulnerable population, People Living with Dementia (PLWD), through *Cracked*, a work of devised theatre created by the research-creative ensemble Collective Disruption that dramatizes the stigma faced by two PLWD and their families. Pia Kontos and Sherry Dupuis, activist-authors of *Cracked*, discuss how theatre can promote transformational cultural change with more immediacy and urgency than academic publications. Dementia care requires what Kontos and Dupuis identify as 'embodied and relational capacities'; theatre, an embodied and relational medium, can directly represent and activate those capacities. Theatre can also depict dementia beyond a purely cognitive framework, showing PLWD in their 'full life context' and as fully sensory, emotive and embodied. *Cracked* makes use of acting and spectacle as forms of research and rhetoric, prompting critical reflection based on immersion, observation, proximity and multiple perspectives. Kontos and Dupuis likewise consider how changing the

[3] Dwight Conquergood, 'Performance Studies: Interventions and Radical Research', *TDR* 46, no. 2 (2002): 146.

theatrical 'genre' of a care narrative can modify perception and thereby treatment: *Cracked* focuses on moments of surprise and humour, moving past a dominant tragedy discourse of dementia to reveal comic richness in the lives of PLWD.

Medical environments are places where patients can feel fixed: in an unsympathetic field of view, in a diagnosis, in a gaze or stare that assesses them for deviations from a medically normative body. Kontos and Dupuis bring the fluidity and 'relational care' of theatre to clinics and residential facilities. Later in this section, Katherine Williams undertakes a different manoeuver, carrying gains in disability awareness and disability knowledge that have, in part, been advanced in clinical care to reform the 'structural ableism of theatre as an institution'. Scholars who work at the intersection of theatre and disability studies have long argued that theatre can offer alternatives to what Petra Kuppers calls the 'spectacle of certainty' that enfolds the lives of people with disabilities. Such spectacles can be crushingly apparent in medical theatres like examination rooms. 'Most disabled people have intimate knowledge of these visual and performative practices of the medical theater: in particular if they have rare congenital impairments, they might have been required to undress in front of doctors and their students, photos might have been taken, demonstrations held over their mute, or even their protesting, bodies.'[4] The insight that many disabled performers have into 'visual and performative practices' from their medical encounters has, however, also been deployed to resist others' certainty about their capabilities and renovate art and activism: they have *un*fixed rigid norms and radically expanded how bodies appear and signify on stage. As Ann M. Fox observes, disability history has been an extraordinarily 'generative, innovative, and creative' influence on modern drama.[5]

In Chapter 15 Williams draws on disability studies scholar Tobin Siebers's conceptualization of disability aesthetics to show how 'disability knowledge' – an understanding of time, space, relationality and what it means to be human in a non-normative body – 'creates new possibilities for dramatic innovation' in Martyna Majok's Pulitzer Prize-winning play *Cost of Living* (2016). In Williams's analysis, disabled performers contributed their specific knowledge of theatre and embodiment to the writing and revision of Majok's play. These actors' most significant contributions to the dramaturgy of *Cost of Living*, Williams argues, contested a productivity-focused, future-oriented temporality of recovery and resolution with a time signature grounded in the rhythms

[4] Petra Kuppers, *Disability and Contemporary Performance: Bodies on the Edge* (Routledge, 2003), 35, 39.

[5] Ann M. Fox, 'Reclaiming the Ordinary Extraordinary Body: Or, the Importance of *The Glass Menagerie* for Literary Disability Studies', in *Disability Theatre and Modern Drama: Recasting Modernism*, ed. Kirsty Johnston (Bloomsbury Methuen, 2016), 132.

of their bodies: 'acts of care in the present, with its attendant frictions and joys' rather than a deferred 'curative imaginary'. By insisting on the 'valuable impediment' of the disabled body within a culture fixated on maximizing efficiency, Williams proposes that disabled actors became co-authors, performing epistemologies and ontologies that rescripted a celebrated play, a hypercapitalist theatre industry and a caregiving industry driven by profit margins.

Chapter 16 offers an approach to medical and theatrical relationships through Indigenous dramaturgy. Matthew MacKenzie, a citizen of the Métis nation of Alberta, talks with two friends, Karen Fricker and Lawrence Switzky, about artistic and communal practices that are 'good medicine'. For MacKenzie, medicine cannot be abstracted from the relationships that it strengthens or diminishes. In this sense, the interview reflects the Opaskwayak Cree writer Shawn Wilson's assertion that 'the shared aspect of an Indigenous ontology and epistemology is relationality (relationships do not merely shape reality; they *are* reality)'.[6] Rather than seeking an abstract definition or series of criteria, the interview creates a shared context in which instances of good medicine might be described in dramas that are meaningful to all the participants: in terms of Matt's life, his plays and finally his relationship with Iris Turcott, a legendary Canadian dramaturg. In his working relationship and friendship with Iris, which became a caregiving relationship at the end of her life, Matt finds a call and response, a seeing and being seen, that was mutual and healing: 'You would talk to Iris and you would feel like someone saw you.'

Every chapter in this section contains acts of reciprocal, renewed and surprised vision, a call to look and look again at what escapes routinized perception or biomedical and ideological abstractions. Researcher and theatre-worker Jill Carter (Anishinaabe/Ashkenazi) makes a distinction between two kinds of seeing, witnessing and voyeurism, that clarifies how seeing well is a way of coming into relationship.

> Witnessing is an intentionally generous act. The witness embodies communal (hi)story in that her body becomes the vessel on which that history is written, her mind becomes the surface on which its details are imprinted, and her voice becomes the vehicle through which that history is transmitted, passed back to those who may have forgotten and passed forward to those who will have to remember ... Voyeurism is an intentionally capricious act: it accepts no responsibility, it requires no somatic engagement, and it is performed without generosity. The voyeur/spectator stands apart from the story, *consuming only what is pleasing* ... and rejecting anything that may

[6] Shawn Wilson, *Research Is Ceremony: Indigenous Research Methods* (Fenwood, 2008), 7.

> unsettle the stomach. In this transaction, she accepts no responsibility to the Other. Instead, she consumes, digests, and expels.[7]

Carter's intensely corporeal metaphors situate relationships fundamentally within a gathering of bodies – their capabilities, their needs and what they can give to and do for each other. That is, as the authors of these chapter contend, where all theatre, like all humane medicine, begins and ends.

REFERENCES

Brecht, Bertolt. *The Messingkauf Dialogues*. Translated and edited by John Willett. Methuen, 2002.

Carter, Jill. 'My! What Big Teeth You Have! On the Art of Being Seen and Not Eaten'. *Canadian Theatre Review* 182 (2020): 16–21.

Conquergood, Dwight. 'Performance Studies: Interventions and Radical Research'. *TDR* 46, no. 2 (2002): 146–56.

Fox, Ann M. 'Reclaiming the Ordinary Extraordinary Body: Or, the Importance of the Glass Menagerie for Literary Disability Studies'. In *Disability Theatre and Modern Drama: Recasting Modernism*, edited by Kirsty Johnston. Bloomsbury Methuen, 2016.

Herzog, Amy. *Mary Jane*. Theatre Communications Group, 2018.

Kuppers, Petra. *Disability and Contemporary Performance: Bodies on the Edge*. Routledge, 2003.

Wilson, Shawn. *Research Is Ceremony: Indigenous Research Methods*. Fenwood, 2008.

[7] Jill Carter, 'My! What Big Teeth You Have! On the Art of Being Seen and Not Eaten', *Canadian Theatre Review* 182 (2020): 19.

13

Bedside Manner

CORINNE MAY BOTZ

I am a photographer, filmmaker and educator, and this essay is an autoethnographic examination of my project *Bedside Manner* (2016). *Bedside Manner* is an eighteen-minute video and a series of twenty photographs that explore the world of standardized patient simulations and the process of learning to 'play' a patient.[1] At the centre of the film is neurologist Dr Alice Flaherty, who plays herself as a doctor, a standardized patient and a real patient. *Bedside Manner* has been shown and studied internationally. This essay was written eight years after the project was released, and it combines reflections on my artistic process and motivations with a personal narrative about my journey through pregnancy and childbirth, which occurred simultaneously with making the film and helped to shape it.

I. BACKGROUND

When I suffered from asthma as a child, my mom would turn the living room couch into a bed and tend to me there, an ideal sickroom scene that led all future ones to pale in comparison. I drew pictures, observed situations outside the window, and made up stories that my mom transcribed. My mother was seemingly always at my bedside, the forever protector of my inner child. The doctors were the villains; they inflicted pain and couldn't be trusted. On one occasion, when my mom brought me to the doctor, he told my mom that I was fine; when she brought me back to the office the following day, the doctor

---

[1] Corinne May Botz, *Bedside Manner* (2016), www.corinnebotz.com/bedside-manner-1.

chided her for not bringing me in sooner. I was occasionally rushed to the hospital in the middle of the night. When I was in kindergarten, I was confined to a hospital bed that was an oxygen tent for weeks. Or, rather, it felt like weeks, but when I fact-checked this text with my mom, I was shocked to learn it was only a few days. I remember each and every detail of those days, including the stack of get well cards my kindergarten class sent me, and forming friendships with other sick children. The rest of my childhood is a happy blur. My mom often said she wished that she could be the one who was sick; I learned that empathy can hurt.

I outgrew asthma, but my general distrust of doctors and unease in medical spaces persisted. In high school, I fainted at the doctor, dentist and optometrist. I was still prone to fainting in my thirties if a needle was involved in the visit. I found the power dynamic of the patient and doctor roles taken on during even the most ordinary check-up to be awkward and uncomfortable. I'm a terrible actor and, when cast in a role against my will, wearing a costume, I can feel my identity fading away.

1. Standardized patients

A standardized patient (SP) is a medical actor trained to portray particular patients with a specific set of symptoms, through these performances providing medical students with hands-on training, thus improving their interpersonal and diagnostic skills. The lessons require everyone to play their part to the fullest, as if the patient really is ill. The practice has become a typical part of medical school training. I was drawn to the role reversal in the SP simulations, especially the way the medical actor or 'patient' snaps out of character at the end of the scenario and provides authoritative feedback to the student, subverting the idea of a passive patient.

I also found the intersection of theatre, illness and film/photography unsettling. Medical practice is innately theatrical, and photographs/films culturally create an idea of illness. The history of Western medicine is connected to issues of spectatorship, display and pathology. I am interested in how visual imagery has been used historically to represent the body and construct medical interactions, particularly relating to women's experiences. I decided to investigate notions of representations through medical simulations in a time-based piece.

Simulations offered a way to explore a larger theme in my work – the perception of reality, which I had explored in prior projects. Embracing the stereotype of female sensitivity to the supernatural, I opened myself to the invisible nuances of a space when photographing and collecting oral stories of sites rumoured to have ghosts in *Haunted Houses*.[2] In *The Nutshell Studies*

[2] Corinne Botz, *Haunted Houses* (The Monacelli Press, 2010).

of Unexplained Death I photographed and wrote about a collection of meticulously detailed miniature crime-scene models from the 1940s and 50s.[3] Similar to medical simulations, they are used as teaching tools and confound the distance between truth and fiction. I considered Frances Glessner Lee, the woman who made the models, my unlikely collaborator and it was important for me to unearth and share the story of this unsung, female pioneer of forensic medicine. In *Parameters*, I photographed the psychologically charged homes and possessions of agoraphobics. In all of my projects, my selfhood expanded through deep identification with another. Although I consider the camera a tool to form connections and relationships, it comes from a history of uneven power dynamics, as reflected in the colonial and medical gaze. I have asked myself if I had the right to tell a story and what constitutes a fair collaboration. A more direct exploration of empathy felt important. Can students learn empathy through medical simulations? Can art teach viewers empathy? These are some of the questions I asked while working on this project.

2. *Conceiving the film*

In the early stages of research for *Bedside Manner*, I reached out to meet with Dr Alice Flaherty, after reading her book *The Midnight Disease: The Drive to Write, Writer's Block, and the Creative Brain*, and learning that she was studying the neuroanatomy of empathy.[4] The writer Marina Van Zuylen suggested during a studio visit five years earlier that I should meet Alice Flaherty, and I had filed this information away for a future time. I had a feeling Alice would be important to my forthcoming project, I just wasn't entirely clear what form this project would take and what her involvement would be. It was during the bus ride from NYC to Boston to meet Alice at Massachusetts General Hospital that I began envisioning a film in which I would reverse the traditional medical gaze from the patient onto the doctor, and edit in a non-linear manner in order to create a sense of mystery and disorientation around the medical encounter. These became the guiding elements. Alice was just as fascinating in person as I had imagined, and much to my surprise and delight, she volunteered to play an SP character in my film.

Five months later, in 2013, I received funding for the film component of the project from the Jerome Foundation. I proposed to film an SP training session at The Ether Dome at Massachusetts General Hospital in Boston and an SP encounter at St. Barnabas Hospital in New York City, with Alice's personal background as both a patient and a doctor interwoven into the

[3] Corinne Botz, *The Nutshell Studies of Unexplained Death* (Monacelli Press, 2004).
[4] Alice Flaherty, *The Midnight Disease: The Drive to Write, Writer's Block, and the Creative Brain* (Houghton Mifflin, 2004).

story. Artistically, making this film was new territory for me. My background is in photography, but I had made a prior film, *Mein Hauptbahnhof* (2008), which focuses on a young woman who is in love with the Berlin Hauptbahnhof train station. *Bedside Manner* was of a greater scope and scale, and I worked with additional camera operators, a sound person and editors for the first time.

The creative process shapes an artwork, and a piece inevitably shifts between the initial concept and the final form. The photography series came as a natural extension of the project, allowing me to explore aspects of empathic looking. I experienced the film shoots as highly stressful compared with taking the photographs, which is a slower, more intimate process that I know and love. It was primarily through the still photography component that I built relationships within the SP community and became friendly with the people running clinical skill centres, developing knowledge about unique details in various simulation labs throughout NYC. When I discovered SP green rooms, I added a scene to the film at Albert Einstein College of Medicine's clinical skill centre, a humorous and surreal waiting room of SPs lounging in hospital gowns as they eat snacks and comment on the medical students' performances. I would eventually add six additional scenes into my initial concept. Alice is so compelling that she perhaps inevitably took on a more central role. To paraphrase her: in the film she is a doctor learning how to be a patient, in order to teach doctors how to be better doctors.

3. *The two-way mirror*

SP encounters are routinely filmed and evaluated by medical professors who observe the interaction of student and medical actor through a two-way mirror. In *Bedside Manner*, the two-way mirror provided me with a visual motif and a metaphor for empathy, and it became integral to both the film and photography components of the work. The distinction between windows and mirrors is often discussed in photography theory. In John Szarkowiski's 1978 MOMA exhibition and catalogue, he described windows as a shorthand for photographers engaging with the world in a more objective/documentary manner, and mirrors belonging to the domain of the personal and abstract. Szarkowiski writes, 'is it a mirror, reflecting a portrait of the artist who made it, or a window, through which one might better know the world?'[5] The two-way mirror is interesting within this context, as it literally combines the mirror and window, and it aligns with my photographic perspective by colliding the real and

[5] John Szarkowiski, *Mirrors and Windows: American Photography Since 1960* (Museum of Modern Art, 1978).

imagined, documentary and fiction. The two-way mirror extenuates the boundary between the viewer and subject, between self and other and between doctor and patient, returning to the question: how does the position from which we view something change the way we construct reality?

My photographs in *Bedside Manner* are studies in empathy, but also in aesthetic distancing. They put the viewer in a surveilling relationship to an SP through a two-way mirror. I want the viewer to be self-conscious during the act of seeing, and to think about the power that doctors wield in the patient–doctor relationship. Compared to the photographic portraits of the SPs through two-way mirrors, the film component of the project is more focused on the patient–doctor relationship and allows the viewer to occupy various positions. The interviews of Alice through the two-way mirror provide important structure and substance for the entire film. I filmed her directly, reflected in the mirror, and through the two-way mirror, highlighting her ability to understand medicine from multifaceted perspectives. She tries to connect with her patient so they are not on two sides of a glass but two people together.

II. THE FILM

Scene 1: Alice as an SP meets with medical students

Influences: Todd Haynes's *Safe*, Steven Soderbergh's *Bubble*, David Cronenberg's *Dead Ringers*, Feminist counter-cinema such as Chantal Ackerman.

How we view each other is vital in medicine, where the stakes can be a matter of life or death. Since there is a hierarchical power dynamic between patient and doctor, I wondered what would happen if I broke that down and turned the camera in the other direction. While they are at their most vulnerable, patients are observed and reliant on a doctor's interpretation and understanding of their body. In the first scene, I enacted a reversal of the traditional medical gaze from the patient onto the doctor in training (see Figure 13.1).

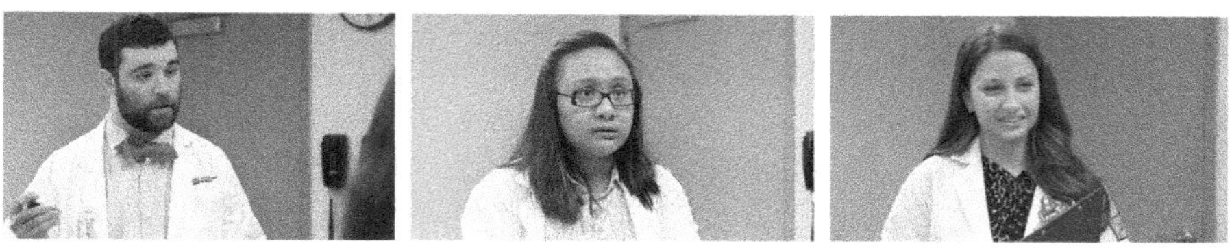

FIGURE 13.1 Stills from the film *Bedside Manner*. Medical students evaluating Dr Alice Flaherty as an SP with delirium.

Prior to the filming, I asked Tony Errichetti, Chief of Virtual Medicine at NYIT College of Osteopathic Medicine, to give me a sense of how this encounter might play out. He replied:

> I'm not sure what the students will do in the room. Although they will be briefed and should have read the material I sent, we won't know until they do it. We could even tell them exactly what to expect (we won't) and they still might not do well. Knowledge provides no help in the short run – it tends to go out the window under pressure – but repeated experience and feedback does make them better. Conversely, students may know what to do, but do it poorly – in the early stages they often look like they're on autopilot, robotically working down a list of things to accomplish.

On the day of filming, the students were nervous as they interacted with the SP – fidgeting, stammering, speaking scripted sentences, displaying stiff and closed postures. Scrutinized with close-up shots, they appear all the more vulnerable. The medical students were sometimes directly challenged by the SP, making the clinical encounter even more difficult. This is one of the purposes of simulations, which provide an opportunity for students to gain self-awareness of their reactions to patient encounters, a skill they will need to hone throughout their career.

The image of the doctor as competent is challenged in this scene as we view student doctors go through the challenging process of becoming an 'authority'. Viewers of the film will not necessarily realize they are watching a simulation rather than an actual medical encounter. Having endowed doctors with so much prestige in our culture, how does this portrayal influence our perception of the power that doctors yield?

It's important that my body isn't absent from this text. I didn't know it at the time, but I was pregnant on this film shoot. As I was filming medical encounters, I was inadvertently preparing to become a full-fledged medical subject myself.

Scene 2: The Ether Dome training session

Influences: 'A Clinical Lesson at the Salpêtrière', painted by André Brouillet in 1887 (Figure 13.3); medical photographs from the Burns archive, historic images of amphitheatres such as The Gross Clinic by Thomas Eakins (1875); Charcot's photographs of 'hysteric' patients, Martha Rosler's 'Vital Statistics of a Citizen, Simply Obtained' and 'Screening the Body' by Lisa Cartwright.

The film moves from the doctor's office in the previous scene to an amphitheatre where Alice is being trained in her delirious patient role by Tony Errichetti,

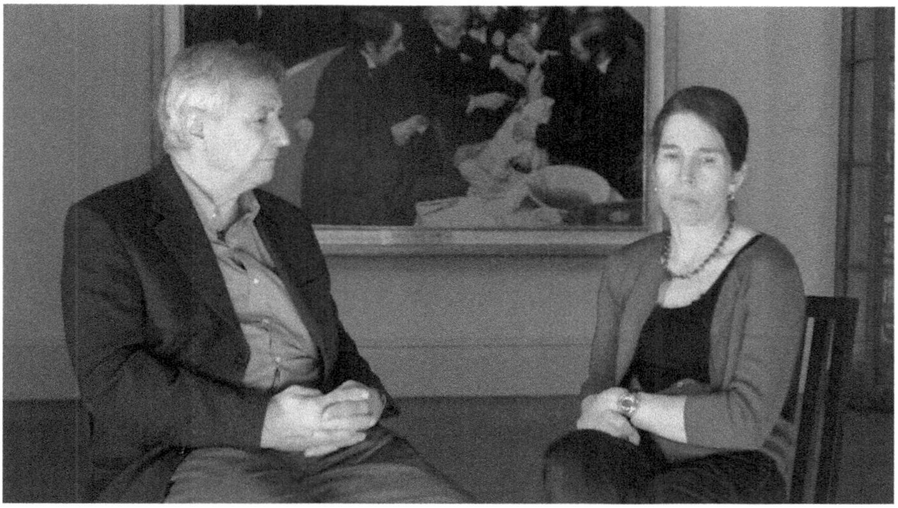

FIGURE 13.2 Still from the film *Bedside Manner*. Tony Errichetti, PhD, and Dr Alice Flaherty rehearsing her SP role in the Massachusetts General Hospital's Ether Dome.

PhD. Unlike the flat light of the doctor's office in the prior scene, the lighting is intentionally lush and cinematic. The amphitheatre is in Massachusetts General Hospital's historic Ether Dome, where anaesthesia was used during surgery for the first time (see Figure 13.2). The scene references the history of medicine, specifically the nineteenth-century French neurologist Jean-Martin Charcot. Charcot presented his female hysteric patients in an amphitheatre, and he spoke of the seminar as a 'theatre' and his most performative patients as his 'stars'. Charcot routinely photographed the patients exhibiting hysterical symptoms that were coaxed by prompts and posing, negatively linking women and pathology.[6] Like a patient who might overact in order to get their illness taken seriously by a doctor, these hysterical patients can also be understood as having enacted their suffering in order to get relief. Most had been sexually or physically abused, and the hospital was much safer for them than their previous lives. The idea of playing sick and playing doctor takes illness outside of an individual pathology and emphasizes societal and cultural norms (see Figure 13.3).

Unconscious bias towards women continues to shape medical experiences. Women's health issues are often dismissed by doctors and misdiagnosed as psychiatric conditions. Women are less likely to be given painkillers in the ER for acute pain, and women are seven times more likely than men to be misdiagnosed

[6] Georges Didi-Huberman, *The Invention of Hysteria: Charcot and the Photographic Iconography of the Salpêtrière* (MIT Press, 2003).

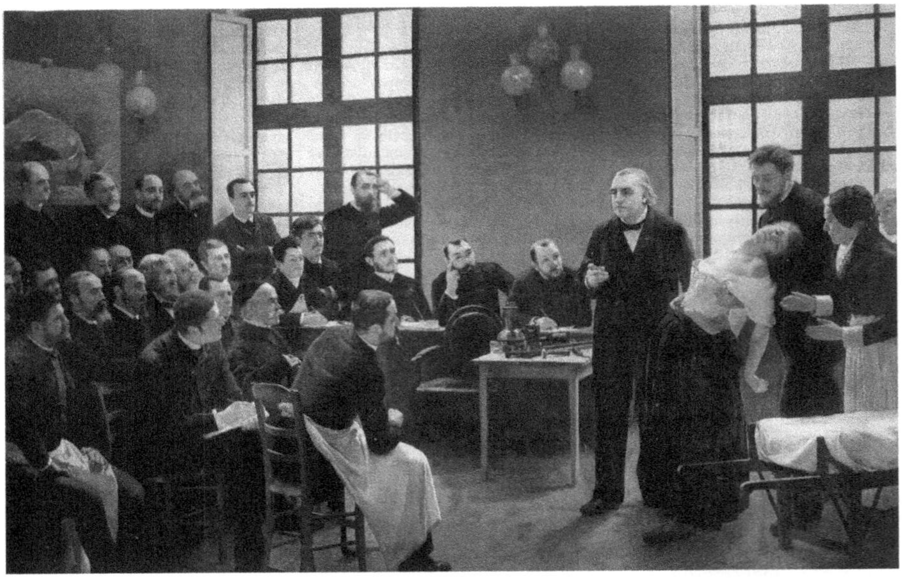

FIGURE 13.3 A painting, *A Clinical Lesson at the Salpêtrière* (André Brouillet, 1887, 114.1 × 169.2 in, Musée d'histoire de la médecine, Paris), showing the French neurologist Jean-Martin Charcot with one of his hysteric patients, who is fainting in a man's arms. Charcot is lecturing to an enraptured all male audience.

and discharged in the middle of having a heart attack. Overt racism and class bias are also factors in diagnosis. African American women are 2.6 times more likely to die from pregnancy-related complications than white women.[7] In light of the history of somatization and psychosomatic illnesses, the central delirium case in the film is key because it is one of the many conditions that stems from a physical cause and produces mental problems; it can be confused with depression, dementia, manic psychosis and schizophrenia.

This is the second scene in the film, but it was the first film shoot. I remember how nervous I was while taking the train to Boston for the filming. I had never worked with a film crew before, and I was not sure if my decision to film in the Ether Dome was a good idea, since an SP training session would never occur in such a location. Maybe it would read as inauthentic and heavy-handed. In fact, I had a disorienting feeling I couldn't shake that I had gotten on a train heading in the wrong direction, and I would never arrive in Boston for the shoot. In the end, I was satisfied with how the space becomes a character in the film.

[7] Emily Baumgaertner and Farnaz Fassihi, 'Racism and Sexism Underlie Higher Maternal Death Rates for Black Women, U.N. Says', *New York Times*, 12 July 2023.

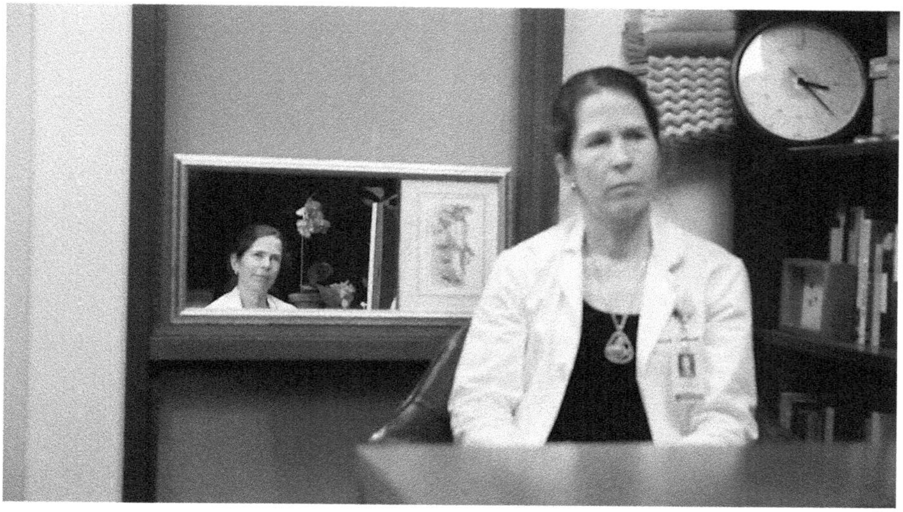

FIGURE 13.4 Still from the film *Bedside Manner*. The mirror scene in Alice Flaherty's office.

Scene 3: Alice's Office

This is my favourite scene in the film. I think of it as my *Twin Peaks* moment; every time I watch the film it somehow catches me off guard. Alice sits in her patient's chair and a mirror reflects her in her office chair (see Figure 13.4). There is an uncanny split between her expressions. Alice told me the mirror was a way for her to monitor her facial expressions when meeting with patients. I will not interpret the scene, as I do not want to shut down meaning for the viewer, but I will note a few key references that inspired and helped shape it. First, this scene is indebted to Laura Mulvey's notion of the woman embodying both spectator and spectacle. Second, there are multiple layers of performance occurring here, as Alice is acting like the doctor who played her on her book's TV show pilot, while also occupying the roles of both patient and doctor. Finally, the mirror scene captures the sense of selves watching selves, with an allusion to the student debrief in the film where the students have to watch and evaluate recordings of themselves, as well as to the multifaceted split between self and other.

This scene relates to the mystery of seeing oneself, and how we can never see ourselves from the outside, only in photographs and mirrors.

If we are talking about the self, where am I?

I was four months pregnant during this filming date. I'm in cameos throughout the film. In the first scene I wheel in medical equipment; my hand can be seen throughout passing notes to Alice through a funny hole in the two-way mirror scene. At the end, my reflection – nine months pregnant – is just visible as I close

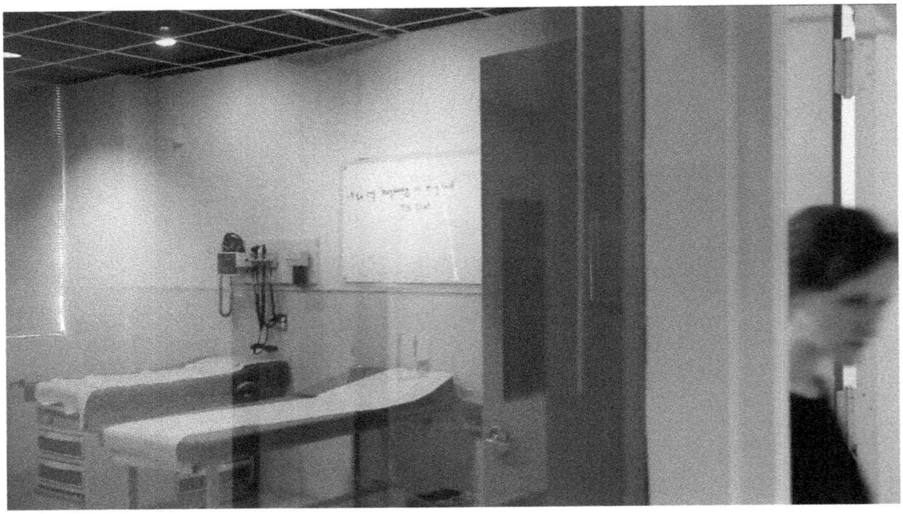

FIGURE 13.5 Still from the film *Bedside Manner*. A glimpse of Botz walking past a clinical skills centre room whose whiteboard serendipitously reads, '"In my beginning is my end" T. S. Eliot.'

a curtain to an SP's room. The cameos are a nod to my presence as the film-maker, they implicate me and acknowledge my subjectivity (see Figure 13.5).

Scene 4: Clinical skills centres

Influences: Michel Foucault's *Discipline & Punish: The Birth of the Prison*; the use of two-way mirrors in police interrogations; Dr Arnold Gesell photographic dome constructed in 1920 at the Yale Clinic of Child Development; Sandra S. Phillips's *Exposed: Voyeurism, Surveillance, and the Camera Since 1870.*

I often use the camera as a licence to enter the lives of others and to access spaces that are usually restricted. When I visited a clinical skill centre for the first time, I noticed how much it resembled a panopticon. The film incorporated the details of surveillance throughout the clinical skills centres to create a sense of anxiety. Photography and film extend the visual field, creating a vast network of seeing and being seen. The policing and surveillance of vulnerable bodies have always disturbed me. The skills centre's central command system records all the clinical encounters, and as the medical professors watch the encounters outside that room through two-way mirrors, the student doctors enter from the periphery, constantly watched and recorded. Both the student doctors and SPs are being evaluated on their performances (see Figure 13.6).

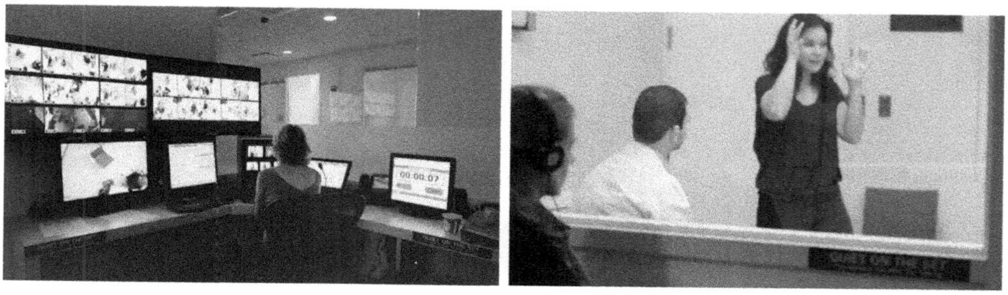

FIGURE 13.6 Stills from the film *Bedside Manner*. The inner chamber of a simulation centre and a two-way mirror at NYSIM in NYC.

Scene 5: The student-doctor

In the film, there's a poignant moment when a medical student comes out of a debrief with an SP early. He looks upset and dejected and needs to pull himself together. Young medical residents must convince patients that they are more competent than they feel. As Errichetti observed, 'medical school is not a very empathic place'. Studies show that empathy plummets during the third year of medical school in the US. According to one article, 'fear of making mistakes, a demanding curriculum, time pressure, sleep loss and a hostile environment have all been described by some students as factors that changed their views about patient–physician relationships'.[8] As Alice discusses in the film, suppressing empathy may also be a form of self-preservation since students are not taught any other way to acquire affect tolerance, which is the ability to manage emotions without becoming overwhelmed by them (see Figure 13.8).

Doctors in the United States are dying at a higher suicide rate than members of any other professional group.[9] More recently, doctors and nurses experienced unprecedented burnout and PTSD during the COVID-19 pandemic, leading many healthcare workers to leave the industry. While we are accustomed to thinking about empathy in regards to the patient, as the project progressed I also began to think about what doctors feel as they struggle to live up to patients' expectations of authority. Empathy began to seep into my portrayal of the 'doctor' in the film. My film began as a study of how doctors learn or unlearn empathy, but ended with my having more empathy for doctors.

When we filmed the student-doctor scene (Figure 13.7), *I was eleven days away from giving birth. I delivered my daughter in another hospital building, just two blocks away.*

---

[8] M. Hojat et al., 'The Devil Is in the Third Year: A Longitudinal Study of Erosion of Empathy in Medical School', *Academic Medicine* 84, no. 9 (2009): 1182–91.

[9] Antonio Ventriglio et al., 'Suicide Among Doctors: A Narrative Review', *Indian Journal of Psychiatry* 62, no. 2 (2020): 114–120, https://doi.org/10.4103/psychiatry.IndianJPsychiatry_767_19.

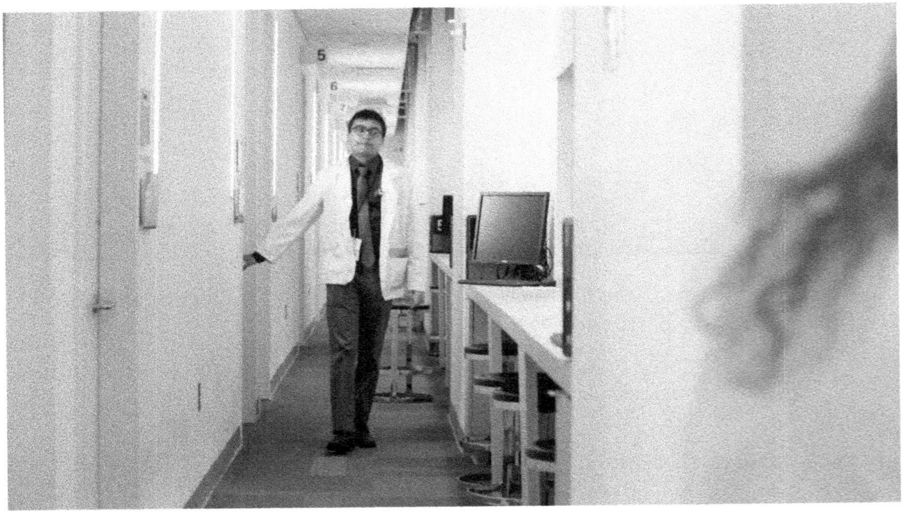

FIGURE 13.7 Still from the film *Bedside Manner*. A medical student exiting an SP encounter early.

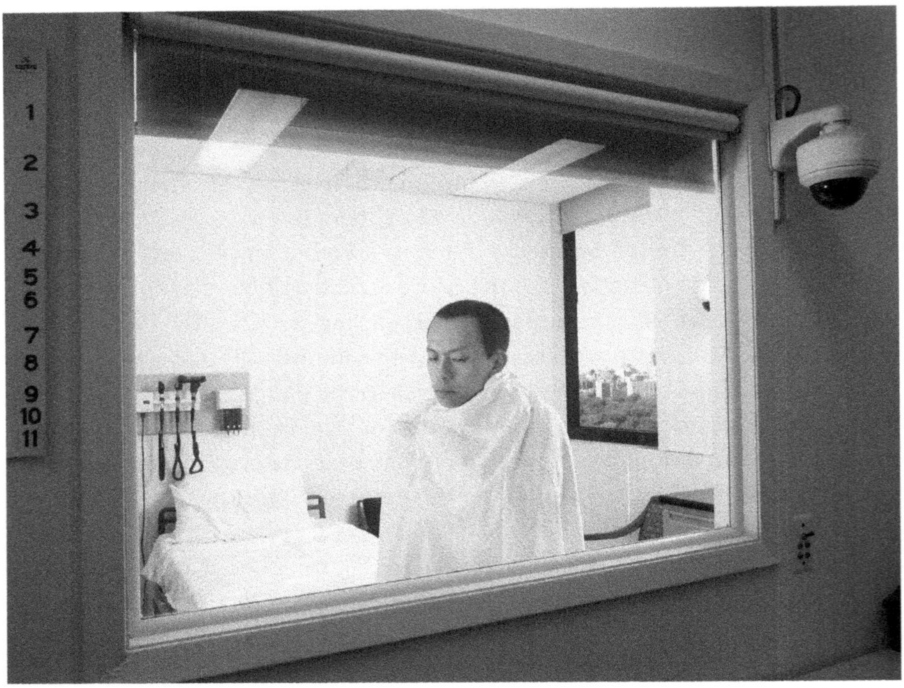

FIGURE 13.8 'Wilton' from the photographic series *Bedside Manner*, 30 × 40 in, Pigment Print.

This was the hardest film shoot to pull off in terms of permissions and I thought it was the last, but everything changed after the birth of my daughter.

III. THE PHOTOGRAPHS

Medical education has come a long way since the nineteenth century when cadavers were stolen from graveyards for dissection, and objectivizing medical photographs of patients were the property of doctors who used them to advance arguments or statistics. One advance in medical training has been SPs. Most of the SPs that I met in New York were professional actors, but many have other day jobs or are retirees. Each SP follows a script and is taught how to convincingly feign symptoms. Over the course of the years I spent working on this project, I photographed simulations of an Ebola case, a teen pregnancy, family violence/abuse, numerous obstetric and gynaecological cases and an end-of-life support simulation in which a couple – who have played this scenario together many times – must make the difficult decision, with the help of a student-doctor, to take their child off a respirator. I was especially interested in photographing psychiatric cases such as borderline personality disorder and depression, partly because of the unsettling history of purportedly representing psychological states with photography (see Figure 13.9).

What does a portrait say about an individual's identity? What do we assume? What is present? These are questions that have always interested me. My portraits of SPs suggest a psychological depth, but the subject matter calls that projection into question. Are the actors fully invested in the character and performance? Is it a projected earnestness? Is emotion shown despite the will of the subject? How do you measure the authenticity of suffering in any photograph? Do the images elicit compassion or pity?

Subjects perform identity to some degree in all photographic portraits, as well as in real life. The portraits are named for the actors, but they are in quotation marks, since they are both themselves and not themselves in my portraits. The medical actors perform illness in my images and medical students are taught to 'play' doctors in the simulated encounters. Even though the SP may be performing, this does not mean the encounter is not also real; acting and staged representations inform the interactions between patients and doctors in important ways. To express their suffering, all patients become – convincingly or unconvincingly – actors in their doctors' offices. Standardized patient encounters reveal the ritual gestures and phrases of medical interactions. Acting can give birth to feeling, and artifice can expose the real. The deeper emotional and psychological implications of these scenarios were never far from the surface – photographing at Bellevue, an SP broke down in tears following a gynaecological encounter with a medical student. When I asked another SP if she could cry for a portrait she said,

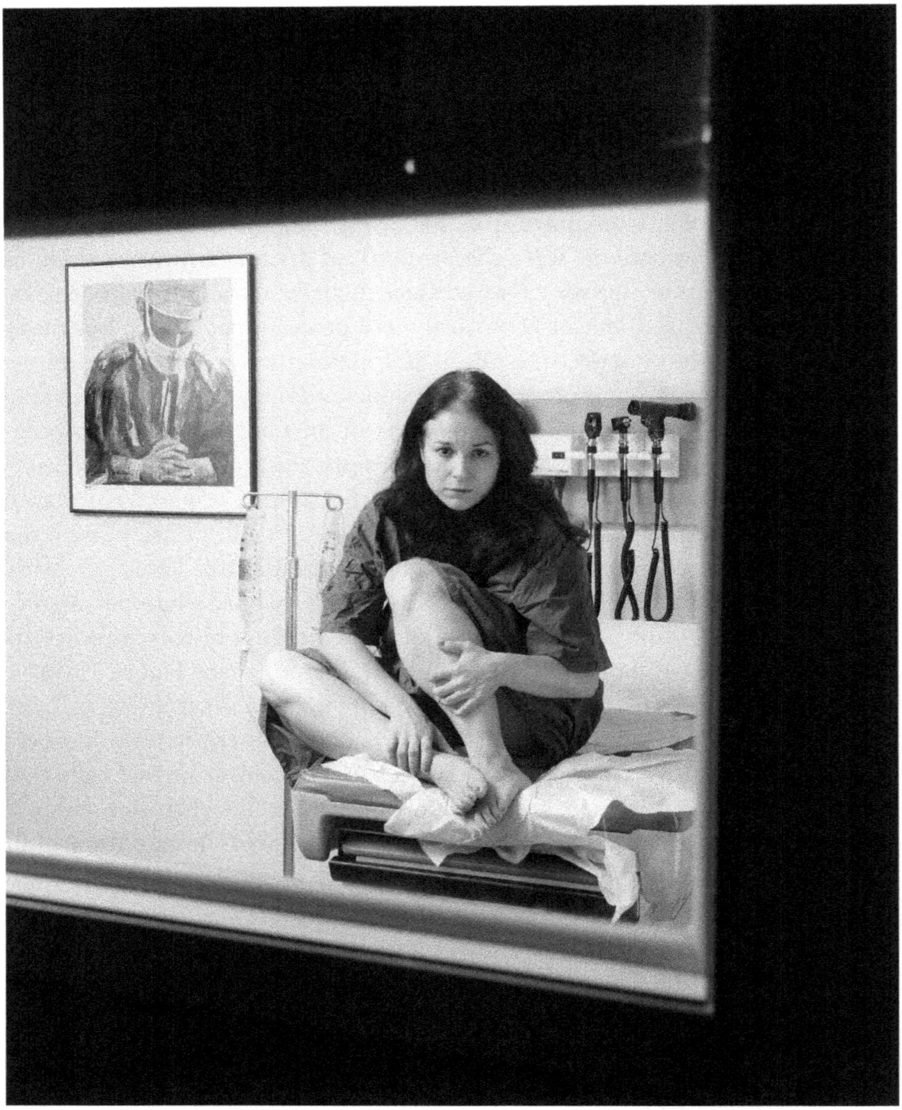

FIGURE 13.9 'Lori' from the series *Bedside Manner*, 40 × 30 in, Archival Pigment Print.

'Yes, that will be very easy for me today.' Who is to judge if her tears were fake or authentic?

I took the photographs in this series from behind a two-way mirror: the subject was looking at their reflection in a mirror, isolated inside a room and acting out a standardized patient role we had previously discussed. There was a periodic interruption by a harsh, bright strobe light when I pressed the shutter button, unseen on the other side of the two-way mirror. While photographers often emphasize eye contact with their subjects, I'm accustomed to taking my best images hidden behind a big camera or disappearing under a photographic dark cloth. I enjoyed the defined parameters of this set-up. These are voyeuristic images taken with the subject's consent.

My photographs document standardized patients and highlight the craft of the staged tableaux: the work gains its power by exposing the way true aspects of medicine are hard to separate from – and sometimes depend on – fictions. It was important that the images contained the artifice of medical simulations (two-way mirrors, microphones and video cameras are almost always apparent). Staging and performance not only relate to the inherent theatricality of medicine, but help to both circumvent and elicit an emotional response from viewers. Viewers are prompted to contemplate their reactions not just to sickness, injury and hospitals, but to the images of human suffering we are inundated with on a daily basis, whether for entertainment or edification. Perhaps the images will lead people to contemplate their empathic processes. 'Photographic empathy' is commonly thought of as different than empathy in real life because it provides a safe place for feelings of empathy: it is easier to feel for someone in a photograph; it does not require action the same way.

To be a 'patient' is to be observed, reliant on a doctor's interpretation and understanding of one's body. The idea of an unreturnable gaze is especially powerful in terms of conjuring the way in which photographs can objectify and dehumanize people. Early medical photography often turned people into objects, and they were the property of the doctors, labelled as a disease rather than with a name. In this context seeing is objectifying and controlling. For instance, the British physician Hugh Welch Diamond photographed female patients in the Surrey County Asylum in his pursuit of a pseudoscience, the physiognomy of mental illness.[10] I wanted to refer to this history in my photographs and have viewers consider the burden of the medical past and the 'spectacle of suffering'. I would never have dared to photograph an actual patient in the hospital: standardized patients were the only way I could make this work without victimization.

The photographs also reflect the isolation I have felt when sick, not just from doctors who might not be able to help, but cut off from life and from friends and family who can feel far away. I see these subjects confined to the netherworld of illness, what Meghan O' Rourke describes in *The Invisible Kingdom: Reimagining Chronic Illness*: 'The patient's identity is thwarted,

[10]Sander L. Gliman, *Seeing the Insane* (Echo Point Books & Media, 2014), 164–78.

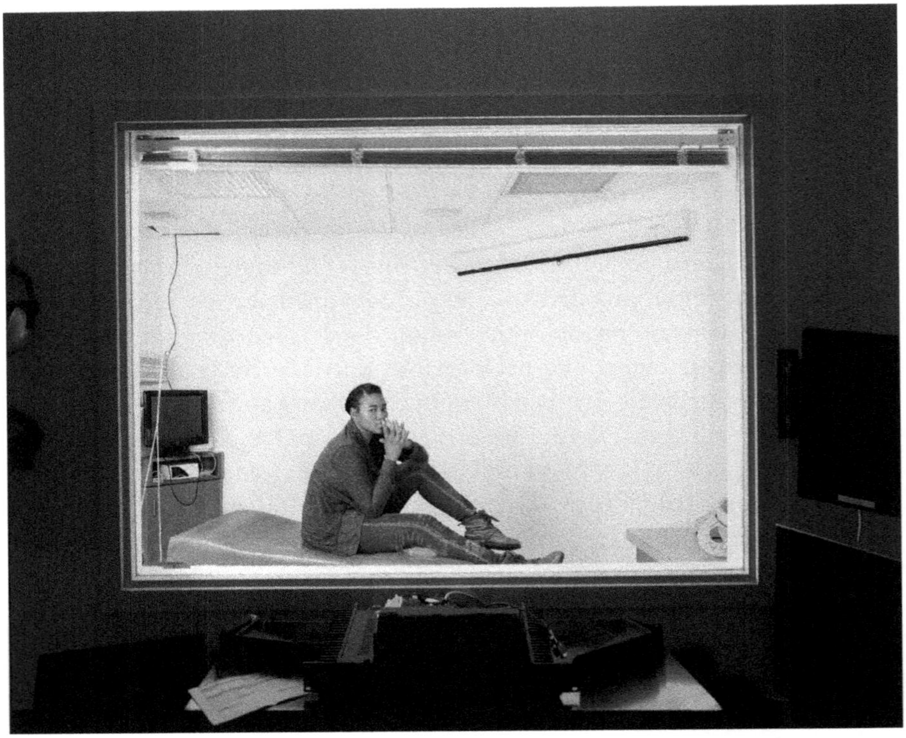

FIGURE 13.10 'Chalise' from the series *Bedside Manner*, 40 × 30 in, Archival Pigment Print.

silenced, distorted in a culture that does not recognize itself in its sick members.'[11]

I have repeatedly used windows as a seeing device in my work – from the very first photograph I took when I was nine years old, of two love pigeons on a snowy pine tree outside my bedroom window, to the photographs I took in college of my family through the dollhouse window I played with as a child, to the photographs of personal belongings taken through car windows following accidents (Repository, 2013).

Perhaps this relates back to how I watched the world when I was sick as a child (see Figure 13.10).

IV. BIRTH

1. I found it helpful to pretend

During my pregnancy, I had photographed and filmed many obstetrical simulations – most memorably post-partum haemorrhages, where blood soaks

[11] Meghan O' Rourke, *The Invisible Kingdom: Reimagining Chronic Illness* (Riverhead Books, 2022), 265.

through the sheets and if a transfusion isn't ordered within a set amount of time the patient dies. There were also episiotomy repairs done on pieces of meat purchased in Chinatown, and a neonatal resuscitation. These rehearsals did not completely prepare me for my traumatic birth experience.

They say the veil is thin when you are close to birth and death. I had the most peaceful labour at home, falling asleep between each contraction and waking to the most distinct sense of another presence beside my bed protecting me. I wondered why I couldn't see them. Arriving at the hospital 8 cm dilated everything was going as planned, but after pushing for over five hours the doctor told me I needed a C-section. I delivered a perfect baby daughter: Echo.

Following the delivery, though, I was in agony with a distended stomach for three days before the obstetricians took my pain seriously and ordered additional testing. (I would later learn that a caring nurse called the attending doctor and told her that someone had to do something and help me). The hospital's CT scan revealed a previously unknown congenital gut malrotation that had caused a life-threatening intestinal obstruction. In retrospect, this explained why, during my last trimester, I had intermittently been in severe stomach pain and threw up green bile – a tell-tale sign of an obstruction. My obstetrician had repeatedly told me I had the flu or indigestion. The doctors put a large tube down my nose into my stomach to suck out intestinal secretions until the obstruction temporarily cleared. I hate hospitals, but when NYU was ready to discharge my newborn and me after a week, I was so scared of my body and something going deathly wrong, that I didn't want to leave. A kind nurse talked me into going home. Two months later surgeons performed a complicated open surgery to reposition my congenital gut malrotation and prevent further obstructions. In the interim, though, a few weeks after giving birth, I had a post-partum haemorrhage because part of the placenta had accidentally been left in during the C-section. That required two more surgeries (they botched the first one) to remove the retained placenta. Those surgeries, in turn, caused Asherman's syndrome, a webbing of scar tissue that blocked my cervix. For that, I needed multiple hysteroscopic surgeries.

During these medical experiences, I found it helpful to pretend that I was an actor in my film, and to think about my experiences as part of my research. It was a distancing mechanism that made me feel more connected to my identity, and it offered an element of play or movement in an otherwise stressful time. If I had been an SP performing a debrief, I would comment on my obstetrician's incompetence and cold disregard for my suffering. I sent a five-page letter detailing my grievances, but without an observing medical professor who would turn their ineptitude into a grade, there was no response. Because patients with intestinal malrotation are so rare, I liked knowing medical students could observe and learn from my operation. While recovering at the hospital from that surgery, I requested that my husband bring my camera from home, and I took photographs of the various 'stage settings', such as the family waiting room.

Five years later, I went to a doctor for diagnosis and treatment of my Asherman's syndrome. After taking my medical history surrounding childbirth he said, 'I'm so sorry.' This surgeon later made a mistake on the first hysteroscopy, which landed me in hospital eight days later with a haemorrhage. He took full responsibility for his error, explained what went wrong (the hospital didn't explain much), and said he was sorry. In a circuitous way, an apology had finally arrived.

2. *Editing*

Viewing an edit of the film at home with my newborn in the midst of my ongoing health crisis, I decided I had to move beyond the ambiguities of playing sick and return to the seriousness of illness and death. Knowing about Alice's previous history of a tragic miscarriage, I asked her if she would be comfortable discussing her experience in the film. She agreed and, on camera, spoke about the death of her premature twins, and how her obstetrician's blank face showed her the necessity of good medical performance. This scene is placed towards the middle of the film so it doesn't function as a reveal at the end. Due to the editing (in the scene prior, Alice lists her wildly varied medical experiences, similar to how the SPs in the film list their many roles), it's unclear if Alice is playing an SP role or talking about a personal experience. This ambiguity calls into question all of the other performances. As my friend, artist Chris Curreri, commented, 'it changes the way everything resonates in the film' (see Figure 13.11).

The structure of the film is paramount to its meaning, and editing proved to be one of the most challenging parts of this project. The editor I hired made important contributions to the film, but our sensibilities were not aligned. Despite the editor's insistence that an ambiguously edited mid-length film would not be accepted into film festivals, I trusted that the structure of the film had to be more non-linear. It became a tiresome back and forth of editing and feedback, and it was as if there were two competing films. I eventually paid that editor and continued to edit the film for months with the invaluable help of a

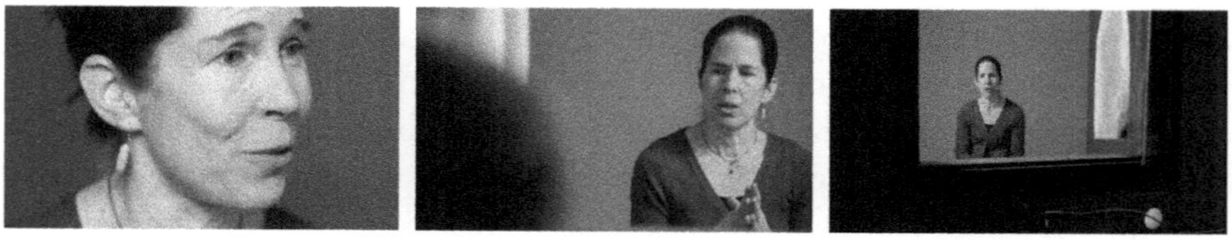

FIGURE 13.11 Stills from the film *Bedside Manner*. Alice Flaherty seen directly, reflected in the two-way mirror, and through the two-way mirror.

new editor, Isabel Freeman. I also added additional shoots at WISER and Albert Einstein. Once I took the film into my own hands, it felt like me. Alice, who watched endless edits of the film and sent me copious notes in response to each edit, described the final cut as 'a little bit orthogonal' in regards to the tension between art film and documentary.

Bedside Manner is not didactic. It invites viewers to become active participants: to enter a world and make discoveries, ask questions and form their own conclusions. Analogous to a medical case in which doctors decide what is true and relevant for diagnosis and treatment, *Bedside Manner* challenges spectators to decipher what is authentic in Alice's narrative. I want viewers to think about what is real and not real, about how confusing perception can be and how the real and imaginary both shape medical experiences. Viewers are compelled to ask which aspects of these scenes are not just true, but relevant to their own medical history.

3. *Project release*

In 2016, I had a solo exhibition of photographs and film from the series Bedside Manner at Benrubi Gallery in New York City. Alice, Errichetti, the simulation lab facilitators, and many of the SPs pictured in my photographs were among those who attended the opening. The work was favourably reviewed and featured in publications including the *New Yorker*, *Wired*, *Hyperallergic*, *TIME* magazine, *Photograph Magazine* and *Museum of the Moving Image: Sloan Science and Film*.

'Bedside Manner' had its theatrical premiere at DOC NYC in 2016, where it won the Grand Jury Prize for Best Short (Oscar-qualifying). The photographs and film have been exhibited at numerous art institutions, and the film made the rounds to film festivals as well as at medical symposiums and medical schools. Alice and I travelled together to many screenings in Europe, the Americas and Asia. The film is part of numerous university collections and I have received notes from professors about how they use it in their courses. I consider the film to be the heart of the project, and the resulting conversations have raised important questions about perception, empathy and the need to humanize medicine.

Elaine Drew, a medical anthropologist at the University of Alaska Fairbanks, wrote the following to me after she screened the film for her medical humanities students:

> We continued to discuss performativity in medicine – from both sides of the equation, the sick role and the provider/healer role ('playing doctor'). The students discussed what it means to 'act' like a sick person and that 'acting' sick doesn't mean a person is 'faking it' ... Dr Alice Flaherty saying 'you are always performing' came up here. From an anthropological lens, we

reflected on how medical education is enculturation/socialization into the cultural system of American biomedicine, which differs in interesting ways from (bio)medical education in other places around the world (e.g., China and Greece).

In a Sheffield Doc/Fest review Matt Turner wrote that the 'film plays upon performance, probing into ideas surrounding empathy and authenticity, and exposing the slim line between reality and artifice, never quite revealing which of what we see is constructed, or what is real, or even whether, in certain contexts there is a difference at all. Just because you feel it, doesn't mean it was there'.[12] A fellow filmmaker, Giselle Minoli, wrote me, 'Even this fourth time watching it, I'm left with this sense of it being this surrealistic painting, and I love that because there are so many places to go with it as a film.' For medical students and doctors, the disorientation sometimes helped make them realize their poor tolerance of ambiguity.

Alice's ability to see from the perspective of both the physician and the patient allows her to approach medicine from a unique angle, breaking down outdated hierarchies and one-dimensional conceptualizations of identity. Over the course of making the film, the role of Alice as subject and consultant blurred into collaborator, mentor and friend (see Figure 13.12).

V. IT LIVES INSIDE ME

Illness drove this essay, though not the way it drove Bedside Manner; it was more akin to the ideal sickbed scene I sometimes experienced as a child. I was isolated as a mild case of Covid slowly made its way through my family, giving me time and minimizing distractions in a way that proved ideal for writing. As with my other long-term projects, *Bedside Manner* lives inside me; I grew and changed along with it. The process of making the work and the conversations that resulted from sharing it were a way of understanding and making sense of my own experiences. Seeing humanity on the other side of the white coat helped to demystify medical encounters, and I'm a slightly better patient now. That said, it's been ten years since I gave birth to my daughter, and I still get emotional every time I talk about my childbirth experience. When I considered having another child, I was haunted by advice I received from a doctor who I didn't even fully trust: 'Whatever you do, don't get pregnant again, you could lose your intestines or die.'

[12] Matt Turner, 'Festival Focus: Sheffield Doc/Fest 2017 – Female Filmmakers', *ShootingPeople*, 26 June 2017, https://shootingpeople.org/blog/2017/06/festival-focus-sheffield-docfest-2017-female-filmmakers/.

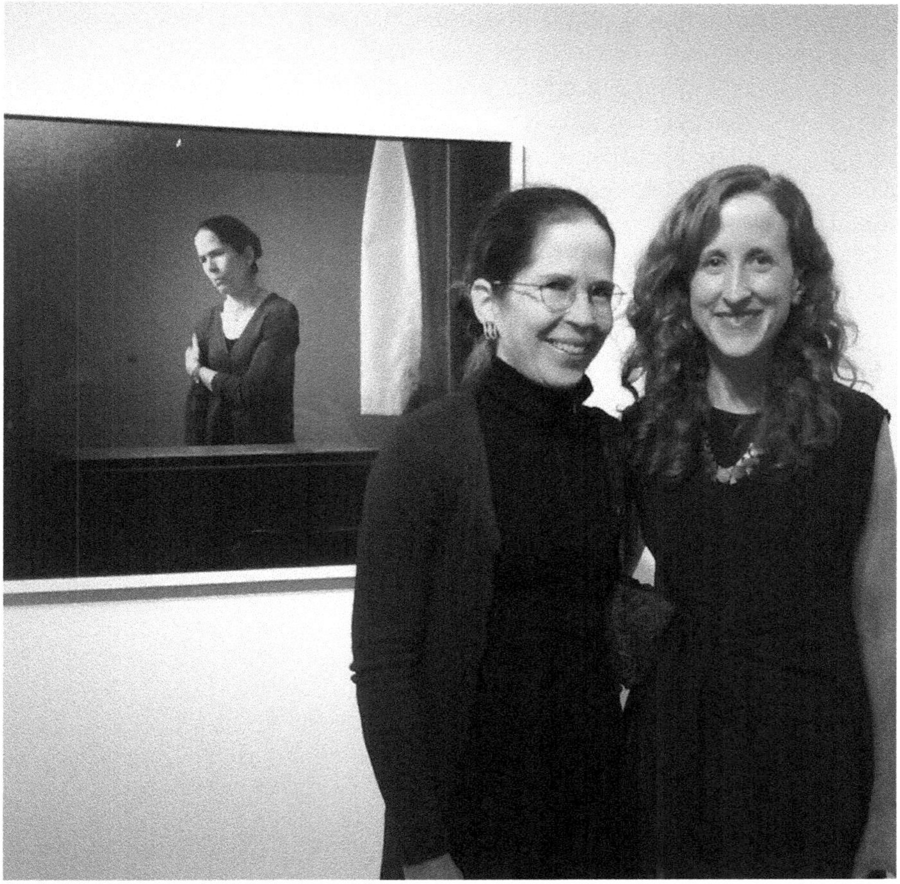

FIGURE 13.12 Botz and Flaherty at the opening of *Bedside Manner* at Benrubi Gallery, NYC.

Following *Bedside Manner*, I embarked on *Milk Factory*, which reflects the shift in identity that occurs in early motherhood. *Milk Factory* is a photography, video, and book project that makes lactation rooms and the invisible labour that takes place there visible. Seldom is any space simultaneously so utilitarian and emotionally charged. The US is the only high-income country that does not offer mandated paid family leave, which causes parents to return to work soon after giving birth, making pumping pervasive. The lactation rooms I photographed were either arbitrary, unconsidered spaces or as sterile as a doctor's office, which reflects the tenuous position new mothers inhabit in the workforce. Continuing the approach that I took in *Bedside Manner*, in the film I used architectural space to help tell the story. The entire film takes place in the bipartisan lactation room of the US House of Representatives, a symbolic location where laws are decided regarding parental policies and reproductive rights. The absence of people in the photographs and anonymous nature of the film highlights how human milk is preferred as a disembodied product in our culture, and the image of a child at a mother's breast is a privilege unavailable to many in a late capitalist society that values productivity over health. *Milk Factory* follows the feminist imperative that a radically different and less binary world is possible.

This essay began with my mom at my bedside caring for me when I was a child, and it feels fitting to close with my project that acknowledges and visualizes a mother's unseen labour. The infant–mother relationship epitomizes the deep dependence of all humans, one that is not separate from historical and cultural circumstances. We all want to feel connected and seen.

The end of Bedside Manner *hints at healing without promising it: a medical student exits the room, we see an older woman get off an exam table, and a medical actor wipes a tear from her face. Alice says 'sometimes getting well is really about unlearning a story'. While viewers have told me the ending of the film is open-ended, it's almost too neat an ending for my taste. I want there to be room for the viewer to step in and out of the story once more* (see Figure 13.13).

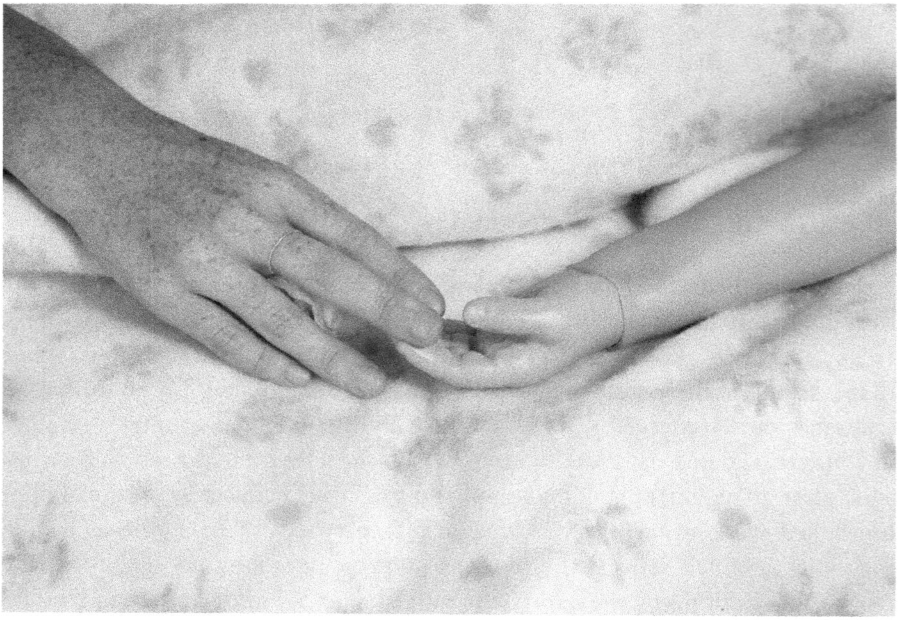

FIGURE 13.13 'Hands' from the series *Bedside Manner*, 18 × 24 in, Archival Pigment Print.

REFERENCES

Baumgaertner, Emily, and Farnaz Fassihi. 'Racism and Sexism Underlie Higher Maternal Death Rates for Black Women, U.N. Says'. *New York Times*, 12 July 2023.

Botz, Corinne. *The Nutshell Studies of Unexplained Death*. Monacelli Press, 2004.

Botz, Corinne. *Haunted Houses*. Monacelli Press, 2010.

Botz, Corinne. *Milk Factory*. Saint Lucy Books, 2025.

Botz, Corinne. 'Bedside Manner'. *Corinne May Botz*. www.corinnebotz.com/bedside-manner-1.

Flaherty, Alice. *The Midnight Disease: The Drive to Write, Writer's Block, and the Creative Brain*. Houghton Mifflin, 2004.

Gliman, Sander L. *Seeing the Insane*. Echo Point Books & Media, 2014.

Hojat, Mohammadreza, Michael J. Vergare, Kaye Maxwell, George Brainard, Steven K. Herrine, Gerald A. Isenberg, Jon Veloski and Joseph S. Gonnella. 'The Devil Is in the Third Year: A Longitudinal Study of Erosion of Empathy in Medical School'. *Academic Medicine* 84, no. 9 (2009): 1182–91. https://doi.org/10.1097/acm.0b013e3181b17e55.

O'Rourke, Meghan. *The Invisible Kingdom: Reimagining Chronic Illness*. Riverhead Books, 2022.

Szarkowiski, John. *Mirrors and Windows: American Photography Since 1960*. Museum of Modern Art, 1978.

Ventriglio, Antonio, Cameron Watson and Dinesh Bhugra. 'Suicide Among Doctors: A Narrative Review'. *Indian Journal of Psychiatry* 62, no. 2 (2020): 114–20. https://doi.org/10.4103/psychiatry.IndianJPsychiatry_767_19.

14

Theatre for social change in the dementia context

A CONVERSATION BETWEEN PIA KONTOS AND SHERRY DUPUIS

We are members of Collective Disruption, a collaboration that brings together interdisciplinary researchers interested in aging and dementia with a range of accomplished performance artists including a playwright/director, musicians and physical theatre creators.[1] Founded in 2013, this research-creative ensemble draws on the humanities, arts and social sciences to challenge dominant and oppressive cultural and social norms and to imagine and affect dementia care through the arts. Central to our efforts is the use of theatre as an innovative approach to pedagogy about stigma and the importance of relational caring to support people to live well with dementia. Relational caring – an approach that focuses on the interdependencies and processes of positive caring relationships – has the capacity to reduce stigma, but has yet to be systematically adopted in care settings despite calls for innovating education about its principles.

One of the outcomes of our collective is *Cracked: new light on dementia*, a research-based theatre project developed with funding from the Canadian Institutes for Health Research with the specific goal of challenging how we come to understand dementia as being irrevocably tragic. *Cracked* is a one-hour

---

[1] For full list of members see Collective Disruption, 'Cracked: new light on dementia', in *ReView: An Anthology of Plays Committed to Social Justice*, ed. Julia Gray (SensePublishers, 2017).

theatre production that follows the stories of two women – Elaine Carter and Vera Nolan – who have been diagnosed with dementia. The play depicts their experiences of stigma, as well as their resistance to stigma through individual and collective action that challenges practices and policies inconsistent with relational caring. The production was performed forty-three times during 2013–17 for approximately 5,000 people in long-term and community care settings, academic and professional conferences and public spaces across Ontario. It was professionally filmed to make the work available to audiences around the world, with funding from the Waugh Family Foundation. Both the live production and film versions have been evaluated with diverse audiences using survey, interview, focus group and observational methods, with funding from the Alzheimer Society of Canada.

Our conversation in this chapter shares reflections, experiences and insights about the impetus for creating *Cracked*, the development process (which included some tensions in our Collective), and the impact that *Cracked* has had on understandings of dementia and caring practices in community and residential aged care settings, as well as other ways that audiences are engaging with the production.

I. WHY THEATRE?

Pia Kontos (PK): Theatre is such a novel means to explore and represent illness experience. What drew you to theatre as a medium to critically explore dementia?

Sherry Dupuis (SD): Directly following my music degree, I was hired to work in a residential aged care setting. I worked closely with people living with dementia (PLWD) and found I could connect with them through music in ways that others could not. I also witnessed conditions within the sector that made it challenging to provide compassionate care because of the focus on body care (e.g. toileting, dressing, feeding) and the harms caused by such objectifying and often inhumane approaches. It made me want to do something to change the culture. I also worked as a director with an amateur theatre company, where I witnessed audience members being moved deeply by what they were seeing on the stage. These experiences stuck with me as I went back to school and became a researcher focused on culture change in dementia care. I quickly discovered, though, that there were structures within the academy that were stifling my ability to support transformative change. What is valued most in the academy are published peer-reviewed articles and academic conference presentations, and I knew it would be difficult to shift the culture with only those outputs.

My work at the Murray Alzheimer Research and Education Program was pivotal for me. When we were planning our first *A Changing Melody* forum, our partners living with dementia talked about how although the focus is typically on the cognitive aspects of dementia, for them dementia was about so much more, including the emotional and social aspects of the experience. They felt strongly that the arts were essential to sharing more authentic and diverse portrayals of experiences of dementia. This led us to intentionally embed the arts (music, visual arts, theatre, dance) in all of our forums as a way to support learning, self-expression, and a fuller representation of life with dementia for all audience members. Then in 2002 I got a call from Dr Christine Jonas-Simpson. She said that she and Dr Gail Mitchell were working on a play about dementia and were wondering if I might want to join them. I jumped at the chance, and the opportunity to work with them on the creation of *I'm Still Here* changed everything for me. From that day forward I found my artistic self again because I was able to bring my passions for art, culture change, and research together; I was able to see the power of the arts for both personal and social transformation. What drew you to theatre?

PK: I can trace my interest back to my doctoral research, in which I conducted an ethnographic study of a residential aged care setting. By attending to the body in everyday life, I was drawn into a social and cultural world of relationships that seemed rather mundane and unexceptional, except when juxtaposed with the dominant tragedy discourse of dementia. There, I found friendships, humour, creativity, conflict, and so much more that challenged assumptions of existential loss with dementia.

As a postdoctoral fellow, I began thinking about how I could help others to see the rich social life that I had encountered in my research and how this could help to challenge stigma and support culture change. I collaborated with director/playwright Vrenia Ivonoffski and we co-created dramatized vignettes based on my ethnographic research. These were staged in residential aged care settings in the context of research conversations with healthcare practitioners, as a way to foster critical reflection about their assumptions and practices and about new possibilities for supporting people to live well with dementia. The vignettes were impactful in how they prompted awareness of the practitioners' own held stigma associated with dementia, supported new understandings of experiences of living with dementia, and effected more humane care practices. This foray into theatre changed the course of my research; I went on to do a number of other projects, including a theatre production about traumatic brain injury that was written and directed by Dr Julia Gray.[2] That was such a

[2] Julia Gray et al., 'After the Crash: A Play about Brain Injury', *Canadian Theatre Review* 146 (2011): 66–86.

successful collaboration that when you, Christine and Gail invited me to join you in the development of a new production about dementia, I too jumped at the chance and invited Julia to join us.

SD: We have both found in our work that theatre communicates research findings in more accessible ways, in sensory, emotive and embodied ways. It also promotes a heightened sense of consciousness, what educational philosopher Maxine Greene calls 'wide-awakeness',[3] that makes us aware of our relational place in the world and the responsibility we all have to making the world a more socially just place for everyone. In doing so, it encourages critical reflectiveness on what is taken for granted and triggers change.

PK: As a critical social scientist, this is why I am so drawn to theatre. It brings voices and experiences often silenced in research to the surface, challenges deeply held beliefs and values, and reflects the complexities of lived experiences by showcasing multiple, contradictory perspectives.

SD: Theatre is able to nurture imaginative capacities and helps audience members to see and hear – to witness – things not seen before, and the harms and suffering experienced by others. There is a scene in *Cracked* where Elaine's daughter and son go to visit her after she moves into a residential aged care setting, and while sitting together the siblings argue with each other about whether visiting their mother makes a difference to her. Witnessing this scene prompted deep emotional reactions, such as for a healthcare practitioner who commented, 'I think that it's very hard before watching the play to understand what it's like to live with dementia, [but] when the two children were fighting and, you know, the mom's sitting there listening to this ... I remember that part, thinking that that'd be awful living with dementia and having that go on.'

What I also love about theatre is that it can help audiences envision possibilities for being and relating differently. One of the scenes in *Cracked* that does this well is the scene where Elaine and her daughter's partner, Alex, are doing the dishes. Elaine stops and it is clear that she suddenly does not know what to do with the dish she is holding. Alex gently touches Elaine's hand that is holding a dish cloth and guides her hand through the motions of washing the dish in her other hand; with this simple touch, Elaine resumes washing the dishes on her own. Audience members talk about the importance of touch and how this scene inspires other relational approaches in their interactions with PLWD. It starts with showing a more complex, expanded picture of dementia from different experiences and angles. In *Cracked*, audience members not only

[3] Maxine Greene, *Releasing the Imagination: Essays on Education, the Arts, and Social Change* (JosseyBass, 1995), 35.

see and hear directly from different characters living with dementia in diverse situations – Elaine is widowed and lives with her daughter, while we see Vera's relationship with her husband Tom, for example – they also engage with the experiences of different family members and healthcare practitioners.

Research participants working in residential aged care settings, who only see PLWD later in the dementia journey, shared how helpful it is to see and hear from PLWD in earlier phases of the journey; they open up to seeing the person in their whole life context and this makes a difference in terms of the ways they care.

PK: I think this is precisely why theatre is well positioned to challenge entrenched and oppressive attitudes, perceptions, institutions and social relations, and help us to imagine and effect more equitable solutions. We have certainly published about stigma[4] – indeed, it has dominated most of our professional and academic careers. But publishing alone is not enough. We need the innovation that theatre offers to address stigmatizing ideologies and associated social injustices to prompt the 'wide-awakeness' so needed in the world.

II. FROM STIGMA TO CARE

SD: We have both witnessed the harms experienced by PLWD, largely due to the stigma associated with dementia. This stigma is deeply entrenched in our cultural imaginary. It is evident in the dominant discourses, metaphors and images used in policy and in popular culture that represent dementia as 'the funeral without end', 'the loss of self', and 'a living death'. These terms perpetuate a deep and pernicious fear of and disregard for the actual PLWD. Stigma is so pervasive that it becomes internalized by PLWD, creating avoidance of social interactions, isolation, feelings of shame, depression, anxiety and even suicidal tendencies.

PK: The harms are significant. The cultural imaginary or collective representation of PLWD as 'non-persons' not only produces stereotypes and prejudices, but enables discriminatory practices such as segregation and confinement to residential aged care settings. As a society, we don't value PLWD and this is reflected in how these settings are sorely understaffed and lack the supportive, relational and enriching environments necessary for flourishing.

SD: As a leisure scholar, who explores how leisure activities and spaces shape our experiences in the world in both positive and negative ways,

[4] Gail Mitchell et al., 'Disrupting Dehumanising and Intersecting Patterns of Modernity with a Relational Ethic of Caring', *International Practice Development Journal* 10, no. 1 (2020); Gail J. Mitchell, Sherry L. Dupuis and Pia C. Kontos, 'Dementia Discourse: From Imposed Suffering to Knowing Other-wise', *Journal of Applied Hermeneutics* (2013).

I have been shocked by how even leisure is implicated in the production and re-production of dominant stigmatizing discourses of dementia. As an example, leisure in dementia care settings is primarily used as therapy, specifically as non-pharmacological interventions with the aim of managing misunderstood 'behaviours', improving cognition and physical functioning and reducing the 'burden of care'.

PK: As Anne Basting says, so many of these programmes amount to little more than 'maintenance entertainment'.[5] Music programmes are often modelled on passive listening rather than active engagement in co-constructing songs or playing instruments. Dance programmes typically emphasize the structured repetition of a set of choreographed movements, rather than encouraging participants to express themselves through movement in their own unique way. As a result, many of these programmes fall short of achieving their full potential to support empowerment, creative self-expression, social inclusion, relational well-being, and so much more of what it is to be human.

SD: There is an urgent need to shift the focus of care from assessing, correcting and controlling the symptoms of dementia to promoting human flourishing, which requires the support of embodied and relational capabilities. We've worked for some time now to develop a relational philosophy and approach to caring grounded in a relational ontology. Rather than focusing on disease and bodies (a biomedical model) or the individual (person-centred care), 'relational caring' focuses on the interdependencies inherent in caring relationships and relational processes necessary to support deep and positive connections: being responsive and emotionally present; being open to the role we play in relationships, to mutual influence and discovery and to vulnerability as a strength; sharing power and working in authentic partnership; and working to remove injustice and inequities that limit opportunities to flourish.

PK: We've also written about 'relational citizenship',[6] which builds on these ideas by emphasizing the citizenship rights and human rights of PLWD, attending to the ways power functions in the dementia context and stressing the importance of recognizing and fully supporting embodied and relational capabilities. These interconnections between individuals and socio-cultural, political and environmental forces really illuminate their role in empowering or

[5] Anne Davis Basting, *Forget Memory* (Johns Hopkins University Press, 2009), 105.

[6] Sherry Dupuis et al., 'Re-claiming Citizenship Through the Arts', *Dementia: The International Journal of Social Research and Practice* 15, no. 3 (2016): 358–80; Pia Kontos, Karen-Lee Miller and Alexis P. Kontos, 'Relational Citizenship: Supporting Embodied Selfhood and Relationality in Dementia Care', *Sociology of Health & Illness* 39, no. 2 (2017): 182–98; Mitchell et al., 'Disrupting Dehumanising and Intersecting Patterns of Modernity with a Relational Ethic of Caring'.

oppressing PLWD. Yet despite the increased interest in relational caring and its benefits, translating the principles of this philosophy and approach to caring into practice has proven difficult – certainly in part because of the limitations of traditional research and pedagogical approaches. This brings us back to *Cracked: new light on dementia.*

III. CREATING *CRACKED*

PK: I recall that much of our initial discussion with Julia [Gray] and the actors focused on the importance of creating space for audience members to engage critically and aesthetically, including emotionally, sensorially and imaginatively. I loved how our theatrical devising process involved all of us – researchers, actors and director/playwright. It was such a collaborative, silly, vulnerable and playful space that embraced what Julia describes as a 'willingness to fail' and 'to step forward with genuine uncertainty'.[7] Our 'rounds' (improvisational exercises), are a good example of this, involving a highly physical and improvisational exploration of all of our material. We arranged ourselves into a semi-circle, and one person at a time would step forward and gesture in some way for a few seconds – a movement, a vocal expression and so on – then return to their place. The rounds were a unique experience for me, because the intention with this exploration was that we link our gestures with spontaneous impulses of desire, vulnerability, surprise, joy, frustration, anger and so on. We were told to work from our 'gut', which definitely took me out of my comfort zone as it was quite different from engaging with our intellect! As academics, we live in our heads and are quite disembodied. I remember having a hard time with the rounds initially, as I was overthinking them. I was trying to be clever with my gestures and it stifled my embodied expressions. I remember Mary Ellen, an actor who led the rounds, would say 'Get out of your head!'

SD: I totally agree, the rounds were liberating and illuminating. With each gesture we were exposing our own embodiment and unique ways of being, and witnessing and exploring the embodiment and uniqueness of one another. This allowed us to slow down and to look closely at some of our own assumptions, while resisting the pressure to move too quickly to a finished product. As the rounds progressed, they became more focused or directed, thinking and experimenting with themes from our research or even direct quotes from interview

[7] Julia Gray, Helen Donnelly and Barbara E. Gibson, 'Seriously Foolish and Foolishly Serious: The Art and Practice of Clowning in Children's Rehabilitation', *Journal of Medical Humanities* 42 (2021): 456.

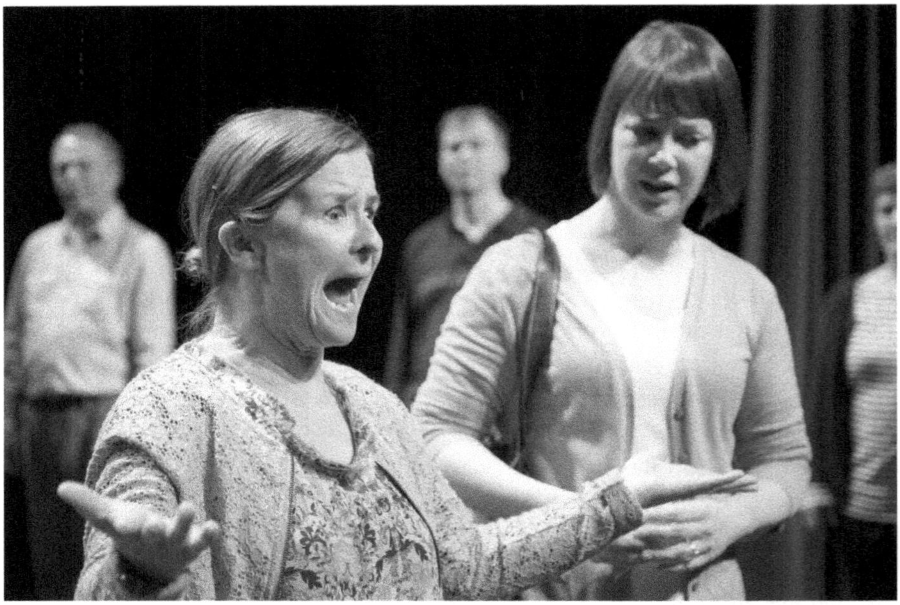

FIGURE 14.1 Administrative hoops in *Cracked*. Foreground L–R: Claire Frances Muir, Lori Nancy Kalamanski. Background L–R: Alan K. Sapp, Tim Machin, Mary Ellen MacLean. Photo by Kelly Kruschel.

transcripts. These 'directed rounds' were like tiny sketches. Sometimes this involved playing out a scene based on the idea or quote without using any language, only bodies and gestures, which might inspire a new idea or an expansion of the scene to try out. I found it interesting how the actors would experiment with different physical aspects of what they imagined of the participants of the research, an imaginative experimentation with voice, breath, gait, gestures. This helped me to see the embodiment and experiences of PLWD in a new way. That was unexpected for me.

In reflecting on our process, I also value how inclusive it was. We as researchers were fully included in the theatrical devising process, but that inclusivity extended to the actors as well, as they were fully immersed in the research that informed the process. I was pleased we were able to arrange for the actors to spend a day in a residential aged care setting interacting with the residents, staff and family. We also had a one-day interactive community arts-based research workshop with PLWD, their care partners, visual artists, and all of the actors and researchers on the team. This provided a unique and creative opportunity for all of us to explore the implications of the tragedy discourse about dementia, and learn from PLWD what they want the world to know about them and their experiences that would challenge the tragedy discourse. These experiences and our discussions about them were powerful in how they highlighted the humanity of PLWD – their humour, creativity, joy, expressed preferences – and also how unsupported PLWD and their family members feel by broader social and health systems, including practices embedded within them. We all were changed after that day.

PK: The ways that stigma is reproduced in the organization and delivery of care was something we discussed and explored a lot. One of the actors brought forward an improvisation based on research I had published about the discordant interrelationship between dementia care practitioners' reflective deliberations and legislative and organizational care mandates.[8] The example was the rules in residential aged care settings against using terms of endearment like 'sweetie' since these are presumed to violate the rights of the residents, despite instances where use of such terms are the expressed preference of residents. The scene involved an actor portraying a healthcare practitioner sitting in a chair in the centre of the stage as two other actors circled around her and questioned her about what she called a resident. It was funny how the interrogators' exaggerated, serious voices and dramatic movements, pointing dramatically and lifting their chins in righteous indignation, were spoofing the film noir style of filmmaking and acting. Their overzealous passion about the imposition of policy regulation and triumph in ultimately getting a confession – 'ha HA! You DID call her sweetie!' – playfully poked fun at this absurdity in practice.

IV. PRODUCTIVE TENSION AND HUMOUR IN *CRACKED*

SD: We came to call these taken-for-granted and inhumane care practices and social policies in care settings 'absurdities'. It was no easy process to figure out how to tackle them in the play without suggesting that we were blaming any particular individuals or reproducing the harms of these policies. In fact, I recall a tension arising in one of our theatrical devising sessions over this. It's hard to forget. You had brought in an article for us all to discuss by cultural gerontologist Julia Twigg, who critiques the clothing regimes in residential aged care setting that standardize modes of dress with polyester easycare fabrics which afford little in the way of style and tactile pleasure.[9] The next time we came together the

[8] Pia Kontos, Karen-Lee Miller and Gail Mitchell, 'Dementia Care at the Intersection of Regulation and Reflexivity: A Critical Realist Perspective', *Journals of Gerontology Series B: Psychological Sciences and Social Sciences* 66B, no. 1 (2010): 119–28.

[9] Standardized clothing of this kind uses only textiles high in artificial fibre, which are often harsh, scratchy and unabsorbent, that can survive the high temperatures of the industrial-sized washing machines. Twigg argues that this standardization restricts residents' expressivity, agency and choice

actors shared a rough sketch that involved a person entering a residential aged care setting. She is approached by a staff person who takes away her purse, her coat and other personal items as part of the admission process. Other residents shuffle in and form a line-up that the new person joins, and they are then spray washed by the staff person, with sound effects and robotic movements evocative of a conveyor belt in a factory. It created a lot of discomfort; there was silence after the actors performed the sketch and then one of the researchers said, horrified, 'I can't believe you made this.' It took some time to talk through what was happening since it wasn't immediately clear to any of us why there was such discomfort with the sketch.

PK: As we talked through the tension, it became clear that what made the scene offensive was that the sketch might have been going too far in how it reproduced the tragedy discourse. It didn't seem to be critiquing it. Having a safe space for that discussion was critical. I recall Julia [Gray] saying that we needed to be able to share things that are rough and difficult, and we needed to be able to respond to these things with the trust that we are all working in good faith. Without the relationships we had developed and nurtured with each other, and without that safe space, we never would have had those conversations or learnings. We had to take real care in how we represented these 'absurdities', and *Cracked* was better because of it.

We decided to return to rounds to explore other ways we might reflect how personhood is threatened in residential aged care settings. In the resulting scene, we see Elaine being assisted with putting oversized and shapeless grey sweatpants on over her more tailored pants to signal her admittance to a residential aged care setting and symbolize the restriction of expressivity, agency, and choice that this so commonly entails. This allowed us to include the element from the original sketch of how policies and practices threaten personhood, in a way that invoked discomfort and concern without offence. A staff participant in our evaluation of the impact of *Cracked* said about this scene, 'It bothered me because it didn't seem like something that she was comfortable in, something that she would wear … It was like wrapping somebody up in a potato sack and, like oppressing them somehow.'

There were other devices that we drew on to critique policies that constrain compassionate care, satirizing those policies and showing them for the absurdities they are. I loved how we poked fun at the administrative hoops in residential aged care settings that family members need to jump through to take their

(Julia Twigg, 'Clothing and Dementia: A Neglected Dimension?', *Journal of Aging Studies* 24, no. 4 (2010): 223–30).

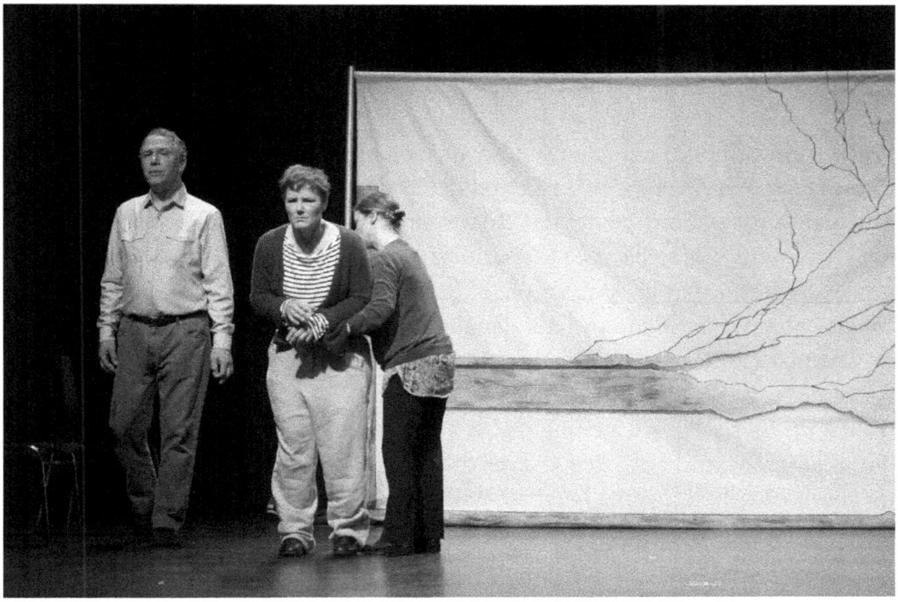

FIGURE 14.2 Sweatpants in *Cracked*. L–R: Alan K. Sapp, Mary Ellen MacLean, Claire Frances Muir. Photo by Kelly Kruschel.

loved one out for lunch, and the strict rules about how staff can acknowledge or celebrate residents' birthdays. So it was good that we worked through the initial tension and figured out how we could critique policies we think are harmful without reproducing the harm.

SD: The production was definitely better because of those conflicts and how we worked through them collaboratively. Having the feedback of PLWD, family members and healthcare practitioners on the developing scenes throughout our creative process also ensured that the scenes would resonate with audience members.

I also loved how we used humour, and not just in the context of critiquing ill-fitting policies. I'm thinking of how humour is evoked in *Cracked* in juxtaposing the tragedy discourse of dementia with joy. PLWD often talk about the importance of humour in living well with dementia. For example, when Elaine joins an advocacy group to lobby for policy changes to address stigma, the group sings their upbeat, joyful theme song for her:

> We've got dementia
> If you get it too
> We can get lost together

The places we can go
The things that we can do
With dementia

Our research on the impact of *Cracked* has highlighted the power of humour to bring joy – and with it surprise and defamiliarization, given how unexpected this is in a play about dementia. Participants talked about how important the use of humour was to balance the seriousness of the play and the deep emotions it triggered. Another great example of this juxtaposition of joy-tragedy is a conversation between Elaine and her daughter where Elaine asks 'where's Frank?' – forgetting that her husband died some time ago. Concerned not to upset Elaine, Caroline conveys the information figuratively by pointing upwards, saying, 'Dad's up there. He's watching us.' It's so funny when Elaine looks up, bursts out in laughter, and says, 'It's just death … it's just coming. Don't get so worked up about it!' – juxtaposing laughter with death. I think these moments of levity also helped audience members to envision hopefulness. One audience member commented, 'I did get the feeling like there was light at the end of the tunnel.'

PK: That is such a funny scene, and I too was struck by the hopefulness that audiences were able to envision. That example demonstrates the extraordinary power of theatrical devices – movement, humour, timing, voice and so on – to shift the tragedy narrative of dementia from loss and decline to hope and new possibilities. There are lots of other great examples of how we drew on the resources of drama to deepen engagement. The 'Tick Tock' scene is a powerful one, when the actors position themselves in a straight line facing the audience and together sing numbers ('1, 2, 3, 4, 5, 6, 7') while moving their arms like the hands of a clock. Elaine steps forward from the line and goes through the motions of being tested for dementia by drawing a clock and counting backwards from one hundred by multiples of seven. Her increasing frustration with not being able to complete the test is amplified by the singing, which begins to fragment into different harmonies, and the actors' gradually more confusing, erratic movements. The scene ends with Elaine facing the audience asking in frustration: 'What does this all mean anyway?'

Many PLWD have shared with us their frustrations with the diagnosis process, including how long it takes and their experiences with the Mini Mental State Exam (MMSE). With the MMSE they specifically mention the clock drawing exercise and counting backwards from hundred by sevens. They describe the shame they feel when they stumble or fail the exercise, and the sadness and confusion they experience when told to go home and get their affairs in order – essentially to go home and prepare to die – instead of being provided with resources to support them. We had so many discussions about these various

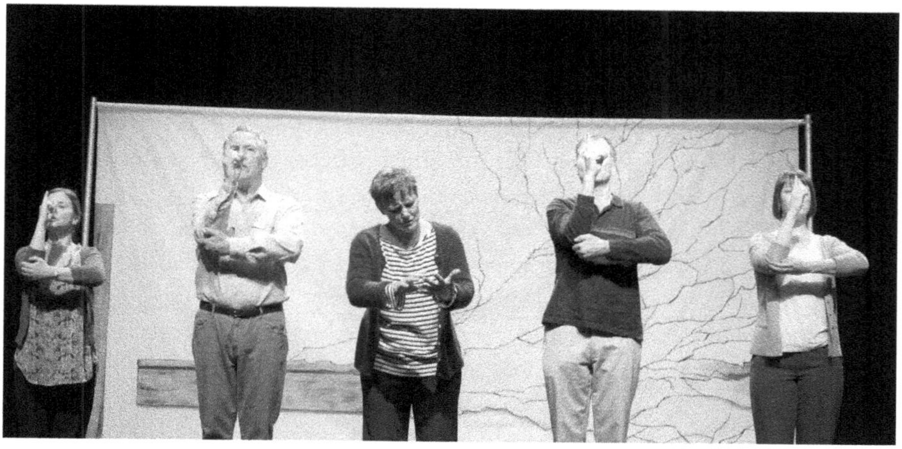

FIGURE 14.3 Counting backwards from one hundred by sevens in *Cracked*. L–R: Claire Frances Muir, Alan K. Sapp, Mary Ellen MacLean, Tim Machin, Lori Nancy Kalamanski. Photo by Kelly Kruschel.

aspects of the screening and diagnosis processes for dementia, and felt it was important to use the play to foster critical reflection and dialogue about these harmful practices.

SD: It was interesting to read in our data how participants sensed that the confusion in the 'Tick Tock' scene was intentional. Many audience members described how that scene helped them to imagine not only what the diagnosis process must be like, but what dementia must feel like for people living with it. It was exciting to hear from audience members how they placed themselves directly in the scenes, trying to sort out for themselves how they might respond in those situations, and in doing so how they were participating in the play by imaginatively co-constructing its meaning. Their experience engendered empathy. One participant was struck by Elaine breaking the fourth wall to talk about her challenges living with dementia: 'They would show just the [PLWD] themselves … talking to the audience … it just gave an insight on what dementia really does for them.' Audiences were immersed, and this is what allowed them to 'see' differently.

V. IMPACTING AUDIENCES

PK: The aesthetics of *Cracked* were essential not only for engagement but for transformation. We saw so much change in understanding and in practice, both immediately following seeing a performance of *Cracked*, and also twelve months afterwards. What are some examples that stand out for you?

SD: Oh my goodness, there are so many. *Cracked* provided an opportunity for audience members to hear the perspectives of PLWD, to hear their words taken directly from our research transcripts. This awakened audience members to the relational nature of care and the interconnections between PLWD, their family members and friends, and the ways relational processes and broader relational patterns shape experiences of dementia in profound ways.

Audience members talked about seeing beyond the disease to the whole person in their life context, not just people with an incurable illness but as vibrant, relational, sexual beings with a life history and a future. Healthcare practitioners talked about seeing the family for the first time, recognizing the complex family dynamics involved and the ways that they have judged family members. They also shared how they were now seeing broader relational patterns, including their own role as well as the ways in which organizational rules, structures, current outcome measures and policies limit relational caring. I especially loved how participants in our research reflected on the hopefulness that they saw woven throughout *Cracked*, and the possibilities for living well with dementia that were conveyed. I will never forget a comment made by a PLWD after a performance in a residential aged care setting attended by residents, family members and staff. This person shared that she had not told anyone except immediate family members about her diagnosis of dementia and then confidently stated, 'I will no longer hide.' She added: 'This is a play about coming out.' Family members and staff saw that there is life after a diagnosis of dementia, and that they have a role to play in supporting it.

PK: These changes in understanding were key to changes in action and expanding the relational literacies of audience members. Audience members were able to imagine and describe, even months after seeing the play, how they would or had already implemented new ways of relating to and being with PLWD, their family members and other staff members. This included being more attentive to the feelings of the PLWD and their family members, being less judgemental, slowing down and being less task-oriented, including PLWD in decision-making, attending to the ways PLWD express themselves and communicate their experiences through their bodies, finding ways to bring joy and meaning to life, recognizing the reciprocities in care and what they get out of caring for others, and being attuned to when colleagues might need support. A particular quote that stands out for me is when a staff member was asked what they might do differently after engaging with *Cracked*: 'Just take a little more time, try not to assume, "Oh, they've got dementia, I know what that's like", and realizing I have no idea what that's like.' Instead of making assumptions about life with dementia, they talked about how they would work hard to understand what was going on from the perspectives of people living with it. They also shared how they now value meaningful connections with PLWD: 'If I'm either running late or if something happens … I'm still going to have that conversation and build, you know … a connection.'

SD: I also get excited about the commitments audience members make to being leaders and strong advocates for the change that is desperately needed in dementia care. We have seen this with administrators of residential aged care settings who have come up to us after seeing a performance and shared that they have the kinds of policies that we critique in the play. They then talk about how they will work with their staff to change those policies; that the play motivated such immediate action is exactly what we wanted to happen.

PK: We also see this commitment in the comments made by other staff members as they see the role they can play in not only advocating for PLWD but also for change for themselves. I remember one quote particularly clearly: 'Whether it's the employee who is trying to ask for that kind of culture change or the broader public, our institutions and our policies come from us. There's something in us that is allowing these things to happen culturally, in the broader culture … We need to advocate for ourselves and for the shift in culture that needs to take place.'

SD: We have also seen in our research that *Cracked* is not always effective for everyone. I think this speaks to how entrenched the tragedy and medical discourses of dementia are in our society and healthcare sector, the embeddedness of certain policies and practices in dementia care, and the certainty of knowledge that is held by some healthcare practitioners. For example, I remember one staff member reflecting on a scene in the play where we critique the absurdity of one-size-fits-all policies and approaches. This scene was inspired by an example described by one of my doctoral students in her research where she found a written policy in a residential aged care setting that aimed to standardize how birthdays were to be celebrated in this particular setting. After seeing *Cracked*, this staff member fervently supported the need for such policies, stating that they could not possibly support the desires and wishes of every resident. They no doubt felt powerless and constrained by the conditions that limit relational approaches and the tailoring of care to the individual preferences of residents; low staffing levels, heavy workloads and emotional exhaustion are just some of these. I remember that this saddened me because of the sense of defiant surrender that was reflected.

PK: This certainly speaks to the hopelessness that practitioners can feel because of the conditions of care that constrain them and their ability to imagine that things could be different. But I think this can also be attributed, at least for some audience members, to their preference for more linear translation of the research than aesthetic interpretation. Reflecting on the 'Tick Tock' scene, while some audience members intuited that the confusion this scene created was intentional – that it was related to how someone living with dementia might experience the assessment process – others experienced the confusion negatively, and this no doubt mitigated the impact of the scene for them. The expectation and preference for more linear translation was also evident in how some audience members literally interpreted heightened theatrical techniques. For instance, some people mistook our humorous depiction of the absurdities of some policies in residential aged care settings as a critique of individual administrators and practitioners; there were some health practitioners who felt we were demonizing these individuals, and by extension them. This too would mitigate impact, particularly any positive transformation.

SD: That the overwhelming majority of audience members and participants from our evaluation of *Cracked* did still engage in aesthetic interpretation speaks to the power of a 'performance aesthetic',[10] and the importance of this for countering traditional modes of engagement (e.g. publications, didactic lectures/workshops) and to fostering critical reflection and culture change.

PK: I totally agree. When theatre and critical health research meet, there's the potential to challenge taken-for-granted understandings and open a space to envision and effect new possibilities. I do believe that this is why *Cracked* is well positioned to respond to urgent calls for culture change, which include reducing the stigma associated with dementia and promoting inclusive and meaningful engagement of PLWD across all levels of society.

SD: What a wonderfully rich conversation this has been. It inspires me to think about our next theatre production!

PK: For me as well. And I do hope it inspires our readers too.

REFERENCES

Basting, Anne Davis. *Forget Memory*. Johns Hopkins University Press, 2009.

Collective Disruption. 'Cracked: new light on dementia'. In *ReView: An Anthology of Plays Committed to Social Justice*, edited by Julia Gray. SensePublishers, 2017.

Denzin, Norman K. *Performance Ethnography: Critical Pedagogy and the Politics of Culture*. Sage Publications, 2003.

[10] Norman K. Denzin, *Performance Ethnography: Critical Pedagogy and the Politics of Culture* (Sage Publications, 2003), 93.

Dupuis, Sherry L., Pia Kontos, Gail Mitchell, Christine Jonas-Simpson and Julia Gray. 'Re-claiming Citizenship Through the Arts'. *Dementia: The International Journal of Social Research and Practice* 15, no. 3 (2016): 358–80.
Gray, Julia. 'After the Crash: A Play About Brain Injury'. *Canadian Theatre Review* 146 (2011): 66–86.
Gray, Julia, Helen Donnelly and Barbara E. Gibson. 'Seriously Foolish and Foolishly Serious: The Art and Practice of Clowning in Children's Rehabilitation'. *Journal of Medical Humanities* 42 (2021): 453–69.
Greene, Maxine. *Releasing the Imagination: Essays on Education, the Arts, and Social Change*. JosseyBass, 1995.
Kontos, Pia, Karen-Lee Miller and Alexis P. Kontos. 'Relational Citizenship: Supporting Embodied Selfhood and Relationality in Dementia Care'. *Sociology of Health & Illness* 39, no. 2 (2017): 182–98.
Kontos, Pia, Karen-Lee Miller and Gail Mitchell. 'Dementia Care at the Intersection of Regulation and Reflexivity: A Critical Realist Perspective'. *Journals of Gerontology Series B: Psychological Sciences and Social Sciences* 66B, no. 1 (2010): 119–28.
Mitchell, Gail, Sherry L. Dupuis and Pia Kontos. 'Dementia Discourse: From Imposed Suffering to Knowing Other-wise'. *Journal of Applied Hermeneutics* (2013). http://jah.journalhosting.ucalgary.ca/jah/index.php/jah/article/view/41.
Mitchell, Gail, Sherry L. Dupuis, Pia Kontos, Christine Jonas-Simpson and Julia Gray. 'Disrupting Dehumanising and Intersecting Patterns of Modernity with a Relational Ethic of Caring'. *International Practice Development Journal* 10, no. 1 (2020). https://doi.org/10.19043/ipdj.101.002.
Twigg, Julia. 'Clothing and Dementia: A Neglected Dimension?' *Journal of Aging Studies* 24, no. 4 (2010): 223–30.

15

Beyond the cost of care: Connection, disability and embodied reciprocity in Martyna Majok's *Cost of Living* (2018)

KATHERINE WILLIAMS

> I like to think of theatre as a place of communication and exploration, of dissent and inquiry: a place of dreaming, of solving, of challenging the present and imagining the future. It's that communal place where we can express all the possibilities of what it is to be human – so why are the majority of representations still so limited in scope and variety, and the potential of those bodies so prescribed?
>
> (Kaite O'Reilly, prologue to *The 'd' Monologues*)

Disabled Irish playwright Kaite O'Reilly has made a career of championing the theatrical possibilities of unlikely bodyminds, a portmanteau in critical disability studies that marks how demands for ablebodiedness and ablemindedness converge.[1]

[1] See Margaret Price, 'The Bodymind Problem and the Possibilities of Pain', *Hypatia* 30, no. 1 (2015): 268–84.

Reflecting on her decades of scripting and making theatre with and for disabled and Deaf artists, the question she poses in the epigraph above reframes the theatre's artistic potential around a pointed observation about the limited range of embodiments that inform representations.[2] Despite the presence of disabled people, and despite the theatre's possibilities for 'challenging the present and imagining the future', representations of disability and engagement with disabled actors are still deeply 'limited in scope and variety'. This capacity to 'express all the possibilities of what it is to be human' suggests how dramatic representations of disability can open up inquiries at the intersection of medicine and theatre, to gesture to this volume's focus. By taking up Martyna Majok's *Cost of Living*, this chapter considers the complex representation of disability as a multifaceted embodied knowledge that goes beyond diagnosis. If the interactions between patient and caregiver may be understood as an ensemble drama, *Cost of Living* foregrounds disabled embodiment as a resource for theorizing human exchanges of care and empathetic identification beyond the necessity of work. Images of caregiving in literary and dramatic depictions range from the utopic (think: Annie Sullivan in *The Miracle Worker*) to the dystopic (think: Nurse Ratched in *One Flew over the Cuckoo's Nest*). Beyond these two poles of fantasy, however, the play's investment in realism foregrounds embodied interaction, refusing a strict binary between non-disabled caregiver and disabled recipient of care. Illuminating how the support required in daily life may offer a vibrant site of reciprocal connection between non-disabled and disabled people, Majok's play also stages the frictions and disparities that threaten fragile connections across lived experience.

My chapter begins with O'Reilly's insistence on opening up theatrical exploration to disabled bodyminds to frame an extended reading of the play because *Cost of Living* features a cast comprised equally of disabled and non-disabled actors. The play premiered at the Williamstown Theatre Festival in 2016, won the Pulitzer Prize for Drama in 2018 and debuted on Broadway in 2022. The play's extraordinary acclaim and successful production history testifies to the significance of foregrounding disability as a facet of experience central to human life. In this chapter, I examine the play alongside insights from actors Gregg Mozgala and Regan Linton who helped to shape in development and even originate (in Mozgala's case) the play's two disabled characters, given that the playwright is non-disabled and incorporated their insights into her artistic craft.[3] Taking up questions of theatrical embodiment from the perspective of critical disability studies, I consider how the play leverages theatrical performance to reshape what disability can mean. Tobin Siebers suggests that

---

[2] Kaite O'Reilly, Prologue to *The 'd' Monologues* (Oberon Books, 2018), 8.

[3] Gregg Mozgala and Regan Linton and I have been working together in The Apothetae Residency at The Public Theater (NYC) since 2023. During this time, I conducted the interviews quoted in this chapter and engaged in informal conversations related to *Cost of Living*.

'disability acquires aesthetic value because it represents for makers of art a critical resource for thinking about what a human being is'; for Siebers, the aesthetic value of disability – or how crafting representations of disability expands the possibility for artistic representations of human experience – means that artistic representation 'enlarges our vision of human variation and difference'.[4] By putting two disabled actors onstage to play two disabled characters, Majok mobilizes theatrical conventions of embodied performance to uncover representational possibilities. While stories about disability in the dominant culture often imagine disability as a site of pity or tragedy, the play insists on the specificity and humanity of its disabled characters, refusing to reduce disability to tropes of diagnosis or cure. *Cost of Living* foregrounds the economic pressures of care and the difficulty of human connection; despite glimpses of possibility the disabled characters are ultimately left behind. The play ends with a focus on the non-disabled characters – a conclusion that threatens to undercut the gorgeous complexity of its disability representations.

One of the epigraphs to *Cost of Living*, from Andre Dubus's book of essays, *Broken Vessels*, asserts that the ordinary act of partaking in a communal meal 'is a sacrament which says: I know you will die; I am sharing food with you; it is all I can do, and it is everything'.[5] The play's opening emphasis on 'sacrament' highlights the invitation to shared vulnerability. Fittingly for this lyrical emphasis on reciprocal exchange, the play follows two couples brought together by the labour of care. In the first character dyad, Ani negotiates life with a newly acquired disability; as a quadriplegic, she is caught in the fraught necessity of dependence on her ex-husband Eddie, a former truck driver, who fills the gap when her assigned aide fails to show. Taking on the role of personal care assistant, Eddie evokes unavoidable reminders of their past. A second strand of the play follows John, a wealthy graduate student with cerebral palsy, who employs Jess, a young woman, as a personal care assistant until the economic logic of work collides with class boundaries and the embodied intimacy of care.

The casting note at the beginning of the play – 'Please cast disabled actors in the roles of John and Ani' (5) – insists that the scripting of disabled characters necessitates disabled actors whose physical presence transforms what disability can mean in the theatre by insisting that disability must be imagined in the theatre in the first place. A vibrant strand of scholarship on disability performance has shown how, in the theatre, visible disability is overdetermined because disability is so often understood as a metaphor or, in David T. Mitchell

---

[4] Tobin Siebers, *Disability Aesthetics* (University of Michigan Press, 2010), 3.

[5] Quoted in Martyna Majok, *Cost of Living* (Dramatists Play Service, 2018), 7. All further quotations from the play are taken from this edition and cited parenthetically in the text.

and Sharon L. Snyder's terms, a 'device of characterization'.[6] In the theatre, disabled characters are almost always played by non-disabled actors who are 'cripping up', or what Samuel Yates calls 'disability simulation'; as a result, spectators typically interpret dramatic characters through the knowledge that they are played by non-disabled actors.[7] Although disability is a complex lived experience, as Rosemarie Garland-Thomson writes, 'representation frequently obscures these complexities in favour of the rhetorical or symbolic potential of the prototypical disabled figure, who often functions as a lightning rod for the pity, fear, discomfort, guilt, or sense of normalcy' of onstage and offstage audiences.[8] Glossing this passage twenty years later, Petra Kuppers underscores how much remains true about audience expectations: 'Disabled characters become foils; they enter into narrative functions that diminish their own complexity.'[9] Disabled characters, in other words, serve stories that are not actually about disability; they often serve as a symbol for deficit – what must be overcome, grappled with, or fixed.

Chief among these 'narrative functions' is what Alison Kafer calls the 'curative imaginary', a key tenet of what the disability rights movement identified as the 'medical model' of disability: the idea that disability can only be imagined as a deficit in need of a correction or intervention.[10] The medical model of disability – and here disability theorists are careful to distinguish the concept from the lived reality of engaging with and benefitting from medical expertise to ameliorate pain or heighten quality of life – understands disability as the tragedy of an individual bodymind rather than as an aspect of identity and valuable human experience. The 'curative imaginary' that derives from a notion of disability as deficit can only imagine some future rehabilitation rather than valuing disability as a lived experience in the present. Writing about what he calls the 'ideology of cure' as it has shaped his lived experience with cerebral palsy, Eli Clare notes that ideas of cure position disability as 'damage, locating the harm entirely within individual body-minds', since the ideology of cure 'seeks to return what is damaged to its former state of being'. Yet in many cases (such as his own), 'an

---

[6] David T. Mitchell and Sharon L. Snyder, *Narrative Prosthesis: Disability and the Dependencies of Discourse* (University of Michigan Press, 2014), 9.

[7] Samuel Yates, 'Choreographing Confinement: *Side Show*'s Fleshy Fixations and Disability Simulation', *Studies in Musical Theatre* 13, no. 1 (2019): 67–78, 68. Much recent critical work at the intersection of disability and performance explores this conundrum. See, for example, Petra Kuppers, *Theatre and Disability* (Palgrave Macmillan, 2017), esp. 11–12; and 'Drama, Theatrical Performance, and Disability', ed. Ann M. Fox and Carrie Sandahl, *Journal of Literary & Cultural Disability Studies* 12, no. 2 (2018): 121–247.

[8] Rosemary Garland-Thomson, *Extraordinary Bodies: Figuring Physical Disability in American Literature and Culture* (Columbia University Press, 1997), 15.

[9] Kuppers, *Theatre and Disability*, 13.

[10] Alison Kafer, *Feminist Queer Crip* (Indiana University Press, 2013), 28.

original nondisabled state of being doesn't exist'; the present therefore becomes a kind of limbo, as if a disabled life is on hold indefinitely.[11] The 'curative imaginary' means that there may be popular support for cure-focused fundraising for medical research, but popular opposition to changes in the built environment (such as the enforcement of building access codes to install ramps). This refusal to value disabled life in the present is, as Kafer puts it, a 'curative temporality', which insists that 'the only appropriate disabled body/mind is one cured or moving toward cure', prompting questions like: 'Were you born that way? How much longer do you have to live this way? How long before they invent a cure? How long will a cure take? How soon before you recover?'[12]

Against a framework of diagnosis (what do you have?) or cure (when will you recover?) that prioritizes a non-disabled future, *Cost of Living* sets its disability representation in the experience of daily life. Majok scripted the roles of Ani and John for disabled actors, whose distinctive embodiments inform the theatrical pyrotechnics of their characters. By foregrounding disability representations and scripting roles for disabled actors – challenging the assumption that the non-disabled actors are merely 'playing disabled', in Kuppers's formulation – *Cost of Living* contests the belief that disability is an unquestioned deficit.[13] The play evokes the capacity of new theatrical representations to challenge the curative imaginary that finds disabled people merely waiting out their disability. As Ann M. Fox argues,

> The play's exploration of care and connection is mitigated through disability; but here, disability does not become the obvious reason for and symbol of isolation. Instead, the play suggests that human isolation (and its attendant causes such as racism, sexism, classism, and xenophobia) cannot be ameliorated without being explored and addressed in ways specifically informed by the knowledge and experiences of disabled people.[14]

Fox brilliantly limns how the play challenges the assumption that disability is the obstacle to human connection, gesturing to how *Cost of Living* allows the disabled characters to complicate ideas about disability introduced by their non-disabled caregiver even as it depicts the necessity and even asymmetry of care. The play represents disabled characters and casts disabled actors while also

---

[11] Eli Clare, *Brilliant Imperfection: Grappling With Cure* (Duke University Press, 2017), 15. On cure as a site of potentially harmful intervention, see also Eunjung Kim, *Curative Violence: Rehabilitating Disability, Gender, and Sexuality in Modern Korea* (Duke University Press, 2017).
[12] Kafer, *Feminist Queer Crip*, 28.
[13] Kuppers, *Theatre and Disability*, 16.
[14] Ann M. Fox, 'Staging the Complexities of Care: Martyna Majok's *Cost of Living*', *Journal of Literary & Cultural Studies* 12, no 2 (2018): 146, https://doi.org/10.3828/jlcds.2018.12.

highlighting disability representations as inevitably social, a matter of interaction with the world including non-disabled characters, played by non-disabled actors. In doing so, it rescripts collective possibilities for attuning audiences to acts of care in the present, with its attendant frictions and joy, rather than deferring to a curative imaginary in which disabled figures are oriented toward future cure.

This first account of the play in my chapter has foregrounded the disabled characters, but there is another way to narrate the plot. The play opens with a long monologue from Eddie, who waits in a bar in Brooklyn while he grieves his ex-wife, Ani, who has died – a death that seems both sudden and recent. The play closes with Eddie welcoming Jess, who was preparing to sleep in her car on a freezing night after she has fled her position as personal care assistant, into the temporary shelter of his home. Between the opening and the closing scenes, we see disabled and non-disabled characters argue, joke and flirt with each other, moving through conflict to intimacy and back again. Yet if the dramatic structure of the play runs from Eddie's loss to a tentative celebration of the fragile care that human beings offer to each other, it is also true that the play uses only the non-disabled caregivers to trace that arc of connection, for the disabled characters never appear outside their homes, and only one lives beyond the end of the play. Ultimately, *Cost of Living* cannot depict disabled characters embracing full lives, capacitated by the care they require – as if the most important aspect of caregiving is the opportunity for empathy such an exchange presents for those who undertake the action.

As this doubled description suggests, my reading of the play's representations of disability is decidedly ambivalent. Like other critics, I find that there is much to celebrate in the play's complex representation of disabled experience. While Fox grants that the disabled characters 'function as narrative catalysts to bring Eddie and Jess together, conveniently disappearing at the play's end', she also insists that the play offers a reminder, 'through the care occasioned by disability, that connecting across identities, including disability, is vital in order to counteract larger systemic oppression'.[15] Building on this insight, I would add that beyond representational content that makes disability central to the play's depiction of social structures, the commitment to authentic casting of disabled actors, who comprise half the cast, models genuinely new possibilities for staging disability. As I explore below, the disability experiences of the actors themselves inform characterizations that offer fresh and specific insights into lived experience. Thus I am aligned with Fox's trenchant observation that 'bodily precarity has a complex and compelling representation in *Cost of Living* not in spite of, but because of disability'.[16]

[15] Ibid., 159.
[16] Ibid., 160.

Yet I also find that critical attention has not fully grappled with how a play might not only employ but rescript possibilities for disabled characters. Some of these possibilities, such as John's invitation to Jess to rethink her own experience of embodiment by encountering his distinctive body, expand the horizons for imagining disability; other dimensions of the disability representations, such as the bathing scene between Ani and Eddie, depart from lived experience to confirm a sense of disability as threat. Majok's scripting practices, as I have noted, orient spectators to the specific embodiments of disabled actors to create new dimensions of characterization. For this reason, by attending to the experiences of disabled artists, I want to insist that it is important to note the play's departures from lived experience too, reading briefly against the grain of the play's embrace of vulnerability as a shared point of connection between disabled and non-disabled people. Ultimately, by tracing the refusal of a curative imaginary of *Cost of Living*, I ask what difference the embodied register of performance – specifically, the virtuosity of the disabled artist – makes for the theatre's representation of disability. And, consequently, how does the play invite spectators to imagine (or not) disability beyond the register of cost? While the play's refusal to stay with the disabled characters troubles the ending, by emphasizing care rather than cure, staging human interdependence and resisting the dominant conception of disability as relegating people to a temporal and existential limbo – a half-life of dependence – the play suggests generative possibilities for moving beyond a biomedical framework to understand disability as an opportunity for powerful connection in the realms of both theatre and medicine.

JOHN AND JESS: THE WORK OF CARE

Midway through *Cost of Living*, a scene invites spectators to witness the apparently unremarkable act of bathing. Scene 5 is set in the Princeton apartment where John resides; a wheelchair user and graduate student, he lives independently. His entrance in Scene 1, in fact, described him as '*beautiful. John has cerebral palsy. A kind of halted way of speaking. Otherwise, he is determinedly polished. Comes from wealth and wears it, undeniably*' (18), while Jess is the '*First generation child of an immigrant. Does not come from wealth, nor does she try to seem it*' (17). Given the distinctive register of their class differences, the play tracks their early negotiations and then, by the middle of the play, lingers on an embodied spectacle that is both intimate and routine. Scene 5 opens with an extended stage direction, which I reproduce here in full to foreground how the play evokes the embodied act of care between these figures:

Jess showers John.
We watch the entire act.
It takes as long as it needs.

Jess wheels John into the shower.
She helps lift him from his wheelchair onto his shower seat.
How this happens: John embraces Jess, who he uses as support.
Jess holds on to John as he pushes himself up and pivots on his toes from the wheelchair to the shower seat.
She undresses him completely.
She runs the water.
Tests it on herself.
Tests it on his arm.
He nods if it's okay.
She washes his hair.
She soaps his body and rinses it off.

Jess picks up a conversation she began earlier.
There is more ease between the two now. (50)

The script insists on a deliberate, unhurried realism in the act of showering – 'it takes as long as it needs' – which underscores the sense that this action is timed around the movement of the actual bodies onstage. The script evokes crip time, a temporality that 'bends the clock to meet disabled bodies', in Kafer's influential formulation.[17] In performance, the actions far outpace the time it takes to read the stage direction, but the lengthy described actions foreground how long the audience is asked to look at two bodies engaged in the daily act of care. Beyond simply putting a visibly disabled body on display, the play foregrounds the dependence required in this scene of care, as Jess initiates actions and John accedes to these actions.

Yet interdependence as a gift of human connection is palpable too. John requires physical care and Jess needs the money that this second job affords. She regales John with stories of bartending, a job that is virtually unimaginable to him not because of disability but because of his class status; when Jess offers an account of a terrible patron and observes, 'Man, fuck rich people. No offense but, heads on sticks' (51), John has no reply (the stage direction reads: '*A moment of silent showering*' (51)). Yet as John and Jess talk while she assists him, it becomes evident that their relationship has evolved beyond the economic logic of its origin to something like friendship, and that Jess has acquired a matter-of-fact acknowledgement that John's body merely demands a version of the labour that all bodies require – for they resume an ongoing conversation that ranges far beyond questions of disability. When Jess hands John the soapy washcloth for his genitals, the stage directions reassure the reader: '*It's*

[17] Kafer, *Feminist Queer Crip*, 27.

not awkward. Routine' (52) and '*The silence of task-doing*' (53). Theatre is an art that depends upon the bodies of actors, and the play moves this medium of embodiment into a distinctly private, even unfamiliar, place for the stage, using the setting of the bathroom to spark curiosity about the spectacle of the disabled body. At the same time, the stage directions frame this embodied encounter as a routine interaction, nothing unusual. The play makes the act of showering suddenly strange however, by presenting disabled embodiment in a setting that the presumptively non-disabled audience member might not expect – not in physical therapy or a medical procedure, but in the intimate space of the home. Yet even as the play depicts John's body as requiring special assistance, the language of the script enumerates these actions with the unremarkable clarity of habitual action. Consequently, although non-disabled spectators are aligned with Jess (the non-disabled character), the act of embodied care in which she engages with John renders this identification surprising.

The easy act of care in the shower scene is particularly pointed, given the play's earlier depiction of the first care interaction between John and Jess. *Cost of Living* ushers non-disabled spectators and readers into an exchange that turns medical symptoms into shared references for embodiment. In an earlier scene that foregrounds the awkward, high-stakes interactions of Jess's first day on the job, the play offers a vignette that blurs the line between actor and character through disability experience. When Jess becomes uncomfortable with John's forceful questions about her personal life, she rushes to begin her task and '*reaches carelessly for John's shirt, as if to undress him*'; as a result, '*the surprising, forceful contact causes John to spasm and splay*' (41). John's involuntary response asserts its own temporal register in performance. While his body enacts the 'spasm and splay' and then recovers from the muscle movement, he explains to Jess:

> My body –
> if you get too close, too fast –
>
> My body overprotects itself.
>
> Anytime I reach beyond myself,
> it's violence.
> You reach and you shake and
> it always feels beyond you.
> So you have to throw yourself – your
> arms, your hands – at what you want. (41)

The moment conflates the body of the actor and character in the virtuosic action of the spasm. In the long description that accompanies John's attempt to calm his body's involuntary movement, he turns to the 'you' to generalize about his experience ('you reach'; 'you shake'; 'it always feels beyond you'). From the possessive of 'my body', his use of the second-person pronoun displaces the action from his body to Jess's. His 'you', where there should be an 'I', occurs at the juncture of 'violence' and it functions to transform his experience into an invitation to his interlocutor. His automatic embodied response of the spasm, productively complicating the line between being and seeming, becomes a potential connection between characters, reorienting the power dynamics of the scene. Although Jess turns to the labour of undressing John to avoid personal connection, he reminds her that such an act of care, though it occurs within the economic transaction of a work relationship, can never be fully abstracted from the specific body of the disabled person. The embodied interaction of care is never neutral or fully objective.

This scene in the play, furthermore, was an addition built around the embodied knowledge that Mozgala, the actor who played John, brought to the role.[18] Majok originally wrote a one-act play, *John, Who's Here from Cambridge* (2015); in the transformation to *Cost of Living*, Mozgala encouraged Majok to add the scene, reasoning that the awkward and difficult interaction between disabled person and caregiver was missing from the arc of their relationship. As he recounted his conversation with Majok, Mozgala observed that he invited her to try out how such muscle tension might feel in her body: 'I described to her what the experience of having cerebral palsy is like in my body. I told her: flex your bicep and let it go, and then flex it again, and put your arm at your side, maintaining the same level of tension – that's the muscle tension I experience all the time.'[19] Just after the lines quoted above, John asks Jess, 'Have you ever been hit?' (41). Making explicit the 'violence' that he names as his experience of embodiment in a moment when his muscles seize up, John asserts: 'That's what it's like. Under my skin. From underneath my skin. Like people hitting me from beneath my skin' (41). 'Like being hit from the inside' (as Mozgala relayed it to me) is knowledge drawn from his own body that inflected the characterization. Across the length of the scene, John turns clinical symptoms – the muscle spasms associated with cerebral palsy – into Jess's, and perhaps the audiences', opportunity to recognize a similar feeling in her own body. Scripting the character's lines around the lived experience of the actor, the play uses the actor's disability experience to inform the character's expression of embodiment.

What I am suggesting here is that the play operates on a logic of characterization driven by what Siebers would call an instance of 'disability knowledges'.[20] This moment between Jess and John relies on the particularity of disability

---

[18] Interview with Gregg Mozgala, 2 April 2024.
[19] Ibid.
[20] Tobin Siebers, *Disability Theory* (University of Michigan Press, 2008), 122.

experience and stages a physical reaction that both is and is not a matter of acting – Mozgala's own involuntary physical response to his scene partner's startling movement offers a resource for theatre-making.[21] And, in the subsequent explanation, the disabled character translates the 'feeling' of cerebral palsy into language that might allow his non-disabled interlocutor and offstage audience to register something like the experience in their own bodies. Disability knowledge creates new possibilities for dramatic innovation – and moments like these enable the theatre to reshape ideas about disability and create imaginative connections between disabled and non-disabled people who share both onstage and offstage spaces.

ANI AND EDDIE: CARE AND THEATRICAL EMBODIMENT

Like the Jess and John plot, the Ani and Eddie plot originally existed as another one-act play, *Care*, before it comprised half of *Cost of Living*.[22] Although the play begins with Eddie's monologue, establishing that Ani has died, *Cost of Living* moves backward in time, introducing the two characters in the middle of an argument: the newly disabled Ani reluctantly allows Eddie, the ex from whom she is separated, to help her when her care assistant has failed to appear. Both figures are drawn as complex, funny, richly specific characters associated with a working-class northern New Jersey world: Eddie is '*an unemployed truck driver*' and Ani's description in the stage directions identifies her acquired disability with great specificity: '*in a wheelchair. Severe incomplete spinal cord injury. Quadriplegic. Though some of the fingers of one hand are partially functioning*' (25). Juxtaposed with the other character dyad, this plot strand flips the gender orientation of roles although it shares a similar concern with the economic demands of care. Ani's disability gestures to a lack of access to disability support services, although the play does not fully explore the specificity of these economic demands – there is no scene in which Ani attempts to navigate the labyrinthine demands of government assistance, though the two discuss insurance plans and the difficult surgeries that she has experienced. Yet the characters are brought together again by Ani's need for help and Eddie encounters her newly transformed life. In a scene that visually recapitulates the action of Jess bathing John, Eddie bathes Ani, and the work of care is inflected by the past intimacy between the two characters. Here, too, humour is a tool for destabilizing spectatorial expectations about disability.

[21] I have explored this idea elsewhere in relation to Mike Lew's play *Teenage Dick* and disability scripting: see Katherine Williams, 'Performing Shakespeare, Rewriting Disability', *Shakespeare Bulletin* 39, no. 4 (Winter 2021): 637–50.
[22] Interview with Mozgala.

While audiences may interpret Ani's first line – 'I fuckin hate this' (59) – as a reference to her acquired disability, her frustration snaps into focus as a lament about their failed marriage: 'Cuz it woulda been good to feel this before. To have had you do this kinda stuff with me before' (59). Although Ani's life is redefined by injury, she is preoccupied with Eddie's past behaviour; her acquired disability is not the affective locus of her exclamation here, as audiences might expect. As the scene proceeds, Ani and Eddie navigate her need for care in relation to their past intimacy and the shape of her present vulnerability; the play explores the currents of their anger, grief and disappointment as human beings.

Here, too, Majok's developmental work prioritized the disability knowledges that actors themselves brought to the role. At one point in the bathing scene, the stage direction reads: '*Eddie's hands in the water are doing something to Ani that she has loved for years. We should not know this has been happening until we hear how he talks to her –*' (62). In an earlier version of the script, actor Regan Linton noted, the subsequent dialogue established the limitations of disabled sex: when Eddie asks Ani whether she can feel him touching her, she replies in the negative. Linton, a paraplegic living with a spinal cord injury, is a wheelchair user and understudied the role of Ani for the Broadway production in addition to playing the role and engaging with the play in the development phase, drawing on her own experience. In conversation with Majok, Linton pointed out the range of possible sensory perceptions available to Ani in the context of an acquired disability. Rather than assuming that Ani's sexual desire and bodily perception was necessarily a binary, 'on or off' model of desire, or implying that Ani's current sensory capacity was permanent, the scripting could be more contingent and more accurately reflect the particularity of disability knowledges. Thus, in *Cost of Living*, Ani complicates her initial 'no': 'I'm not sayin I don't. Or I won't. I could' (62), and she asserts 'I feel that ... kind of feeling. It's just not on that part of my body' (62). Importantly, the actor's lived experience does not diminish but expands the possibilities for dramatic representation. The play, now sharper and more precise about embodied sensation through the disabled actor's own experience, offers a rendering of character newly attuned to the complexity of sexual experience.

Though my analysis focuses here on the disabled character in particular, I want to highlight the importance of reciprocity, following Fox's explication of the play's emphasis on connecting across isolation. As the play depicts Eddie's encounter with unexpected bodily intimacy beyond sex, disability is not just a matter for the disabled actor but a nuanced possibility for interaction with the non-disabled actor. This second bathing scene in *Cost of Living* is elongated, dwelling on the vulnerability of the disabled character receiving care from her ex-husband, and activating the memories of past intimacy in the fraught intimacy of bodily exposure. In the middle of it, Eddie departs for the kitchen while Ani remains; she '*sits with herself in the tub*' and utters a thought addressed to Eddie, who is offstage. When she, unthinking, turns her head to call out to him, the play punctuates theatrical time through a disability jump scare. The stage direction reads:

> *Suddenly, she slips down into the tub.*
> *Not intentional.*
> *Becomes submerged.*
> *We hear yelling from underwater.*
> *From off, we hear rummaging in the kitchen.*
> *Eventually, Eddie returns, holding a plate for an ashtray. He drops the plate and reaches into the tub to retrieve Ani. She gasps for air.*
> *He holds her against him.*
> *She gasps.* (70)

The scene ends with Ani's frantic protests in the terrified aftermath of rescue while Eddie comforts her: 'You can't leave me in the –' and 'You can't leave me in –' (70). In this bathtub scene, the theatre's capacity to simulate experience, the 'as if' that theatrical representation offers, implicates the real bodies in the room. The actual seconds ticking away for audience members are measured in the sound of Ani's flailing body in the water, as she struggles with limited capacity to lift herself up to breathe.

I saw the play at Manhattan Theatre Club (the Off-Broadway premiere) in 2017 and again on Broadway in 2022, and both times audience members around me gasped while watching this moment. Quick intakes of breath, audible expressions of surprise, one audience member half-rising from her seat as if to rescue the character: this moment intends to shock watchers into horrified awareness. If earlier in the scene non-disabled audience members are asked to think about what both Ani and Eddie have lost through Ani's acquired disability, this moment shifts the perspective through the feeling of threat it represents – or, more accurately, implies (since the actor is not visible in the tub, and the audience hears the character's struggle). The theatrical gimmick – a startlingly imaginative exploitation of the theatre's formal work with bodies – evokes existential threat.[23] Yet what I want to underscore is that the moment of identification with Ani depends upon understanding the experience of disability as one

[23] I have argued elsewhere that such a 'disabling', a moment of temporary fixing in which disability representation operates more like a verb than a noun, is foundational to the early modern theatre's use of disability as a formal aesthetic: see Katherine Schaap Williams, *Unfixable Forms: Disability, Performance, and the Early Modern English Theater* (Cornell University Press, 2021), esp. 1–22.

of both vulnerable exposure and stark helplessness: what would it feel like if it were *you* in the bathtub, unable to get out?

This question is one addressed to non-disabled audience members because it refuses the specificity of a disability knowledge of a quadriplegic. In a play that so deftly animates a sense of the fragility of human life, this moment of disability representation in *Cost of Living* crucially departs from lived experience. For starters, as Linton observes:

> Leaving Ani, a quadriplegic, alone in a bathtub where she could easily slip under the water is an amateur mistake. Anyone who has actually been quadriplegic, or cared for someone who is, would recognize this as a basic-level 'don't'. The fact that the character is in a clawfoot bathtub in the first place, and sitting upright without a support mechanism, is laughable. My quad friends could tell you the end result of a quad in a conventional bathtub is calling to the fire department to get out, and a conclusion of 'never again'.[24]

Linton observes that a further irony of the play's casting of Ani is that this moment requires significant hand dexterity, a capacity pointedly unavailable to Ani, who is scripted with very limited movement in one hand: 'Very few people with Ani's disability could actually be in the play because [the bathtub scene] is so dangerous.'[25] To be sure, many disabled people can navigate and enjoy the experience of a tub bath but Linton's point has broader implications for the play's insistence on disability and theatrical authenticity. This observation is not merely posing a question about 'realistic' scripting (why would Ani choose a tub rather than a sponge bath, and how does she get into the bathtub in the first place?) in a play that has foregrounded theatrical realism in the bath scenes. Nor does this objection only highlight the inaccessible conditions of the built environment of the theatre; Linton notes that there is no designated worker responsible for the backstage support of the disabled actor who requires assistance getting into and out of the bathtub in the scene, since the IATSE (The International Alliance of Theatrical Stage Employees, Moving Picture Technicians, Artists and Allied Crafts of the United States, Its Territories and Canada) contracts for stagehands do not cover disabled actor assistance. Although the play lays claim to a representational realism rooted in the rhetoric of 'authentic' casting, here the script abandons the disability knowledge of the actor to land a moment of spectacle.

---

[24] Regan Linton, 'Not My Disability Play', unpublished reflection, dated November 2022, 2.
[25] Interview with Regan Linton, 10 April 2024.

WHOSE COST?

Beyond the technical and formal problems of characterization, Ani's bathtub scene troubles the disability politics of vulnerability. For Linton, the question becomes: Who suffers from *Cost of Living*'s notion of disability as cost? Linton writes:

> The marketing of the show at Manhattan Theatre Club leaned heavily into storying the play around 'care', not disability. (Which in itself feels a bit ableist and afraid to name the hard fact that disability is the basis for the caregiving connection of the characters). But there, too, the play fails, painting care as mired in *cost*: loss, heartache, loneliness, and at worst, exploitation. These unfortunately *can* be realities of caregiving. But so, too, can joy. Connection. Growth. And deep love. Disability and caregiving are not solely experiences that cost ... much is gained through both.[26]

As Linton notes, the play's emphasis refuses to imagine that disability might be a benefit, an asset, an enhanced and expansive perspective on life. Instead, the economic language takes stock of 'the impact and effect that these relationships with disabled people have on the non-disabled caregivers'.[27] Linton's reading of the title underscores how the play upholds the sense that caregiving is primarily a burden to be avoided rather than a potential site of interdependence or connection. Thinking with Fox alongside Linton, we might also note that the final scene of the play suggests that Eddie and Jess are able to connect across difficulty precisely because they have been changed by their experiences of caregiving.

The nuanced disability representation and performance of care in Majok's play, which works both with and against the bodies of disabled actors, underscores the theatre's power to create representations that change how a concept – like 'disability' itself – may be understood. Locating the action in two domestic spheres marked by a contrast in economic status, the play offers a welcome challenge to the assumption that a disability play must be set in medical institution or structured by a curative imaginary. For both John and Ani, cure is the wrong way of thinking about the disability they experience in the present and foresee in the future; indeed, by going home with the disabled characters, audience members benefit from a disability representation that dwells on the likeliest quotidian scene of care: the daily act of being bathed.

The theatre's depiction of care demands that we ask what the cost of living without disability would look like, for Eddie and Jess, and for non-disabled

---

[26] Linton, 'Not My Disability Play', 2.
[27] Interview with Linton.

spectators outside the world of the play. *Cost of Living* charts new possibilities for disability representation to foreground the labour of disabled actors through authentic casting. Yet this depiction is no mere reduction of actor to disabled embodiment, as if the fact of their disabilities were the most important thing about John and Ani, or as if 'disability' meant the same thing for both characters. Through deftly detailed moments that expand audience perceptions of disability as a facet of rich and complex experience, the play offers instead an unhurried realism that invites audiences to witness interactions between disabled and non-disabled bodies. In the bathing scenes, the theatrical production slows down to make meaning of the actors' bodies that make theatre happen – defamiliarizing the act of care and demonstrating the value of disability as a source of personal, interpersonal and theatrical reinvention. The play requires the disability knowledges that disabled artists possess and invites audience members to understand their own bodies differently. The play's disability politics are also complicated by the frame of 'cost' that registers disability as a kind of threat, or risks reinforcing the asymmetry of caregiving as burden: by the end of the play, Ani dies, with no clear explanation, and Jess leaves John's employment after he refuses her the temporary shelter she needs. Yet *Cost of Living*, by imagining experiences of disability that resist a curative imaginary to dwell in the present, also prompts new possibilities for living with and through acts of care beyond the question of cost.

ACKNOWLEDGEMENTS

I am grateful to Marlene Goldman, Lawrence Switzky and Alice Flaherty for superb editorial guidance, to Joel Faber for careful close reading, and to Regan Linton and Gregg Mozgala for their willingness to explicate their artful virtuosity.

REFERENCES

Clare, Eli. *Brilliant Imperfection: Grappling With Cure*. Duke University Press, 2017.
Fox, Ann M. 'Staging the Complexities of Care: Martyna Majok's *Cost of Living*'. *Journal of Literary & Cultural Studies* 12, no 2 (2018): 145–61.
Garland-Thomson, Rosemary. *Extraordinary Bodies: Figuring Physical Disability in American Literature and Culture*. Columbia University Press, 1997.
Kafer, Alison. *Feminist Queer Crip*. Indiana University Press, 2013.
Kuppers, Petra. *Theatre and Disability*. Palgrave Macmillan, 2017.
Linton, Regan. 'Not My Disability Play'. Unpublished reflection, 2 November 2022.
Majok, Martyna. *Cost of Living*. Dramatists Play Service, 2018.
O'Reilly, Kaite. 'In Water I'm Weightless'. In *The 'd' Monologues*. Oberon Books, 2018.
Siebers, Tobin. *Disability Theory*. University of Michigan Press, 2008.
Siebers, Tobin. *Disability Aesthetics*. University of Michigan Press, 2010.

Yates, Samuel. 'Choreographing Confinement: *Side Show*'s Fleshy Fixations and Disability Simulation'. *Studies in Musical Theatre* 13, no. 1 (2019): 67–78.
Williams, Katherine Schaap. *Unfixable Forms: Disability, Performance, and the Early Modern English Theater*. Cornell University Press, 2021.
Williams, Katherine Schaap. 'Performing Shakespeare, Rewriting Disability'. *Shakespeare Bulletin* 39, no. 4 (2021): 637–50.

16

'Knots that I can't seem to easily undo': Playwright Matthew MacKenzie on making illness dramatically interesting

AN INTERVIEW WITH MATTHEW MACKENZIE

Matthew MacKenzie is a citizen of the Métis Nation of Alberta, a distinct Indigenous people in Canada with mixed First Nations and European ancestry, and he approaches the intersections between theatre and medicine as an Indigenous playwright. He serves in a number of roles, including as Artistic Director of Punctuate! Theatre, an Indigenous-led professional theatre company based in Edmonton, Alberta, as a founding member of the Pemmican Collective, which supports new Indigenous dramatic writing throughout Turtle Island, and as Canadian Liaison of the Liberian Dance Troupe. Several of MacKenzie's plays, including the Dora Award-winning *Bears* (2018), reflect his experience tracing his family's Métis, Cree and Ojibway heritage, featuring characters awakening to a personal and cultural past that has been repressed by their families and societies.

In this interview, conducted collaboratively by Lawrence Switzky and Karen Fricker, MacKenzie explores theatre's capacity to be 'good medicine' – a multifaceted idea that encompasses both communal and artistic health. Many of his characters are caught in cycles, stuck in 'knots', or refuse to see the realities in front of them, all conditions which resemble forms of illness. But he does not see his plays as therapy. In that sense, MacKenzie questions the overlap between medicine and theatre, particularly medicine's tendency to offer pat and prescriptive solutions to complex problems, and thinks through the problem of how to make illness theatrically compelling as a communal event rather than a self-report from an individual. Instead, MacKenzie looks to 'way[s] of knowing' and 'fram[ing] a world' as sources of illness and recognizes theatre's capacity to challenge the cycles of unwellness that entrap his characters.

MacKenzie refers to a number of his plays, many of which are set in the Canadian province of Alberta, including *The Particulars* (2008), *Sia* (2012), *Benefit* (2014), *Bears*, *After the Fire* (2019) and *First Métis Man of Odesa* (2022). He also discusses the healing nature of his relationship with Iris Turcott, a legendary Canadian dramaturg and the end-of-life companionship he shared with her. During her final two weeks, MacKenzie acted as a caregiver and confidant to Turcott, an experience dramatized in his solo play *The Situation We Find Ourselves in Is This* (2021). In MacKenzie's account, Turcott 'dramaturged many aspects of her own death', arranging her affairs and legacy with the same incisiveness she brought to supporting writers with the structure and meaning of their plays. Her advice and example act as 'slow-drip medicine' that infuses his plays.

I. GOOD MEDICINE

Lawrence Switzky and Karen Fricker (LS/KF): What does the relationship between theatre and medicine suggest to you?

Matt MacKenzie (MM): Theatre as medicine is something an Indigenous Elder would say. The work that we do, as Indigenous artists, is medicine for ourselves and medicine for our communities; that's where my mind would initially go.

LS/KF: How do you understand that phrase, 'medicine for ourselves and our community'?

MM: That it's a good thing, an important thing. That it has an impact larger than you might imagine. You might affect one person, but hopefully that effect ripples through other areas of their lives and their communities. You're tackling certain challenges as a group that you might get stuck on by yourself. It's a good thing for all aspects of your health, both as the creator and as the person receiving it, if it's good medicine. I've been taught by my Elders, Jerry and

Jo-Ann Saddleback, that the most important thing is that an artist do no harm with their work.

LS/KF: How would you be able to tell if art – and theatre in particular – was not good medicine?

MM: From an Indigenous perspective, I think you should ask an Elder about that. From a theatre practitioner standpoint, an example would be an actor who's feeling it all on the stage and leaving nothing for an audience to feel, that sort of self-indulgence. A frequent critique of Canadian theatre is that we write plays about the bad things that have happened to us and explain why it hurts, ad nauseam. That's not particularly interesting on a dramatic level, and I wonder whether an Elder would consider it good medicine either.

In terms of sharing Indigenous stories, just to be able to be heard is pretty important, so that Indigenous people can see other Indigenous people succeed. In traditionally white spaces – the regional theatres that get the most resources – having someone like Sheldon Elder [who has performed in MacKenzie's plays *Bears* and *After the Fire*] on stage in a lead role is very exciting because he's Indigenous, playing both non-Indigenous and Indigenous roles. To an Indigenous kid or Indigenous person seeing him perform, that means a lot.

I think the bar is set a little differently for communities that are historically shut out from theatre, or have been used and then discarded as we're seeing right now after the pandemic – all the 'charitable' Indigenous programming is falling away. We're seeing where most institutions' values really lie, values which are not aligned with Indigenous artists or Indigenous communities.

From a community standpoint, a piece of theatre is good medicine if it isn't just being written for trauma porn purposes or shock effect, or to claim to be part of or have allyship with a community that you in fact have no relationship with.

LS/KF: A number of the characters in your plays experience themselves as unwell in some sense. Very often they're surrounded by various kinds of sickness and it does often seem like they're looking for some kind of healing. I'm wondering whether you understand your playwriting this way.

MM: I don't think I'd have ever come to that myself. I describe the ideas and stories that really stick with me as knots that I can't seem to easily undo. That becomes dramatically interesting to me, and hopefully to an audience.

LS/KF: When I think of the character of Ty in *After the Fire*, a Métis man who has lost his job as well as his wife and family while working in the oil sands in Alberta, he's trying to think about what being well would mean.

MM: If I'm being honest, that doesn't sound too dramatically interesting to me. If I was hearing that a character was unwell or a narrative was centred around someone in our community being unwell, I don't know if that would be of interest in a play to me.

But yes, Ty is dealing with addiction, and he's also an obvious human representation of our addiction to oil. But he does have an idea, or he can see a horizon he could get to where he would be well. I don't know if we can say that he gets well or will get well. I don't know if he's that far along in the journey, or if he'll just continue in the addiction cycle, like we are with oil.

LS/KF: Why do you feel that someone being unwell doesn't sound dramatically interesting?

MM: I guess it could come across, as I was saying, as 'this is what happened to me and this is why it hurts'. It becomes an attempt at therapy for the person who's writing it, or trying to teach an audience a lesson. That sounds like theatre jail.

II. DRAMATICALLY INTERESTING ILLNESS

LS/KF: One of the strengths of your work is that you're not giving diagnoses. You're not saying 'here's how you get from a state of trouble to a state of resolution'. People have to live with complexity and, very often, with a lot of pain.

MM: I'm interested in people who find themselves on the margins or between the margins of what would be called normal, and what got them there. Were they born feeling on or between the margins, or did something occur that led them there?

Also, how do we break cycles? Ultimately, in *Bears*, I think Floyd [a Métis oilsands worker fleeing a workplace accident] breaks the cycle. I always imagine that, when he's shot by the RCMP at the end, Floyd's being is suddenly in the heavens and the stars. I don't think he's dead-dead.

There's definitely a kind of cycle, and maybe it's a cycle in myself that I find … I don't want to say self-loathing, but a lack of self-love. And in *Bears*, it's a lack of, or a forgetting of our love for the earth.

LS/KF: Following on your point about forgetting our love for the planet: is a positive relationship with nature good medicine in your work?

MM: Yes, I think so. Before I wrote *Bears*, I had a total crisis, something close to a nervous breakdown. I guess you could say I returned to the land. I was in

Canmore [Alberta]. I knew two people in the mountains, and I walked every day, and that was my therapy. Maybe real therapy would've helped me get through it all faster, I don't know. But then maybe it wouldn't have become a play. I think that that Floyd has the same thing where he stops working in the patch, he gets back to the land; this transforms him, and he remembers. He remembers what he was, he remembers his culture, he remembers his mother.

LS/KF: One thing that comes up in *After the Fire*, a play you wrote after *Bears*, is that not being able to see clearly is also a kind of illness – you're asking what happens when an entire city like Fort McMurray [Alberta] can't see.

MM: Yeah. What interests me so much about human psychology is how we can see something right before our eyes and then somehow – whether because it's too upsetting, or it's too much for us to handle at that time – we don't see it. Everyone who I've talked to who works in Fort Mac, or who works in the oil industry generally, knows quite a bit more about the effects of what's happening to the environment than arm-chair environmentalists.

My play *Benefit* is the story of a children's charity that is having a big fund-raising event in the Rockies. During this event, allegations come to light that the head of this charity is a paedophile. Exploring the nuances of paedophilia is not of interest to me – what's super interesting to me in this play is the paedophile's wife, Cynthia.

When we first did an iteration of the play, the actor who played Cynthia said, 'I don't believe that it would be okay if she had any inclination that her husband was a paedophile.' And I said, 'Well, I don't think you look at it that rationally.' So many of these men who committed these horrible crimes are married or have a partner. In a place where someone is not guilty as a perpetrator, the question is not so much what they knew or what they did not know. It's more like, what's their way of knowing? How do they frame their world? What happens when they're forced to look at things irrefutably, when they've been obfuscating before? What does it say about our society that we don't want to think that women are capable of the same evil that men are?

I haven't realized it yet to my satisfaction, but in that play there is a character who is faced with having to speak directly in a controlled situation to the acts of her husband. That to me is very dramatically interesting.

LS/KF: Acknowledging that theatre is not therapy for you, have there been times when making theatre was a kind of medicine in your life?

MM: The first play that I finished was *The Particulars*, which is sort of the story of almost killing myself. The story of *The Particulars* is that the central character, Gordon, has lost who he sees as his true love due to a tragic accident.

That was different from me, as I just went through a breakup. But I did have that problem, where I suddenly could not understand why I should go on living without my true love, and came very close to taking my life. I then spent seven years in my twenties, during and after theatre school, single and basically celibate.

In terms of theatre as medicine, I would definitely say that *The Particulars* was that for me. It helped me to – I don't want to say, to mythologize, but sort of dramatize what I was going through. Whereas if I had just talked about it with a therapist, or just journaled or something, I don't think I would have come to the same conclusions. The first few times we did it, I was still in that world, so the subtext in the play for me was pretty hot. But now I have distance from it. We did *The Particulars* last four or five years ago, and I know the place it comes from, and that that place is still inside me, but I'm quite removed from that place.

At the same time I wrote *The Particulars*, I was trying to write *Sia* [a play about a former Liberian child soldier who takes a University of Alberta student hostage], and if a psychologist looked at the process of me doing that – I did not look well. I rewrote the same twelve-line scene again and again, like 300 times, in multiple journals. And then when [dramaturg] Iris [Turcott] came along, she just cut the scene.

It's the same thing with Gordon in *The Particulars*: he repeats the same actions, just repeat, repeat, repeat. Being caught in cycles where you're not well, be it as a person or as a society, and then asking how we actually break out of those cycles, that is something that sticks with me.

III. THE DRAMATURG

LS/KF: You're a playwright who works very intimately with dramaturgs. If we think of theatre as medicine as a metaphor, what role does the dramaturg play who advises about the development of a script? Are they the person who gives you, the playwright, a diagnosis?

MM: Some people have called dramaturgs doulas. That's a very gentle term for Iris.

LS/KF: Can you talk more about how Iris worked with you on your plays, starting with that example of her cutting the scene from *Sia* that you were obsessing over?

MM: Well, I want to say that she knew there was something in me that wouldn't let that play go, because you hear that from dramaturgs: 'Oh, you need the playwright to write that one play and get it out of their system, and then they can go on and write other plays, and it won't be as hard, and they probably will be a lot better.'

But she knew that there was some sort of reason why I could not let that play go. And she started a system with me where I had to finish the play; I had to find the final notes. She knew – and I've learned this now as a writer – that once you find the final notes you want to hit in a piece, it's much easier to find the notes that get you there. Whereas to just keep trying to write the notes to find the ending is like trying to write music in outer space.

When I finally found the ending, it was like, 'Ding, ding, ding, ding!' After that, I didn't fight it that much when she then cut the scene I'd rewritten so many times. As long as I'd created whatever I needed to find that final note, then I was satisfied.

Iris had an incredible ability to understand the subtext of why a writer was writing something, or why a writer was writing at all. The level of investment, the level of writing, made realizing stories, exploring stories with her a higher calling, a higher purpose. Even if you were making no money, if everyone in your life thought you were a joke, you would talk to Iris and you would feel like someone saw you.

Some people describe dramaturgs as muses, but that's not accurate with Iris at all. It's like all of her playwrights were her muses, and she would dance with each of them.

LS/KF: It sounds like working with Iris on your writing was a form of good medicine. At the same time, your relationship with Iris raised questions and emotions that you needed to work out dramatically. You described your motivation to write plays and the relationship of that to unwellness before as trying to undo a knot. Was there some knot that led you to write your play about Iris and being with her before her death, *The Situation We Find Ourselves in Is This*?

MM: I'm still undoing that knot. Iris knew many people who are more capable and knew her a lot better than me, but she asked me to come and be with her as she was preparing her affairs before she died [in 2016]. I don't think she believed that I would be with her when she actually died, because she sort of dramaturged many aspects of her own death.

LS/KF: In that part of your relationship with Iris, you were performing a sort of palliative care; you were in a role that's often given to a medical professional. You may not have been in a traditional caregiving role where you were washing her and bringing her things she needed, but you were actually serving the function that an end-of-life caregiver would give.

MM: Yes, for sure. But our conversations were...well, they were about her life, but also lots about me. I think Iris told me things she'd never told anyone, and I told her things I'd never told anyone. It's interesting talking to someone who you know is going to die right away, because you can really tell them anything. It was an incredible gift to be there.

Other people have said, 'That was very inappropriate for Iris to do that. It really traumatized you.' And yes, it's still taking me time to make sense of it all, but those people who've made perfect sense of death, keep them away from me ... that's creepy.

I lived in the mountains for four years on and off and never felt lonely. After Iris passed, I went back to the mountains, and for the first time, I felt lonely. And I thought, 'I only know two people here. Why did I never feel lonely before?' It was because Iris, from Toronto, thousands of kilometres away, would help you believe in the universe you're creating with the stories and your writing. And when she was gone, I had to kind of rebuild that.

LS/KF: When you were in that final time with Iris, how did you understand the care you were giving her? Did you think of it as care?

MM: Well, it was only two weeks. It was very fast. And she didn't let me do anything physically for her until the last night, hours before she died, when I did wash her face and her back, and then her face again before she died. But before that, she was fiercely independent, violently independent. It all happened so quickly that I don't think I really had time to think about it. It was overwhelming.

I know that she had already said her goodbyes to people she knew a lot better than me. And so, it felt like she'd made it only a few people she was talking to at the end.

LS/KF: So you thought of yourself as somebody who had to come to talk with her and exchange aspects of your lives?

MM: Yes – and not to make it about me. I know I can be incredibly self-involved, but I think that, for whatever reason, at that time at least, she saw me as one of the artists she worked with who could do something and not make it all about me. She loved certain artists, but they did not have the ability to get out of that mode. She asked me to write about her. So that's also why I've tried to write *The Situation We Find Ourselves in Is This*, because she asked me to write one of my dance plays about her.

She wanted me to write the stories of her art – about the thirty-six pieces of art that she owned, some that she painted and some that she collected. I think she wanted to sort of paint a picture, but not necessarily a story about herself and her life. She asked a number of the playwrights she worked with to create artworks for her son, Merrick, and this was part of that.

I never heard the story of all the pieces of art because she died so quickly. So the play became a little bit more about those two weeks, because so few people knew what had gone down. [Canadian theatre artist and arts leader] Brendan Healy called it an unburdening. I shared it with people in the community.

I told my dad, 'Iris saw something in me that I don't know what it is.' And he just joked, 'Oh, it must be that she saw you had a strong disassociative state.' That sounds so harsh, but I do find it funny.

LS/KF: *The Situation We Find Ourselves in Is This* is a solo piece which you perform. Was it part of Iris's request that you be the performer?

MM: It's funny now that you say it. She didn't say for me to perform in the piece. I guess it's sort of like with *First Métis Man of Odesa* [a play written and performed by MacKenzie and his wife Mariya Khomutova about their courtship and marriage in the context of the COVID-19 pandemic and the war in Ukraine] – if you have a profound experience then I think it's something that people want to hear about from the source. I wanted to write *The Situation* for Iris's people – for [her son] Merrick, and for the Toronto and Canadian theatre community. In that world, it should be me.

LS/KF: What do you think you have learned from Iris? What kind of legacies did she leave you in terms of thinking about theatre as medicine?

MM: Iris said dramaturgical stuff about my plays that I figured out years later, or that I'm still trying to figure out. I figured out a moment in *Bears* two years after she died. It was a slow-drip medicine.

I'm working on a show now, *Takwahiminana*, which is about a character who assists her Elder to pass. That's very much tied to my time with Iris, and I feel like it will maybe lead me back to writing about her and the literal things that occurred.

At the end of her life, Iris felt that she had gotten away from the work that was important and had been working on projects that one might term bad medicine, whether it was an ego project for an individual, or a project going to some heights without getting to the heart of the thing. She said that 98% of people are only about their own self-aggrandizement, and that the trick is to work with the 2% who are about something more. So I really try to think about why I'm doing something, who I'm doing it with, who I see myself doing it for. It's a constant question.

Conclusion: A performative future for healthcare

MARLENE GOLDMAN, LAWRENCE SWITZKY AND ALICE FLAHERTY

Theatre and medicine can seem like worlds apart. The play of masks, the uncertain line between seeming and being, the claim that artifice and convention are vehicles to reveal truth, all can appear very distant from the life-and-death stakes of diagnosis, treatment and care. The chapters in this book have outlined the field of performative medicine, which asserts that medicine always already has elements of theatre – an art form that takes the human body as means and message – and that embracing and refining those elements can lead to more receptive, responsive, inventive, compassionate and playful medical care.

These two adjacent arts share more than the body as common ground. Illness and theatrical enactments are both events that stand outside everyday experience: they are spatially separated (in clinics, hospitals, rehabilitation centres, or a sick bed; on a stage, or platform, or on ritual grounds) and ontologically demarcated (sickness, like acting, indicates that one has entered a special and, in many senses, heightened state of being). As we noted in the introduction, critic and dramaturg Elinor Fuchs encourages readers of plays to view them not as literature but as 'small planets', 'another world passing before you in time and space', in which language is only one component.[1] In theatrical worlds, attention is concentrated, and nothing is 'without significance'. Clinics, hospitals and doctors' offices are likewise places where the signifying body is examined carefully, and where no bodily performance is presumed to be accidental or unimportant.

Seeing medical worlds through the lens of theatrical worlds can make us more attentive to how those former planets have been constructed and might be remade. It can also call attention to how the charged zones where healing occurs, like theatres, are also places where normative conduct is suspended and various forms of play – some liberating, some troubling – are permitted. Theatre audiences generally know not to interpret a fight on stage as a real act of aggression (even though actual violent feelings can be summoned in both actors and audiences) and to clap and speak only at designated moments. Likewise, exceptional relationships to the body are required in medical environments. An understanding of medicine's longstanding relationship to theatre as well as its inherent theatricality allows those relationships to be scrutinized and discussed. As folklorist Lisa Gabbert notes in her study of the 'medical carnivalesque', medical students regularly signify their sense of the licensed transgressions in medicine by engaging in humorous performances to cope with the fact that they 'break every boundary and taboo imaginable with respect to the body'.[2] Even after examining and manipulating bodies has become second nature to experienced physicians, they turn to black comedy to bracket their usual professional rigour and authority and acknowledge the vulnerability and ambivalence they feel.

Viewing medicine as a fellow traveller with theatre also brings to the fore another shared feature of the two arts that many of our contributors discuss: both are fundamentally concerned with metamorphosis. Medical environments and theatres are places where bodies change, sometimes drastically and irrevocably, with concomitant changes to the self and its attachments to personal control and coherence. These alterations can be painful, confusing, even shattering; but they can also open up possibilities for renewal, where the self, its circumstances and its embodiment become sites of amazement.

Theatre historian Martin Meisel identifies transformation as one of the 'primal attractions' of theatre and includes both spectacular transformation (an actor is made to fly, a theatre stage suddenly becomes a battlefield) and personal virtuosity (one person flawlessly impersonates another, a human body sings or dances with extraordinary power and grace). Transformations of the

[1] Elinor Fuchs, 'EF's Visit to a Small Planet: Some Questions to Ask a Play', *Theater* 34, no. 2 (2004): 6.

[2] Lisa Gabbert, *The Medical Carnivalesque: Folklore Among Physicians* (Indiana University Press, 2024), 5.

somatic body in medical care are likewise not only transitions marked by catastrophe or abjection but also calls to create a different person who can inhabit partially or radically modified conditions of embodiment. Physicians and carers can help to recognize and prop up the patient's self during transitions and can suggest characters and scenes that a transformed self can inhabit in its search for accommodation; they can also model survival across transformation through their own theatrical and affective suppleness. As Arthur Frank comments, the crisis of illness is also an occasion to reflect on the dynamism of the body and to reclaim wonder from the 'bureaucratic rationalizations of institutional medicine': 'Being available to yourself ultimately means having the ability to wonder at all the self can be.'[3] 'Playing sick' is thus a multidimensional act, a guided and mutual exploration that is at once existential, social and epistemological.

Contributors to this volume have adopted this spirit of multidimensional exploration, identifying opportunities for honing our approach to the ensemble drama of illness. The tenets of performative medicine will have been new to some, familiar to others, and, we hope, enlivening to all our readers. Historically, a new and complex play in the theatre has required the services of a *souffleur* or prompter: an officer who reminds actors of their lines, cues and placement on the stage from a hidden position offstage.[4] In this final scene, we offer patients, doctors, caregivers, scholars and theatre the following 'prompts' that we have distilled from *Medicine as Theatre: Theatre as Medicine*, a collection of brief observations and provocations about what performative medicine is and has been, where it's going and how to do it.

USE THEATRE TO CONVEY AND ALIGN OBJECTIVES

Following the lead of sociologist Erving Goffman and more contemporary theorists such as Judith Butler, we take the position that people are inherently embodied performers. Some remain unconscious or resist an awareness of this dynamic; for them, the narrative of illness is all that matters. But if that were true, then patients could simply write their doctor a letter describing their history, symptoms and fears and desires. And while verbal communication certainly plays a role in the clinical encounter, the ensemble drama of illness recognizes that doctors glean crucial information from their patient's bodies and vice versa – and this goes beyond the quantitative data of the medical exam.

[3] Arthur Frank, *The Wounded Storyteller* (University of Chicago Press, 2013), 68.
[4] Philip Oltermann, 'Why Is the Prompter Strolling Around the Stage? Meet the Secret Heroes of German Theatre', *The Guardian*, 26 September 2023, www.theguardian.com/stage/2023/sep/26/meet-the-secret-heroes-of-german-theatre.

Caregivers' gestures and tone of voice tell patients if what ails them is prosaic or truly dreadful, for example, and there is ample potential for dissonance. A chasm may well lie between what one says and how one acts.

In the clinical encounter, there are always at least two dramas occurring. The first is explicit and instrumental: a patient might ask for drugs. But in the parallel, unspoken drama the patient may also be asking, 'Will you care for me, or will you abandon me?' In the first drama, the physician may write a prescription. In the second, his tone of voice and gestures assure the patient that the doctor is well and truly present for whatever transpires. Only when both dramas are played with expertise and compassion can patient and doctor align and convey their objectives.

MAKE SPACE FOR THE INVISIBLE

Theatres, like clinics, are spaces of transformation that rely on spoken and unspoken, embodied modes of communication. They are both also places of seeing, of bringing the invisible – the interior of a body, a hidden or unknown past, a network of relationships – into view. But there are important dimensions of medical and theatrical experience that resist sight. Illness has an elusive subjective register. Medical performances in the present are shadowed by and contain performances in the past. Medical policy, which determines how one body relates to another body in a clinic, is shaped by the actions of countless dispersed bodies.

In drama, Andrew Sofer calls the pull of what is not or cannot be seen on what does appear a kind of theatrical 'dark matter'.[5] Performative medicine brings what's hard to see into the act. Exposing 'dark matter' might involve revealing the effects of the hidden curriculum; it might also entail reframing healthcare issues, often perceived as individual problems, as communal or even national concerns.

BUILD UP A WIDE AND FLEXIBLE REPERTOIRE

Actors may become known for a single role, but they play many roles over their careers. In fact, actors seek out parts, plays and scene partners that will allow them to develop breadth and technique. The capacity to modulate performances isn't a form of inauthenticity, but rather a way of exploring the

[5] Andrew Sofer, *Dark Matter: Invisibility in Drama, Theatre, and Performance* (University of Michigan Press, 2013).

vastness of who you already are; as playwright Bernard Shaw once wrote, 'We are all striving to get cast for the part which most fully realizes us.'[6]

A physician, like an actor, needs to be prepared to play comedy as well as tragedy, and to find both in a single scene, since no play and no life is ever only one or the other. Shifting the genre in a clinical encounter can crucially change approaches to illness and to treatment. Likewise, performers in medicine and on stage bring everything and everyone (and the specific knowledge everyone has) into the act. That makes a scene – and every medical consultation is a scene, as drama and TV writers have long realized – meaningful and particular to patient and carer.

RECOGNIZE THE ROLE OF PATIENTS AND CARERS AS PERFORMERS

Doctors need to recognize their role as performers, and this also holds for patients. The latter need to read the room, as it were, and determine how best to perform their symptoms to obtain optimal treatment. Strange as it may seem, 'ailers' (to use Alice Flaherty's term) do better when they learn how to regulate their instinctive responses and act unnaturally so as to convey their distress in ways that recruit potential carers. This role can be terribly demanding since, in some circumstances, ailers may need to express their pain and simultaneously convey that they are not the sort of person who signals pain too often.

Ideally, carers' performances complement those of ailers – for example, helping ailers navigate the demands of their role by describing the ailers' pain to the doctor. The often-repetitive gestures of care also draw on healing rituals that transcend our modern quest for a cure.

BE OPEN TO VULNERABILITY, ERROR AND FAILURE

Attuning to patients – who seek care precisely because something seems strange or wrong – necessitates experiencing humanity's bounded, mortal existence, and, with that, accepting vulnerability, error and failure. While failure can feel to carers like falling without a net, it can also be part of a collaborative process that offers crucial information. When experienced and accepted, failure can in fact provide a necessary step toward arriving at a solution or a diagnosis. Alternatively, failure may not be useful or instrumental or anything more than itself.

[6] Bernard Shaw, 'Acting, by One Who Does Not Believe in It', in *The Drama Observed*, vol. 1, ed. Bernard Dukore (Penn State University Press, 1991), 98.

Whereas in the medical context failure can be professionally and legally catastrophic, when portrayed on stage, it can be socially beneficial. By encouraging vulnerability and viewing error and failure as opportunities for learning, performative medicine develops confidence in all the actors in the ensemble drama of illness.

GO BEYOND THE CURATIVE SCRIPT

Clinging to curative scripts when patients fail to get well can lead some physicians to abandon their patients. This is a particular problem for patients living with ongoing pain, chronic illness and disability. In these cases, healing is instigated and maintained by the caregivers' willingness to collaborate with the patient in the diachronic, performative labour of articulating and assimilating the embodied and affective changes associated with illness, disease and disability.

RECOGNIZE CAREGIVERS AS FELLOW ACTORS IN THE ENSEMBLE DRAMA OF ILLNESS

Because doctors dart in and out of sickrooms, the doctor's clinical gaze only captures static snapshots in the drama of any illness. Although doctors' heroic struggles capture the public's imagination, in reality, depending on the illness, its duration and its trajectory, patients and doctors share the stage with a host of actors ranging from specialists to home care aides. As we note in the preface to George Anderson's interview, 'over 90% of patient care comes not from doctors but home caregivers and nurses, but to date the medical humanities have shamefully neglected their perspectives'. Performative medicine corrects this oversight by challenging the implicit hierarchy it maintains and demonstrating the importance of daily rituals of care. Recognizing caregivers as fellow actors and learning the art of respectful collaboration greatly enhances the healing process.

FINALLY, PLAY!

For many sick people, play is vital to complement what Marcus Coates terms 'the medical contract', the tacit understanding that medicine relies on reason and empirical evidence to arrive at a diagnosis and, ideally, a cure. Healing works best when the medical contract is counterbalanced by an alternative 'imaginative contract'.

Theatrical restagings of illness can counter the diagnostic and often pathologizing, shaming and stigmatizing medical gaze that reads transformation as deviance. Think, for example, of Tony Kushner's fantastical play about the AIDS epidemic, *Angels in America,* where the theatrical context allows for reinterpretations of illness-induced transformation. Revisioning valium addicts and AIDS patients as truth-tellers and prophets helps forge rather than fracture intra- and interpersonal identities. As contributors to the volume demonstrate, there is a crucial difference between relying on empirical reasoning to arrive at a diagnosis and using one's intellect and imagination to help people to feel more at home in the world.

REFERENCES

Frank, Arthur. *The Wounded Storyteller*. University of Chicago Press, 2013.

Fuchs, Elinor. 'EF's Visit to a Small Planet: Some Questions to Ask a Play'. *Theater* 34, no. 2 (2004): 5–9.

Gabbert, Lisa. *The Medical Carnivalesque: Folklore Among Physicians*. Indiana University Press, 2024.

Oltermann, Philip. 'Why Is the Prompter Strolling Around the Stage? Meet the Secret Heroes of German Theatre'. *The Guardian*, 26 September 2023. www.theguardian.com/stage/2023/sep/26/meet-the-secret-heroes-of-german-theatre.

Shaw, Bernard. 'Acting, by One Who Does Not Believe in It'. In *The Drama Observed*, vol. 1, edited by Bernard Dukore. Penn State University Press, 1991.

Sofer, Andrew. *Dark Matter: Invisibility in Drama, Theatre, and Performance*. University of Michigan Press, 2013.

INDEX

www.ingramcontent.com/pod-product-compliance
Ingram Content Group UK Ltd.
Pitfield, Milton Keynes, MK11 3LW, UK
UKHW050943290926
15470UKWH00005B/1614

9 781350 460720